GONIOSCOPY AND THE GLAUCOMAS

GONIOSCOPY AND THE GLAUCOMAS

Barry M. Fisch, O.D.

Chief of Optometry
Brockton Division of the Brockton/West Roxbury Veterans
*   Administration Medical Center*
Brockton, Massachusetts
Associate Professor of Optometry
New England College of Optometry
Boston, Massachusetts

Butterworth–Heinemann

Boston   London   Oxford   Singapore   Sydney   Toronto   Wellington

Every effort has been made to ensure that the drug dosage schedules within this text are accurate and conform to standards accepted at time of publication. However, as treatment recommendations vary in the light of continuing research and clinical experience, the reader is advised to verify drug dosage schedules herein with information found on product information sheets. This is especially true in cases of new or infrequently used drugs.

Recognizing the importance of preserving what has been written, it is the policy of Butterworth–Heinemann to have the books it publishes printed on acid-free paper, and we exert our best efforts to that end.

Library of Congress Cataloging-in-Publication Data
Fisch, Barry M.
  Gonioscopy and the glaucomas / Barry M. Fisch.
    p.   cm.
  includes bibliographical references and index.
  ISBN 0-7506-9049-6 (ppc : alk. paper)
  1. Glaucoma—Diagnosis. 2. Gonioscopy. I. Title.
  [DNLM: 1. Glaucoma—diagnosis. 2. Gonioscopy—methods. WW 290
F528g]
RE871.F57 1993
617.7'410764—dc20
DNLM/DLC
for Library of Congress   92-48238
                                                              CIP

British Library Cataloguing-in-Publication Data.

A catologue record for this book is available from the British Library.

Butterworth–Heinemann
80 Montvale Avenue
Stoneham, MA 02180

10 9 8 7 6 5 4 3 2 1

Printed in the United States of America

Contents

Foreword

Only once in a great while does the need for a medical book remain unfulfilled for an extended period of time. Such is the case for an in-depth text on gonioscopy. After having stimulated an original flurry of innovation and investigation of clinical applications, the gonioscope languished as an esoteric instrument for the glaucoma specialist and as a screening device for the general ophthalmic practitioner.

Two developments occurred that rekindled interest in observing the angle structures of the anterior chamber. First, argon laser trabeculoplasty, using a gonioscopic delivery system, gained widespread acceptance as a treatment for open-angle glaucoma, and general ophthalmologists became interested in offering this mode of therapy to their patients. At about the same time, optometrists acquired the right to diagnose and treat a variety of anterior segment conditions. After initially learning gonioscopy to screen narrow angles prior to pupillary dilation, they began examining abnormal angles to diagnose the cause of many types of anterior segment disease. Mastery of these skills led to slit lamp ophthalmoscopy using the three-mirror lens to examine retinal details stereoscopically and under high magnification.

A number of authors have written excellent tutorials and articles on the various uses of gonioscopy. For several decades, however, there has not been a comprehensive reference source describing, in detail, the instrumentation, the techniques, and the interpretation of findings. This textbook provides new knowledge for both experienced gonioscopists who want to fine-tune their skills and newer users who need guidance in technique and evaluating findings.

Barry Fisch has melded his love of teaching, his passion for excellence, and his attention to detail in producing this clinically oriented book. His students and associates are constantly impressed by his diagnostic talents. Some of it, in part, is due to his innate observational skills. Those who know him well, though, recognize that this ability is the result of many hours of diligent study. His mind is a resevoir of current clinical information; his interests are wide ranging. Here, in a relatively few chapters, you will garner the fruits of his efforts.

Clifford Scott, O.D., M.P.H.
Paul White, O.D.

Preface

Since my graduation from optometry school in the early 1970s, the role of the optometrist has broadened considerably. At that time, gonioscopy was an examination technique unfamiliar to me. Optometry was virtually a "drugless" profession, and examination techniques requiring pharmacologic agents were not ordinarily used in optometric practice or routinely taught in optometric colleges. After my graduation, I was required to implement diagnostic pharmacologic agents and the examination techniques the agents allowed, such as applanation tonometry, gonioscopy, and indirect ophthalmoscopy. It provided a means for me to care better for the total visual needs of my patients. I became interested in gonioscopy because it provided an important first step before dilation as a means of assessing whether an eye was at risk for angle closure from the dilation. It was also clear that gonioscopy had a major role in the diagnosis and management of the glaucomas. This made it imperative for me to apply this technique in all patients at risk for or diagnosed with glaucoma.

Approximately 10 years ago, along with my colleague and friend Clifford Scott and with the assistance of Damon Pouyat, I started to lecture and run workshops at the Ellerbrock meetings at the American Academy of Optometry. I have also had the opportunity to examine many thousands of patients using the gonioscope during the past 20 years of optometric practice. Gonioscopy has allowed me to observe an area of the eye otherwise hidden from my view. Because of the large variation among eyes and the numerous subtleties encountered, my interest grew, and it continues today. I am continually surprised at the variations encountered when studying the anterior chamber.

The idea of a book on gonioscopy was developed because of my desire to provide optometric students, residents, and colleagues the information I had gathered in order to make the general principles and the intricate details of gonioscopy readily available. What I had spent many hours and years learning and teaching could be passed on to others. Because of the close association between gonioscopy and the glaucomas, it was decided to expand the original concept for this book, away from an atlas of gonioscopy and toward a book that also discusses the role of gonioscopy as it relates to the glaucomas.

My goal is to provide a foundation for students, residents, and practitioners so that they can use this technique in routine practice with ease and confidence. I hope that, after reading this book, clinicians will have a better understanding of the techniques and instruments involved in gonioscopy, the ability to differentiate between the normal and abnormal anterior chamber, and the ability to recognize the subtleties of the gonioscopic appearance of the eye. The unique gonioscopic findings in the glaucomas, which directly affect the diagnosis and management of these disorders, is also covered, along with how these findings may influence the management of this condition. An understanding of the anterior chamber anatomy, its gonioscopic appearance, and its role in glaucoma diagnosis and treatment will aid my colleagues in caring for patients. The appropriate diagnosis and treatment of the glaucomas most often hinge on the results of the examiner's observation and interpretation of the gonioscopic examination.

A number of people helped with this book. Barbara Murphy, editor, and Kathleen Higgins, assistant editor, were persistent and patient. My past students, especially the optometry residents I have had the opportunity to work with over the years, have stimulated me to grow as an optometrist, an educator, and a person. I value our time together.

A number of other people deserve thanks as well: Ernest Barsamian, Chief of Staff, and Shukri Khuri, Chief of Surgery, who have been very supportive of me in my role at the Brockton/West Roxbury VA Medical Center; the administration and faculty at the New England College of Optometry, for providing me with the opportunity to teach; the many optometrists and ophthalmologists with whom I have worked over the past 20 years who have taught me much; my teachers and classmates at the Massachusetts College of Optometry; the library staff at the New England College of Optometry who were extremely helpful in gathering materials; Dotti Bilodeau who was helpful with some last-minute typing of tables; Rodney Gutner, who supplied support and many many slides; Sam Baron for his encouragement; Chuck Foltz and Brian Botehlo, for their illustrations; Lisa Fancuillo, for reading the manuscript, and Judith Gimple, for her persistance.

Paul White has been a teacher, mentor, and friend. He has always been supportive of me, and I extend particular thanks to him for all he has done for me over the years. Clifford Scott is a special person, friend, and colleague. We have worked together for the past 10 years, and I value that time as he has provided me with considerable professional insight and personal friendship.

My family is most important to me. I am fortunate to have a wonderful, caring, loving, and supportive wife, Nancy, who has been very understanding over the past 25 years, especially during this project. Jonathan and Jeffrey I love as my sons and respect and admire as people. Whenever I asked if their studying was done, they would respond with, ''Is your book done?'' It took me longer to write this book than for them to finish their studying. I also acknowledge my sister Ina, a remarkable woman, who I look up to and who has displayed great faith in me.

I dedicate this book to the memory of my parents; my father, Solomon, my first and greatest teacher and the finest man I have known, and my loving mother, Dorothy, always providing unquestioned support. I miss you both.

GONIOSCOPY AND THE GLAUCOMAS

Chapter 1

History

The modern era in gonioscopy arrived with the development of the coaxially illuminating and viewing slit lamps and their wide availability in the 1960s. With the use of these modern slit lamps and indirect-type gonioscope lenses, we can observe the angle structures stereoscopically under high magnification, with bright illumination and with optic sections. The view of the anterior chamber structures is enormously more detailed and accurate than the early pioneers, like Trantas and Salzmann, could experience (Table 1.1).

In the field of ophthalmology, gonioscopy became a very important clinical technique specifically in relation to the detection, diagnosis, and treatment of the glaucomas. Interestingly enough, it was not a procedure widely used as we now know it, until the late 1950s and the 1960s, although Barkan had demonstrated as early as 1936 that congestive glaucoma was the result of the iris closing the anterior chamber and recognized the need of gonioscopy to observe angle closure (1). It was during the late 1950s and the 1960s that Posner, Gorin, and others were teaching the modern method of gonioscopy at the annual meetings of the American Academy of Ophthalmology; however, as recently as 1977, comments appeared in the ophthalmology literature lamenting the fact that the procedure, even at that time, had not been universally appreciated (2) and more recently still that it was used too frequently for specific indications only; thereby some cases of chronic angle closure were not identified (3).

Prior to the 1970s, optometry was a drugless profession and gonioscopy was done without the use of a topical anesthetic. Techniques using contact lenses or prism-adapted swimming goggles filled with saline were described as alternative methods (4,5,6). These techniques were awkward, cumbersome, and somewhat optically inadequate for routine optometric implementation and therefore not often used.

Today, virtually all optometrists in the United States utilize diagnostic pharmaceutical agents and many are licensed and certified to prescribe therapeutic agents in caring for their patients. This greater emphasis and responsibility placed on disease detection and management within the optometric profession makes the utilization and understanding of this examination technique mandatory for the optometrist.

Gonioscopy is a necessary and valuable part of the examination of patients considered suspect for open-angle glaucoma and patients with open-angle glaucoma in order to differentiate the primary and secondary forms of this disease. It is also necessary for patients at risk for angle closure glaucoma based on examination signs and/or symptoms. Patients with abnormalities of the anterior chamber, and patients with disease processes that may interfere with the anterior chamber, such as inflammatory disease or anterior segment tumors or cysts, and patients who have suffered trauma and require gonioscopy. Some practioners suggest gonioscopic evaluation in routine examination.

The Early Years

The word *gonioscopy,* derived from the Greek, means to view the angle. The term was first used in a paper published in 1915 by Alexios Trantas. Just prior to this, Trantas had developed a technique to observe the ciliary and retrociliary area of the fundus. His method consisted of direct ophthalmoscopy with digital pressure or pressure via a Lang transilluminator in the retrolimbal area. He positioned himself lateral to the eye, and by pressing firmly over the outer limbal area, with the aid of high plus lenses, he was able to view a portion of the angle (7). Angle viewing with his technique, however,

TABLE 1.1
History of Gonioscopy

Year	Person	Event
1900–1936	Trantas	First used term *gonioscopy.* Viewed retrociliary area with direct ophthalmoscopy, and digital pressure.
	Salzmann	Correlated anatomic structure to clinical observation. Published observations. Used indirect ophthalmoscopy to view angle. Used contact lens to negate critical angle. Observed blood in Schlemm's canal.
	Mizvo	Used water to negate critical angle. Viewed inferior angle.
	Koeppe	Designed lens still utilized today. Used binocular microscope.
	Thorburn	Noted most glaucomas had open angle. Pioneer of gonio-photography.
	Curran	Noted relationship of posterior chamber and angle closure.
	Troncosco	Devised first gonioscope and popularized term. Made gonioscopy a useful clinical technique.
1936–present	Troncosco	Published text on *gonioscopy.*
	Barkan	Developed goniotomy. Improved technique of direct gonioscopy still used today. Defined glaucoma on basis of gonioscopy (open- or closed-angle glaucoma).
	Goldman	Developed indirect lens system for gonioscopy.
	Allen	Developed prism four-mirror lens.
	Posner-Gorin	Taught technique of indirect system. Text on gonioscopy.
	Shaffer	Text on gonioscopy grading system.
	Schie	Grading system for gonioscopy.
	Forbes	Introduced techniques of indentation gonioscopy.
	Brandreth-Saladin	Use of adapted swimming goggles to view angle.
	Spaeth	New grading system for gonioscopy.
	Krasnov	Introduced laser surgery for open-angle glaucoma.
	Wise and Witter	Refined ALT technique.
	Kimbrough	Iridopathy
	Simmons	Goniophotocoagulation.
	Sussman	Developed hand-held four-mirror lens.

Adapted with permission from Spaeth GL. Gonioscopy uses old and new—The inheritance of occludable angles. *Trans Am Acad Ophthalmol Otolaryngol* 1978;85:222–232. Published courtesy of *Ophthalmology.*

was limited to eyes with deep chambers and prominent corneas.

His first mention of any anterior chamber observation was made in 1907 in a published case report of keratoglobus (8). He had actually described his techniques and findings as early as 1899, therefore claiming a priority in the technique of examining the anterior chamber.

At about this same time, Maximilian Salzmann was also interested in the examination of the anterior chamber. He is credited with laying the groundwork of gonioscopy (9). He was able to correlate his observations in the living eye with the normal anatomic structures of the angle that he had observed in microscopic sections (7). Working independently and not knowing of Trantas's work, he found the use of indirect ophthalmoscopy a better method for examining the anterior chamber. He even called it "ophthalmoscopy of the chamber angle"(8). He came to realize that the use of a contact lens with a smaller radius than that of the cornea would make the task of examining the anterior chamber easier and more practical. Originally he used Fick's contact lens with a radius of 8 mm and later a contact lens produced by Zeiss with a radius of 7mm, which made gonioscopy less troublesome (10). He altered the curvature of the lens to reduce astigmatic distortion and produce clearer images. Without the use of a contact lens, he was able to observe only those angles in deep-chambered eyes with convex corneas. In shallow-chambered eyes, where it is often more critical to observe the angle, the angle could not be readily observed without a contact lens (8).

At best, these methods allowed fleeting glimpses of the angle. Salzmann, however, was able to describe a number of pathological conditions, such as peripheral anterior synechia and angle recession, and he was able to identify the trabecular meshwork as a grayish band but thought it to represent Schlemm's canal. He also observed that peripheral anterior iris synechia does not always cause increased elevated intraocular tension. He was the first to observe the presence of blood in Schlemm's canal in certain conditions (4). He published his accurate observations in 1914 and 1915, along with color plates, which represented the first extensive study of the angle (8).

After the publication of Salzmann's work, a controversy developed between Trantas and Salzmann as to who made the first observation of the angle. Trantas even wrote to Salzmann, claiming priority in the observation of the angle. Gorin (11) has suggested that Trantas be noted as the originator and Salzmann as the developer of gonioscopy.

Around this time, a third pioneer, Mizuo, also reported on viewing the angle (12). He observed the lower chamber angle by everting the lower lid and instilling water into the cul-de-sac. With the cornea surrounded by fluid, its refracting characteristics are eliminated, and direct observation of the angle is possible. This was an impractical technique, however, because only one quadrant could be viewed and the fluid would run off quickly (12). Others have tried to duplicate this technique using a flashlight illumination and a 5x or 10x loupe or by adapting swimmers' goggles (13,14).

Salzmann's use of the contact lens was the first step in making the examination of the angle of the eye a practical endeavor. According to Barklan (1), it was Fick who in 1897 was actually the first to use the contact lens and the direct ophthalmoscope to view the anterior chamber, but it was Salzmann who was to refine the technique later (1). Moreover, Salzmann provided the anatomic and scientific foundation of the examination of the anterior chamber (15).

Salzmann's realization that without the use of a contact lens on the cornea, light rays emanating from within the anterior chamber angle will be totally internally reflected is based on critical angle and total reflection. The concept of critical angle is important in gonioscopy because it is this optical principle, along with the existence of a prominent corneoscleral overhang, that prevents direct observation of the angle.

Critical Angle

A critical angle occurs when light from an object passes from a medium of higher index of refraction (denser) to a medium of lower index of refraction (rarer). The angle of refraction in the rarer medium increases more rapidly than the angle of incidence. At a certain angle of incidence, the angle of refraction will be 90 degrees; thus, the refracted light will run parallel along the surface. This angle is known as the *critical angle*. The light hitting the surface at an angle greater than the critical angle will not enter into the second medium and will be reflected at the surface; thus, the light striking the media interface at the critical angle will pass along the interface. If the light rays create an angle of incidence greater than the critical angle, the light rays will be internally reflected. In the eye, the light rays from the anterior chamber strike the anterior corneal surface at an angle greater than the critical angle, estimated at 46 degrees to 49 degrees and, as such, are totally internally reflected. The index of refraction of the aqueous and posterior cornea are similar so as not to produce any significant deviation; therefore, the interface of importance is the one between the anterior cornea and air. When a contact lens in the form of goniolens is placed on the eye, the air interface is replaced by the lens surface, with an index of refraction similar to the index of refraction of the corneal tissue. Once the differences in the refractive indexes are minimized, the critical angle is eliminated because the light is refracted by the steep curved outer surface of the contact lens. At this point, the light rays from the anterior chamber can be directed to the examiner's eyes by means of simple refraction as in the direct viewing systems, or by reflected rays, as in the indirect viewing systems (16) (Figure 1.1). Salzmann is given credit for recognizing this concept, and by utilizing the lens constructed by Zeiss, which was more convex than Fick's, and thus he was able to observe the angle in eyes with shallow anterior chambers.

Attempts at Clinical Application

With the development of the first Zeiss slit lamp in 1920, Koeppe made gonioscopy into a clinical tool. The Koeppe-type lens design is still used today for direct nonmirrored gonioscopy. With the use of the binocular stationary microscope and slit beam, he was able to observe closure of the angle in glaucoma and studied the trabecular layer covering Schlemm's canal (1). He was the first to observe the appearance of pigmentation to the trabecular area and

attributed this with pathological significance (17). (We now know this is a normal occurrence in many nonglaucomatous eyes and is probably an age-related phenomenon.) He obtained a stereoscopic magnified view. He mathematically calculated a contact lens that was thicker and overcame astigmatic problems of the prior lenses. His lens had a recessed area in the outer convex portion, where a knot of a strip of bandage was placed to hold the lens in place (7). His observations were limited to the nasal and temporal areas of the anterior chamber, however, because the examination was done while the patient was sitting upright. Ascher refined Koeppe's technique by examining the patient in a supine position, which allowed for examination of the superior and inferior angle (18).

In the early 1930s Trantas reported on a method using a slit lamp and a Koeppe lens, which allowed him to view the angle in optic section (8). He could view the superior and inferior angles by having patients tilt their heads while he tilted the microscope, but he had difficulty observing the lateral angles.

Observation of the angle nevertheless was still very rudimentary and difficult. The slit lamps lacked a coaxial illumination and observation axis, so they were cumbersome when focusing the microscope and illumination systems, since each was done separately. The light sources were also weak.

In the following decades, interest in gonioscopy was sustained by Trantas and Manuel Uribe Troncosco. In 1925, Troncosco had devised an instrument he called the gonioscope, and thus he popularized the term *gonioscopy* (1). He found the illumination and magnification of the ophthalmoscope inferior and thus devised a self-illuminating direct-view monocular gonioscope united in one instrument. He attached a rotatable prism periscope to the objective, which allowed examiners to view the angle quadrant closest to themselves (9,18). He also modified the Koeppe lens: he used acrylic plastic, changed its shape by making the outside surface more convex, and added the ridge around the outside of the lens to allow the lid to hold the lens in place (8,18). Additionally, he devised a head band; it held a shaft with a ball at its end, which was placed into a hole of the contact glass to hold the lens in place (9). He and Castroviejo were credited with providing important information on the comparative anatomy of the angle (20). In 1942 he developed a combination binocular direct-vision microscope and illumination system that made gonioscopy less cumbersome and provided a binocular view (7). In 1947 he published the first text on gonioscopic identification and deserves credit for clearly describing the anatomy of the angle and its correlating gonioscopic identity (18). He is credited with making gonioscopy a useful clinical technique (9).

Glaucoma and Gonioscopy

Troncosco's interest in gonioscopy stemmed from his interest in glaucoma, but the first investigator to concentrate on gonioscopic findings in glaucoma was Thoburn. He utilized a Koeppe lens with the patient supine and with an external illuminating source and 4x loupe magnifier. In 1927 he published a paper describing peripheral anterior synechia and its relation in glaucoma and noted changes in angle depth with changes in the size of the pupil (2,18). He concluded that in most cases of glaucoma the angle is open. He was also a pioneer in goniophotography, later expanded on by Castroveijo, Bogart, and Sugar (7).

It was actually earlier, in 1920, that Curran had first recognized that closure of the angle may have some relationship to glaucoma. He thought that the anterior chamber became shallow because of retention of aqueous in the posterior chamber, and this caused the iris to balloon forward, implicating relative pupillary block as the mechanism for shallow anterior chambers. He performed peripheral iridotomies to reestablish communication between the anterior and posterior chambers (18). His ideas were not universally accepted at the time.

It was not until Barkan published his studies in 1936 and described goniotrabeculotomy that gonioscopy became a true clinical procedure with significant practical application. Barkan critiqued the earlier methods, noting, among other things, that the magnification was insufficient; the systems were monocular; the illumination was not bright enough and it produced shadows, creating false appearances; the examination in the upright position prevented lateral angle observation and in the supine position, the poor illumination and magnification resulted in poor images; and with the exception of Koeppe's methods, the earlier techniques caused light, shadow, and colors that led to false interpretations. His goal was to develop a method that produced a magnified stereoscopic view with slit lamp illumination that could easily be used to view the entire angle within a short time frame and with patient comfort (1). He realized he would need high magnification, bright illumination, and stereopsis to perform accurate examination of the anterior chamber. To accomplish this, Barkan utilized a Zeiss binocular microscope suspended from the ceiling, a Koeppe contact lens, and a powerful carbon Vogt arc slit lamp, thus introducing the technique of direct gonioscopy still used today.

Because of the bulkiness and weight of the instruments, gonioscopy remained a cumbersome procedure. Barkan described his system as combining the rigidity of the Koeppe system utilizing the slit lamp and lens, with the flexibility of the Troncosco method using a portable microscope. He avoided their respective limitations: the requirement that the patient sit upright and the lack of binocularity. He also developed a lucite lens with optical principles similar to those of the Koeppe lens with a 1.5x magnification (10). Until that time, the lenses had been made of glass, and there was concern that the lenses were too heavy to be allowed to remain on glaucomatous eyes for long periods of time, for fear they would increase vascularity (21). (See Figure 1.1.)

Barkan provided a "definitive classification of the types of primary glaucoma based on microscopic gonioscopy" (13). He recognized the usefulness of transillumination as a technique to examine the angle; noted that the angle is more narrow superior than inferior; classified glaucoma into open- and closed-angle glaucoma; and introduced the idea of surgery

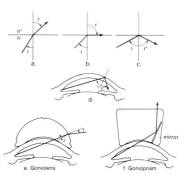

Figure 1.1 *Principles of gonioscopy. (a) Light ray is refracted when angle of incidence (* i*) at interface of two media with different indices of refraction (* n *and* n'*) is less than the critical angle. (b) Angle of refraction (* r*) is 90 degrees when* i *equals the critical angle. (c) Light is reflected when* i *exceeds the critical angle. (d) Light from the anterior chamber angle exceeds the critical angle at the cornea-air interface and is reflected back into the eye. (e, f) Contact lenses have an index of refraction (* n*) similar to that of the cornea, allowing light to enter the lens and then be refracted (goniolens) or reflected (gonioprism) beyond contact lens-air interface. (Reprinted with permission from Shields MB. Textbook of glaucoma, 3d ed. Baltimore: Williams & Wilkins, 1992.)*

for congenital glaucoma utilizing the gonioscope to maintain visualization of the angle, the importance of gonioscopy as a technique in the diagnosis of adult glaucoma, and recognized that increased pigmentation of the angle, particularly in the inferior angle, was normal (8).

In 1940, Gradle and Sugar attempted to quantify the nature of the anterior chamber and the angle depth. They termed the measurement of the angle depth *goniometry*. They recognized the important clinical value of observing the angle depth as a means for predicting future angle-closure glaucoma, thus emphasizing the clinical importance of gonioscopy in glaucoma (22).

Indirect System

It was clear that observation of the angle required a contact lens, an appropriate fluid to fill the interface between the lens and the cornea, a magnification system, and an illuminating system. Improvements in lens type, illumination, and magnification occurred in 1938 when Goldmann popularized gonioscopy as we know it today with the design of a mirrored gonioscope lens to be used with the newly manufactured Haag-Streit slit lamp and thus introduced indirect gonioscopy. The lens design incorporated a plano anterior surface that eliminated corneal refraction as a factor. The light rays are reflected to the front of the lens by an enclosed mirror tilted at an angle of 64 degrees, thus allowing the observer to view the angle structures from in front of the patient (15). This design permitted the anterior chamber observation while the patient remained seated upright.

A number of mirrored lenses have been introduced since that time, but it was the development of coaxially illuminated and viewing slit lamps with binocular observation and variable illumination that brought us to the modern era of gonioscopy. With these slit lamps, the microscope and light source can remain focused at the same location and thus free the gonioscopist to maneuver the lens with one hand and move the microscope and light source with the other.

More recent advances in lens designs and materials provide greater flexibility and more choices. The gonioscopist has the option of choosing from a number of specialty lenses depending upon the clinical needs. Early designs included a self-illuminated Koeppe-type lens developed in an attempt to improve angle visibility. The forerunner of the modern four-mirror lens was developed as a four-sided contact prism lens made in acrylic resin instead of glass in an attempt to facilitate examination of the anterior chamber (23,24,25). Low-vacuum-style direct and indirect lenses have been designed as a means to enhance flexibility by allowing the examiner's hands to remain free. Dual-observation gonioscopy lenses have been proposed as a means of providing a simultaneous examination of opposite-angle sections based on the principle of total internal reflection, where rays from the two angle sectors travel the same path and converge on a single reflecting surface. Therefore two-thirds of the angle can be examined at one time (26). More recently, a pigment gradation lens was designed and manufactured with a color scale built into the lens to help in the grading of trabecular meshwork pigmentation. The development of the flatter, curved, smaller-diameter four-mirror gonioscopy lenses simplified and shortened the time required for routine screening of the anterior chamber, and these lenses are also used for differentiating peripheral anterior synechia from iris apposition by performing dynamic compression gonioscopy. Another specialty lens designed to use without methylcellulose is a bubble-free goniolens, a modification of the single mirror gonioscopy lens in which the lens has a flat base curve radius of 8.4 mm and an intermediate peripheral bevel of 9.5 mm and thus does not compress the cornea; the single mirror is positioned in one-third of the lens cone, thus producing a large field of view. It is considered a good lens choice for children and adults with small palpebral apertures.

Gonioscopy and Glaucoma Therapy

In 1973 and 1974, Krasnov reported on the use of laser surgery in glaucoma (27). His early treatment consisted of creating holes in the trabecular meshwork to increase outflow. In 1979, Wise and Witter (28) reported on the effects of evenly spaced nonpenetrating laser burns to the circumference of the trabecular meshwork, and since that time argon laser trabeculoplasty (ALT) has been an accepted mode of therapy for lowering the intraocular pressure. In the same year, Kimbrough and associates described iridoplasty treating 360 degrees of the iris through a gonioscopy lens (29). In 1977 Simmons and associates reported on the treatment for neovascularization of the angle with laser, a procedure termed *goniophotocoagulation* (26). The advent of laser therapy for the treatment for glaucoma has spurred the development of lenses used for this therapeutic mode, creating a new role for gonioscopy as a means of delivering the laser energy to the appropriate treatment site. As an example, the use of contact lenses with different magnifications provides the necessary options for treating various conditions. In an eye with a shallow chamber suffering angle closure, a wide-angled beam provided by a convex lens will be required because it will prevent the laser light from being absorbed by the cornea (30).

The systems we use today are not error free. Although we assume that when the gonioscope lens is placed on the eye, we are observing the anterior chamber free of mechanical or optical distortion, that is not the case. Any unwanted pressure placed against the eye with the lenses can cause distortions and angle characteristic changes. Each lens design has advantages and disadvantages, and the examiner should be aware of the different views provided by each lens.

References

1. Barkan O, Boyle SF, Maisler S. On the genesis of glaucoma. *Am J Ophthalmol*. 1936;19:209–215.
2. Spaeth G. Gonioscopy: Uses old and new: The inheritence of occludable angles. *Ophthalmology*. 1978;85:222.
3. Greenidge KC. Angle-closure glaucoma. *Int Ophthalmol Clin*. 1990;30(3):177–186.
4. Eskridge JB et al. Erickson goniolens system. *J Am Opt Assoc*. 1978;49:395.
5. Forgas LS et al. Gonioscopy without the use of corneal anesthetics. *J Am Opt Assoc*. 1974;45:258.
6. Richmond PR, Saladin JJ. Gonioscopy using the Brandreth-Saladin goniochamber. *Am Opt Assoc*. 1978;49:761.
7. Troncosco MU. *A treatise on gonioscopy*. Philadelphia: FA Davis, 1948.
8. Gorin G, Posner A. *Slit lamp gonioscopy*. Baltimore: Williams & Wilkins, 1967.
9. Becker S. *Clinical gonioscopy: A text and stereoscopic atlas*. St. Louis: CV Mosby, 1972.
10. Barkan O. A diagnostic contact lens made of lucite. *Arch Ophthalmol*. 1940;24:798.
11. Gorin G. Gonioscopy. In JG Bellows, ed. *Glaucoma: Contemporary international concepts*. New York: Masson Publishing, 1979.
12. Cowen J. Pool gonioscopy. *Am J Ophthalmol*. 1957;43:619.
13. Brandeth R. Biomicroscopy Multimedia Communications Center, School of Optometry Communication Center, University of California, Berkeley 1973.
14. Sokolic P. Utilization of saline solutions for examination of chamber angle etc. *Acta Ophthalmol*. 1968;46:725.
15. Becker S. Critique of gonioscopy. In Becker B, Drew RC. *Current Concepts in Ophthalmology*. St. Louis: CV Mosby, 1972.
16. Gray L. Fundamentals of gonioscopy. *Rev Optom*. October 1977.
17. Hobbs HE. The trabecula in chronic simple glaucoma with special reference to the gonioscopic appearance of blood in the canal of Schlemm. *Br J Ophthalmol*. 1952;34:498.
18. Dellaporta A. Historical notes on gonioscopy. *Surv Ophthalmol*. 1975;20(2):137–149.
19. Troncosco MU. Gonioscopy and its clinical application. *Am J Ophthalmol*. 1925;8(6);433–439.
20. Adler FH (ed). Ophthalmologic reviews Sugar H.S. gonioscopy

and glaucoma. *Arch Ophthalmol.* 1941;25:674–717.

21. Boyd TAS. Gonioscopic abnormalities in open-angle glaucoma. *Trans Ophthalmol Soc.* 1962;25:206–220.

22. Gradle HS, Sugar HS. Concerning the chamber angle. III: A clinical method of goniometry. *Am J Ophthalmol.* 1940; 23:1135–1139.

23. Friedman B. Self-illuminated goniolens. *Am J Ophthalmol.* 1966;61:1541.

24. Kapetansky F. A bubble-free goniolens. *Ophthalm Surg.* 1988;19(6):414–416.

25. Lee A, Obrien CS. Gonioscopy simplified by a contact prism.

Arch Ophthalmol. 1945;34:413–414.

26. Simmons et al. Goniophotocoagulation for neovascular glaucoma. *Trans Am Acad Ophthalmol Otolaryngol.* 1977;83:1.

27. Kranov MM. Laser puncture of anterior chamber in glaucoma. *Am J Ophthalmol.* 1973;674.

28. Wise JB, Witter SL. Argon laser therapy for open angle glaucoma: A pilot study. *Arch Ophthalmol.* 1979;97:319.

29. Kimbrough et al. Angle-closure glaucoma in nanophthalmos. *Am J Ophthalmol.* 1979;88:572.

30. Schirmer KE. Argon laser surgery of the iris, optimized by contact lenses. *Arch Ophthalmol.* 1983;101:1130.

Chapter 2

Anterior Chamber Anatomy and Landmarks: Gonioscopic Correlation

Gonioscopy permits a detailed clinical examination of the anatomy of the anterior chamber, which is otherwise hidden from view (Plate 7). The primary anatomic structures available for observation are the pupil border; the iris; the wall of the anterior chamber, which includes the ciliary body, the scleral spur, the trabecular meshwork, and the area of Schlemm's canal; Schwalbe's line, which is the internal limit of the cornea; the posterior corneal surface; and in some instances the ciliary processes and posterior chamber (Table 2.1).

Anterior Chamber Formation

The precise mechanism for the formation of the anterior chamber angle is not completely confirmed, but it is thought to be a progressive deepening that initiates at month three to four of gestation and continues after birth possibly as long as four years after birth (1) (Figure 2.1).

Earlier theories proposed that the anterior chamber deepened by either atrophy or rarefaction and reorganization of mesenchymal cells. Without evidence of atrophy, later theories proposed the role of cleavage into the tissue; this has been opposed, however, on the theory that this observation is the result of artifacts that occur when tissue is prepared for histological examination (1).

TABLE 2.1
Gonioscopic Landmarks

Pupil border
Iris contour, surface
Iris root
Ciliary body (CB)
Scleral spur (SS)
Trabecular meshwork (TM)
Schlemm's canal (SC)
Schwalbe's line (Schw)
Posterior cornea
Ciliary processes
Posterior chamber

According to Anderson (2), based on his light and electron microscopy of 10 eyes with infantile glaucoma and 40 normal eyes, at five months gestation the ciliary body is within the uveal tissue at the same level of the trabecular meshwork and faces the trabecular meshwork. The progressive deepening of the angle is the result of posterior movement of tissue, so that the ciliary body, including the muscle and processes, ends up at a position posterior to the trabecular meshwork. The repositioning of the tissue is probably related to the differences in growth rate of the different tissues. "In normal development,

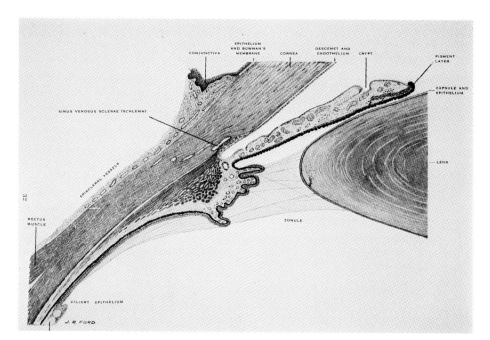

Figure 2.1. Normal anterior chamber anatomy. (Reprinted with permission from Wolff's anatomy of the eye and orbit, 6th ed. Philadelphia: WB Saunders, 1968.)

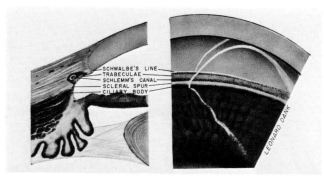

Figure 2.2. Drawing showing the anatomical angle structure on the left and the corresponding gonioscopic counterpart on the right. Gonioscopically Schwalbe's line represents the internal limbus at the termination of the internal cornea and the anterior limit of the trabecular meshwork. Schlemm's canal is located in the posterior portion of the trabecular meshwork. From Gorin G, Posner A. Slit lamp gonioscopy, *3d ed. Baltimore: Williams & Wilkins, 1967.*

the corneoscleral coat grows faster than the uveal tract during the last trimester, leading to a posterior migration of the ciliary body attachment from Schwalbe's line (fifth month) to the scleral spur (ninth month) and then to a location behind the scleral spur [postnatally] (2).

At birth, the apex of the angle, formed by the insertion of the iris along the anterior chamber wall, is located posterior to Schlemm's canal, at the level of the scleral spur. The angle at this time has more uveal meshwork anterior to the ciliary muscle and lies in front of the scleral spur (1). Maldevelopment of the irido-corneal angle can be the result of heredity or sporadic embarrassment (3).

Spaeth reported on a group of 1432 individuals (non-ophthalmic). He found that in the child, the angular approach is wider, there are more iris processes (Plates 28 and 29), peripheral curvature of the iris is flatter, and pigmentation of the trabeculum is less than in the adult (Plate 41). He also noted the membrane that covers the angle in the newborn could still be seen (4). This membrane, according to Barkan (17), is transparent with a surface shagreen and, according to Anderson, is probably transparent trabecular tissue (2,5).

In the adult eye normally, the iris inserts into the ciliary body (Figure 2.2); above the ciliary body, the sclera can be visualized as the scleral spur. Fitting into the spur is the trabecular meshwork, which runs superior to the posterior cornea. Located in the posterior third of the trabecular meshwork is Schlemm's canal, the opening through which the aqueous filters from the anterior chamber. The trabecular meshwork runs superiorly to Schwalbe's line, which is actually the internal location of Descemet's membrane and the internal demarcation between the sclera and the cornea.

The gonioscopist should evaluate and comment on the appearance of (Table 2.2):

- The pupillary margin.
- The iris and the location of the iris insertion, the contour or curvature of the iris along its course to the wall and just before its insertion, and the angular approach of the peripheral iris and angle recess.
- The ciliary body.
- The scleral spur.
- The trabecular meshwork.
- Schwalbe's line and the wall above Schwalbe's to the clear cornea.

In addition to angle depth determination, these structures should be evaluated for normalcy in each quadrant (Table 2.3).

TABLE 2.2
Angle Width

Finding	Condition
Wide	Normal, myopia, and aphakia
Intermediate width	Normal
Narrow	Hypermetropic, eye at risk for angle closure
Excessively narrow	Angle-closure glaucoma
Closed	Angle-closure glaucoma
Irregular narrowing	Anatomical narrowing superiorly
	Chronic or subacute angle-closure glaucoma
	Dislocation of lens
	Cysts or tumors of iris or ciliary body
	PAS
	Plateau iris
Irregular widening	Traumatic recession of angle
	Dislocation of lens
	Cyclodialysis

Adapted from Epstein DL. *Chandler and Grant's Glaucoma*, 3d ed. Philadelphia: Lea & Febiger, 1986.

TABLE 2.3
Iris Contour

Finding	Condition
Slight convexity	Normal, physiologic
Excessive convexity	Hypermetropia
	Malignant glaucoma
	Angle-closure glaucoma (pupil block)
Plateau iris	Angle-closure glaucoma, secondary to plateau iris configuration
Concave iris root	Myopia
	Aphakio
	Pigment dispersion syndrome
Irregularity of contour	Dislocation of lens
	Cyst or tumor
	Pupillary block in aphakia
	Segmental atrophy
Segmental atrophy of iris	Previous acute glaucoma
	ICE (iridocorneal endothelial) syndrome
	Herpes zoster
Pigment sprinkling	Exfoliation syndrome
	Pigmentary dispersion syndrome
	Malignant melanoma
	Cyst of iris or ciliary body
Pigmentation abnormality	Nevus/Melanoma
	Heterochromic cyclitis
	Glaucomatocyclitic crisis
	Hemangioma
	Neurofibroma
	Siderosis or chalcosis
	ICE syndrome

Adapted from Epstein DL. *Chandler and Grant's Glaucoma*, 3d ed. Philadelphia: Lea & Febiger, 1986.

Pupil Border and Iris Contour

Anatomically, the iris consists of an anterior and posterior portion. The posterior portion is of retinal or ectodermal origin, and the anterior portion is of mesodermal origin and consists of two zones: the pupillary zone and the ciliary zone

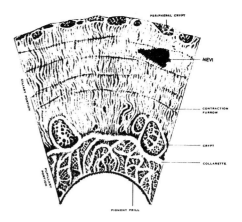

Figure 2.3. Normal iris anatomy. (Reprinted with permission from Wolff's Anatomy of the eye and orbit, 6th ed. Philadelphia: WB Saunders, 1968.)

(Figure 2.3). The demarcation of the two zones is determined by the collarette of the iris, usually located 1.5 mm from the pupillary zone.

The pupillary zone undergoes atrophy of the anterior stroma after birth, and remnants of this tissue are noted as persistant pupillary fibers. The atrophy in this area is also responsible for the formation of Fuchs' crypts. At the margin of the pupil, there may exist a physiologcial ectropion of the iris (6). The sphincter muscle is located in the pupillary zone. The dilator muscle is located in the posterior portion of the iris and continues to the iris periphery.

The ciliary zone of the iris consists of two stromal layers; longitudinally, it is divided into three parts. The portion closest to the pupil is the *collarette*, a peripheral area with contraction furrows, and the most peripheral portion is the *iris root*. The iris root inserts into the *ciliary body* and is the thinnest portion of the iris. Iris processes originate from the anterior iris surface in this region. Gorin has suggested that the peripheral portion of the iris contains ciliary crypts formed by progressive atrophy of the anterior stromal leaf of the iris. These peripheral crypts are often not seen gonioscopically because of the oblique observation of the peripheral iris, and thus the crypts are hidden by iris surface irregularities. Gorin believes that these crypts may prevent angle closure in some eyes because they prevent a complete seal of the peripheral iris against the angle wall (7).

Gonioscopic observation should start at the iris pupil border and the more central areas of the ciliary zone. Abnormalities in this area—such as deposition of exfoliative material, ectropion uveae, iris atrophy, iris cysts, and rubeosis—can be observed. The examiner then should move fixation along the iris surface, noting the contour of the iris plane—whether it is flat, concave, or convex—and noting any irregularities of the surface. In the normal adult, there may be a slight convexity of the iris at the pupil zone as the pupil zone is normally 0.6 to 1.0 mm anterior to the iris root (8). This is the result of the anatomical lens pushing the iris forward. There may be a slight physiological peripheral bowing as well from normal amounts of resistance of aqueous flow from the posterior chamber.

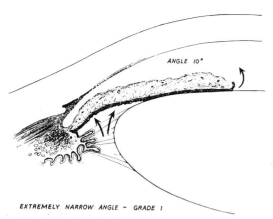

ANGLE 10°

EXTREMELY NARROW ANGLE - GRADE 1

Figure 2.4. Example of relative pupil block in narrow angle. Peripheral iris bows forward from increased pressure in the posterior chamber, narrowing the angle created between the peripheral iris and the trabecular meshwork. (Reprinted with permission from Hoskins HD Jr, Kass MA. Becker-Schaffer's diagnosis and therapy of glaucomas, 6th ed. St Louis: CV Mosby, 1989.

In cases of significant pupillary block, more significant iris bombé forms in the peripheral zone (Figure 2.4 and Plate 38). The bombé in these cases is from the resistance to the aqueous flow created by the iris and lens contact, making it more difficult for aqueous to flow from the posterior chamber to the anterior chamber. This creates a pressure difference: the pressure in the posterior chamber becomes greater than that in the anterior chamber, resulting in the bowing or bombe of the mid-peripheral portion of the iris. In addition to the bombe, these eyes will have shallow chambers both centrally and peripherally, which can be detected on slit lamp examination. With wide dilation in some of these eyes, the iris will be moved beyond peripheral to the crystalline, the anatomical lens, and beyond the position of relative pupillary block. Thus, the iris will no longer be pushed forward by the posterior chamber pressure or the anatomical lens. This explains why the chamber in some dilated eyes appears deeper than they are when the eye is undilated. When the pupil constricts back to its normal position, the iris will again be positioned against the lens, pupil block will resume, and the peripheral iris will bow forward, narrowing the angle. Thus, a dilation-provocative test in an eye at risk for relative pupillary block may be misinterpreted as negative if the pressure and angle are evaluated while the pupil is fully dilated. Testing should be done while the pupil is in the position of greatest pupillary block: at mid-dilation with the pupil going up or more so when it is more lax and coming down (8).

Although the depth of the chamber is genetically determined by polygenic inheritance, there are normal variations that will influence the depth of the chamber and the iris contour. The examiner should keep this in mind while examining the eye. The depth of the chamber is known to have a diurnal variation, being shallowest in the late afternoon (9). Differences in refractive error also contribute to differences in chamber depth and iris contour. As most myopic eyes have deep chambers and flat iris planes, whereas most

hyperopic eyes have shallower chambers and a more convex iris plane.

When examining patients, the examiner should consider the age of the patient. The iris plane is relatively flat and the chamber depth shallower in newborns. Over time, the continued growth of the crystalline lens causes iris bowing and shallowing of the chamber. Thus, older patients (above the mid-50s) tend to have a more bowed iris and a shallower chamber than young or middle-aged adults. This is less pronounced in myopic patients, particularly high myopes (10). Males tend to have a slightly larger anterior chamber than females, and this correlates with the fact that women have a greater incidence of angle closure than men (9). As for the risk for angle-closure glaucoma, clinical statistics indicate that the incidence of narrow angles is between 2% and 5% and occludable angles at 1.64%; however, the incidence of angle-closure glaucoma is only 0.09% in the general population. This demonstrates the rare incidence of angle closure in the occludable population and is even more rare in the general population (7).

Peripheral Iris, Iris Root, and Normal Blood Vessels

The peripheral iris provides the site of insertion of the iris onto the inner wall of the anterior chamber. In general, the more posterior the iris inserts, the wider is the angle created between the mid-peripheral iris and the angle wall. This angular measurement is the basis of the Shaffer system of chamber grading (11) (Figure 2.5). This angular notation does correlate in most cases with the openness of an angle; however, it does not adequately describe the true configuration of the recess of the chamber angle because it does not adequately describe the configuration of the most peripheral portion of the iris—whether it angulates posterior (just prior to insertion) as in plateau iris, whether there is a prominent last roll of the iris, or whether the iris bows forward before insertion. It also does not consider the axial depth of the

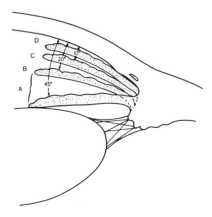

Figure 2.5. Shaffer's gonioscopic classification of the anterior chamber. (Angle: A = wide open, B = moderately narrow, C = extremely narrow, D = partially or totally closed.) (Reprinted with permission from Shields MB. Textbook of Glaucoma, 3d ed. Baltimore: Williams & Wilkins, 1992.)

chamber or the actual point of insertion of the iris onto the anterior chamber wall. These are additional features that should be considered in determining whether an eye has an open angle or is susceptible to angle closure. The examiner must remember that the space bounded by the iris, ciliary body, and the wall of the anterior chamber is not a true angle in the geometric sense (12). In the Shaffer system, an angle of 20 degrees or less is considered narrow and capable of closure. This correlates with a van Herick estimation of 1/4:1. That is, an angle deemed as 1/4:1 and/or 20 degrees indicates that gonioscopy should be performed, and certainly prior to dilation. In most instances, the iris root will cover the ciliary body to a certain extent. In some shallow-chambered eyes, a normal prominent last roll of the iris, located before the iris root, may interfere with the gonioscopic view of the angle wall.

The iris root is the only movable anatomic landmark along the wall of the anterior chamber; therefore, its structure may have a significant influence on the configuration of the angle and, thus, the closability of the angle. Spaeth's grading system for gonioscopy accounts for this variability in the peripheral iris configuration, as he recommends not relying solely on the angle dimension or most posterior visible structure when determining the occludability of an angle. His system grades a number of iris configuration variables, including location of iris insertion, contour of the iris before insertion, and contour of the iris in the mid-peripheral zone. He feels that the characteristic with the greatest correlation to primary angle-closure glaucoma is the amount of convexity of the peripheral iris (4).

Iris Root and Normal Vasculature

In most instances the iris root normally will cover the ciliary body to a certain extent. When the iris root is thin, the angle recess is deep and wide, and when the iris root is thick and short, the angle recess will appear shallow and the iris inserts more anterior (12). In normal eyes, the last roll of the iris—the roll of Fuchs—usually does not obscure the view of the peripheral iris zone and the iris root. The iris root is usually smoother and lighter than the rest of the iris because of a thinning of the anterior leaf of the stroma (12). Iridodonisis of the iris root may be observed when doing gonioscopy on a supine patient. It is also seen in myopia and pigment dispersion syndrome and after blunt trauma to the eye.

The inherent characteristics of the iris may influence the incidence of angle closure. When the pupil dilates, the peripheral iris forms circumferential folds, which can be located close to the limbus. The direction of the iris folds is variable; in some eyes, it may fold directly into the angle recess and promote an angle closure, and in others, it may fold away from the angle recess. Folding of the iris and its relation to the angle vary from eye to eye. The folding of the iris generally increases its thickness, and texture and thickness may influence the onset of angle closure. A flaccid iris is more likely to bow forward into a convex shape; a rigid iris is less likely to take that shape (13) (Figure 2.6).

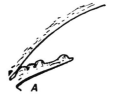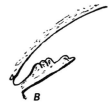

Figure 2.6. Variation of iris folding. (A = The iris folds peripherally and occludes the narrow angle. B = The iris folds away from the angle toward the ridges, and in the absence of increased pupil block, the angle widens.) (Reprinted with permission from Lowe RF. Primary angle closure glaucoma. Singapore: PG Publications, 1989.)

The root of the iris may exhibit many bumps and undulations, sometimes allowing visibility of the normal vascular circle that runs circumferentially and radially. The vascular layer of the iris is continuous with the ciliary body. At the juncture of the ciliary body and the iris, the blood vessels may undergo sharp angular deviations. This occurs at the ciliary margin of the iris behind the scleral spur. These normal blood vessels are most often seen in a light iris, when vessels are congested, or in deep anterior chambers with a posterior insertion of the iris. They are also visible in cases of iridodysgenesis, where there is abnormal cleavage of the angle wall. Henkind (14) noted that on gonioscopic examination of 200 consecutive patients, he found three unique types of vessels (Figure 2.7): circular ciliary band vessels (circular iris root vessels), the most common; radial iris vessels; and radial ciliary body or trabecular vessels, the least common. These normal angle vessels were found in 26% of the eyes examined—more so in blue-eyed wide-angle patients, possibly the result of increased visibility in deep angles and increased contrast in light-colored eyes. This is consistent with Shihab's finding of an incidence of 21%. These vessels usually do not bleed; however, Shihab reported two cases of spontaneous hyphema associated with these vessels and anterior chamber intraocular lens–induced chronic trauma. He recommended avoiding anterior chamber angle fixed lenses in angles with prominent circular vessels (15).

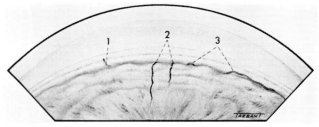

Figure 2.7. Composite drawing of normal angle vessels. (1) Radial ciliary body. (2) Radial iris vessel. (3) Circular ciliary band vessels running circumferentially. Angle vessels in normal eyes. (Reprinted with permission from Henkind P. Angle vessels in normal eyes. Br J Ophthalmol. 1964; 48:551–557.

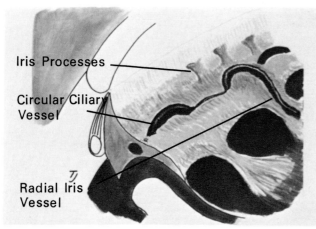

Figure 2.8. Artist's representation of common circular ciliary band vessels. (Reprinted with permission from Jerndal T et al. Goniodysgenesis: A new perspective on glaucoma. Copenhagen: Scriptor, 1978.)

These normal vessels emanate from the major arterial circle and its radial branches and should not be confused with abnormal neovascular vessels. They are thicker than neovascular vessels, are found in nondiseased eyes, tend to run in deeper portions of the iris, occasionally rising to the iris surface, and are not associated with fine surface vessels radiating back to the pupil margin (Figure 2.8).

The circular ciliary band vessels are the major arterial circle of the iris and are formed by branches of the medial and lateral long posterior ciliary arteries and the anterior ciliary arteries. They run circumferentially around the angle. Gonioscopically, the vessels are usually red, with visible segments sheathed or unsheathed. They are located either within or on the ciliary body or slightly anterior to the ciliary body, behind the last roll of the iris, and they may appear to run along the iris root. They undulate along their course and are visible in the deepest sections of the angle; they are more easily noticed in the inferior quadrant and can be seen to have radial iris vessels running off them.

The radial iris vessels, which can be seen at the iris root, run off the circular ciliary vessels. They are surrounded by a white sheath and disappear into the deeper peripheral or mid-zone of the iris. This differentiates them from neovascular vessels, which usually arise from the pupil border, are thin, are not sheathed, and run along the surface of the iris.

The radial ciliary body or trabecular vessels are the least common normal-angle vessels. They may be most easily confused with neovascular vessels because of their orientation; they run perpendicular to the plane of the iris. However, they are thicker than neovascular vessels, they cannot be seen connecting to another vessel, and they do not run along the length of the iris. According to Henkind, they are probably branches of the arterial circle in the area of Schlemm's canal or branches of the deeper scleral plexus (14). Chatterjee described the presence of this type of vessel in 11 of 50 eyes he examined with iridocyclitis. He did not

feel they represented neovascularization but was unsure of their significance (16). The radial vessels become more apparent in eyes that have suffered angle recession (6). A fourth type of normal vessel (Plate 48) may be seen on gonioscopy. It is located on the ciliary band that extends perpendicular to the ciliary body, courses along the wall, and disappears directly into the sclera. This probably represents the ciliary artery on the inner surface (8).

Iris Processes

Gonioscopically, iris processes may be observed along the inner surface of the uveal meshwork (Table 2.4). The processes usually lie close to the ciliary body, but they may bridge the angle. They appear as thin, fine, lacy fibers or a coarse, dense, interlacing network or membrane attaching at the level of the trabecular meshwork. They have been described as akin to wall ivy, with the terminal edge having many fine tendril-like branching terminations (8). In the iris root area, this layer of tissue representing iris processes is usually atrophied; however, in blue eyes with deep chambers lying on the juncture between the iris and the ciliary body, sometimes an amorphous billowing residual mesodermal tissue (iris processes) can be seen (17). Boyd described a fine-textured woolly substance in this location in normal eyes and in eyes with open-angle glaucoma. He noted that, to an examiner using a finely focused slit lamp, they may appear as white strands, and in other eyes they may have a cotton wool appearance, located between the iris root and the angle wall and may be confused for the ciliary body giving a false appearance of angle recession. This substance can have a teardrop configuration (18).

Anatomically and embryologically, iris processes were thought to be vestigial phylogenetic remnants of the pectinate ligament in animals. They were first studied in horses by Hueck in 1839 and were given the name *pectinate* because of their similar appearance to a comb. In the early literature,

TABLE 2.4
Iris Processes

Finding	Condition
Network of grayish strands, variable amount	In blue-eyed adults
Network of brown strands, variable amount	In brown-eyed adults
Uneven pigmentation	Corresponding to uneven iris pigmentation, nevi, post inflammation
Greater amount nasally	Common normal finding
Disruption of defects, baring underlying structures	Result of tear by blunt trauma or cyclodialysis
Separation of sheet or shelf	Result of blunt trauma
Abundant and dense	Congenital or developmental angle anomalies
	Pigment dispersion syndrome

Adapted from Epstein DL. *Chandler and Grant's Glaucoma*, 3d ed. Philadelphia: Lea & Febiger, 1986.

there was some confusion regarding iris processes; the term was used to describe the entire meshwork by some and the uveal portion by others. Lichter (18) noted that the terms *mesodermal remnant, pectinate fiber,* and *iris processes* were used to describe the same structure and concluded that if the structure was iris tissue running from the iris to the angle wall (which it is), it was more accurate to use the term *iris processes.* He explained the presence of iris processes as the result of improper cleavage of the mesodermal tissue of the angle during development, where a persistent adherence of the mesodermal tissue to the trabecular meshwork after cleavage results in the iris processes. Incomplete cleavage is associated with infantile glaucoma and mesodermal dysgenesis. Lichter further proposes that the presence of extensive iris processes with high iris insertion may be a sign of abnormalities of the deeper levels of the trabecular meshwork. Spaeth, however, noted that the presence of iris processes may simply be representative of the youthful eye, not an abnormality (18), and their presence varies with iris color and age, appearing more frequently in younger patients with brown irides. This later information agreed with Lichter's earlier observation.

According to Tripathi and Tripathi (1), iris processes are actually a bridge between the iris root and the uveal meshwork, and morphologically, the base of the process is similar to the iris stroma. At their attachment to the angle wall, they resemble the inner uveal tissue. Gonioscopically, especially in the adult eye with indirect gonioscopy, the examiner is visualizing iris processes as the uveal meshwork is not usually gonioscopically apparent; although, some (8) continue to differentiate gonioscopically between iris processes and uveal meshwork.

Gonioscopically, Lichter defined iris processes as "tissue connecting the iris to the angle wall either bridging or wrapping around the angle recess. The tissue had to be distinct from the insertion of the iris or, in cases where this distinction was difficult, had to insert at the level of the scleral spur or higher" (18). Barkan, using his direct gonioscopy method, noted that iris processes vary in number and extent in different portions of the same eye and from person to person (19). They are usually similar to the iris stroma, appearing brown or yellowish in dark irides and gray or white in blue ones. With the indirect Goldmann-type system, they appear darker and sometimes can have a slight reddish-brown coloration. In some instances, they may be mistaken as neovascular vessels. This is more likely to occur when they are isolated and attached high onto the wall, at the level of Schwalbe's line. The nonprogressive nature, lack of iris neovascular vessels, and presence in an otherwise healthy eye helps differentiate these as iris processes. In older individuals and in anterior segment inflammatory disease, they become more prominent, possibly the result of collected pigment granules adhering to the processes.

Contrary to Lichter (18) and others (1,5), Gorin and Posner (11) differentiated gonioscopically between iris processes and remnants of the pectinate ligament. They described iris processes as embryonic remnants that bridge the angle from the iris periphery to the ciliary body or any portion of the angle wall. They observed them to be dark brown in dark eyes and gray to light brown in light eyes. They noted that the remnants of the pectinate ligament are coarser structures, and with time they become thin and lose their continuity. When that occurs, they may be seen as a short stump at the iris periphery, with a pigmented spot on the angle wall opposite the stump.

Lichter (18) graded the iris processes in 340 eyes of volunteers or routine refraction patients. Most patients were younger than age 30 years. He graded the angles in terms of the abundance of iris processes in the entire angle. Grade 0 meant no processes were present, and grade 4 meant dense processes were present throughout the angle. Eyes with many processes confined to a small area with few elsewhere, were grade 1 or grade 2, with a statement to indicate the presence of a dense clump. In the 340 eyes he studied, 92% had grade 2 or less, with 55% of eyes showing some processes. Most eyes without processes were blue. In the blue eyes where processes were detected, they appeared as wisps of white thread against a pale background, and these eyes had a loose, fluffy, whitish tissue in the recess of the angle. Generally, the iris processes were most dense nasally, and the two eyes frequently mirrored each other in regard to location and density of processes. He also noted that they tended to insert at the same location for a given eye, and in some cases they did not bridge the angle but actually wrapped around the angle recess.

Iris Processes vs. Synechia

Sometimes iris processes (Plate 30) can be confused with peripheral anterior synechiae, which are forward adhesions of the iris tissue to the angle wall (Figure 2.9). Unlike iris processes, which are tree branch–like figures that bridge the angle recess, synechiae tend to be full-thickness attachments of actual iris tissue that rarely bridge the angle. A synechia is actually the anterior iris face attached to the wall. It is more uniform and solid in appearance than the open, lacy-appearing porous network of iris processes (8). An area of iris processes will probably transilluminate between the lacy network; a peripheral anterior synechia will not, as it obscures the wall behind it. Compression gonioscopy can be useful for differentiating between the two. A synechia will continue to hold against the wall sometimes referred to as *tenting of the synechia* (20), where the network of iris processes will become lacier in appearance, exposing the angle wall behind them. According to Epstein (8), synechiae are never found in primary open-angle glaucoma or pure exfoliative or pigmentary glaucoma. Their presence indicates another abnormality.

Synechiae result from the iris being placed abnormally against the angle wall (Plates 4,11,23, and 31). Often there is pigment scattering along the angle wall when there is evidence of synechia. This is characteristic in cases of postinflammatory conditions such as uveitis or acute angle-closure glaucoma.

Depending on the etiology, peripheral anterior synechia (PAS) may have different characteristics (Table 2.5). For

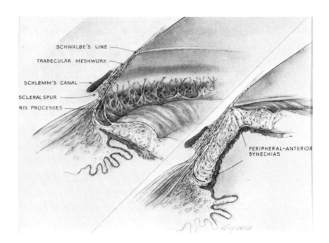

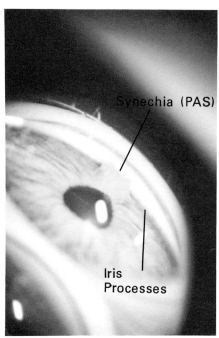

Figure 2.9. Artist's representation of iris processes versus peripheral anterior synechia. Top left: Iris process. Bottom right: Iris adhesion to the angle wall. (Reprinted with permission from Hoskins HD Jr, Kass MA. Becker-Shaffer's diagnosis and therapy of the glaucomas, 6th ed. St Louis: CV Mosby, 1989) B. Slide showing synechia and iris processes in the background along the angle wall. Photo courtesy Rodney Gutner, O.D.

TABLE 2.5
Peripheral Anterior Synechia

Condition	Finding
Angle-closure glaucoma	Usually broad
	Synechia at all levels but not to cornea and not bridging angle structures
Absence or excessive shallowing of the anterior chamber after surgery	Synechia to all levels—sometimes to cornea, sometimes bridging angle
Glaucoma secondary to iridocyclitis or KP (keratic precipitates) on the trabecular meshwork	Typically tents and columns to all levels but not to cornea
Neovascular glaucoma	Broad synechia to full width of angle, with new vessels
ICE syndrome	Synechia advancing on the cornea, sometimes obstructing trabecular meshwork
After laser trabeculoplasty	Small, irregular synechia to scleral spur, occasionally to posterior trabecular meshwork

Adapted form Epstein DL. *Chandler and Grant's Glaucoma*, 3d ed. Philadelphia: Lea & Febiger, 1986.

Although the iris processes do not interfere with outflow, abundant iris processes may be an indication and evidence of an underlying angle anomaly that could cause outflow disturbances. Lichter and Shaffer (24) reported on 104 patients referred for glaucoma evaluation who were examined for iris processes. They categorized the patients with grade 3 to 4 iris processes and found that the incidence of abnormal iris processes in the primary open-angle glaucoma and the ocular hypertensive group was higher than in a series of normal patients and still higher in a group of patients with pigmentary glaucoma. They felt that the presence of abundant iris processes was an indication and evidence of underlying anomoly of the angle that may manifest in glaucoma and in cases of pigmentary glaucoma, the presence of pigmentation was an additional insult to the eye, over and above the basic underlying angle anomaly present in those cases.

In summary, the appearance of iris processes in an eye or quadrant of an eye can be quite variable. The iris processes can appear individually or in sheets; they can be thin or thick, short or long, light or dark. They may bridge the angle and insert as high as Schwalbe's line, or they may undergo atrophy, with only the presence of a remaining stump attached to the root of the iris or trabecular meshwork. They may be so dense that they hide the angle wall structures, as in cases of incomplete embryological separation of the iris from the angle wall. In these instances, transillumination of the angle wall (Figure 2.10) will often help to identify the scleral spur in the areas with less dense processes. Most of the iris processes lose their pigmentation at the level of the scleral spur and merge with the uveal meshwork (23). In general, it is rare for them to attach anterior to the scleral spur, and when they are numerous or thick, it should be considered an anomaly. They have been included in descriptions of developmental angle anomalies

example, after laser trabeculoplasty, it may be more tooth shaped. In the ICE syndrome (Plate 23), they typically terminate higher along the wall than in other forms. The quadrant location may vary also depending on the etiology. In primary angle-closure glaucoma, it tends to be located in the superior angle; in inflammatory disease, it tends to be located in the inferior angle (21). PAS can be an attachment to the ciliary body, or it can be as high as Schwalbe's line or any structure between the two. The low, broad-based attachments may be difficult to recognize but are critical for identifying early chronic angle-closure glaucoma (22). PAS interferes with aqueous outflow, whereas iris processes do not interfere with aqueous outflow (23).

associated with glaucoma (18). Histologically iris processes are similar to iris tissue and not similar to uveal meshwork. References to iris processes should be reserved for iris tissue remnants and not the uveal meshwork, which is difficult to observe and distinguish on indirect gonioscopy. References to iris processes as pectinate ligament or pectinate is also incorrect as these are fibers forming a prominent pectinate ligament acting as a suspensory ligament found only in animals (8).

Wall of the Anterior Chamber

Ciliary Body

The vault of the so-called angle of the anterior chamber is formed by the ciliary body, which consists of the ciliary muscle and ciliary processes (Table 2.6). Normally the iris insertion into the ciliary body is observable on gonioscopy; however, in some normal eyes, the anterior surface of the iris root may have some knobby elevations that interfere with the visibility of the ciliary body and produce variable views. The thickness of the iris root may also affect the actual width of the ciliary body. In normal wide angles, the iris inserts 0.5 mm behind the scleral spur. In eyes with thicker iris roots, the iris inserts closer to the scleral spur, and this zone will be less then 0.5 mm, making the ciliary band appear narrow. This normal variation should be differentiated from other causes of narrow-appearing ciliary bands.

In dark brown eyes, it may be difficult to tell where the iris ends and the ciliary body begins. Iris processes may also interfere with observation of the ciliary body in the normal eye, as they may lie over the ciliary muscle. In some dark-colored eyes, the ciliary margin of the anterior leaf of the iris stroma may have a thick, tongue-shaped extension projecting on the ciliary body surface, which will also obscure the ciliary body. Gorin and Posner (12) describe these as dark-colored triangular fringes of iris tissue that are different gonioscopically from iris processes, iris processes being thin, with club-shaped endings. Often iris fringes and iris processes are present in the same eye; both are derived from the anterior mesodermal layer of the iris. As such, most clinicians do not differentiate between the two but rather clump them together as the same process and label them as iris processes, in one instance noting them to be thicker and

TABLE 2.6
The Ciliary Body

Finding	Condition
Very light gray, reddish-gray	Normal in white race
Darker gray, traces of brown	Normal in dark races
Darker, slate gray	Melanoma
Whitish cobwebby	Tear into the muscle or deep open angle
Scleral whiteness, cleft behind the spur	Tear through the muscle or cyclodialysis

Adapted from Epstein DL. *Chandler and Grant's glaucoma*, 3d ed. Philadelphia: Lea & Febiger, 1986.

more predominant than in another. The ciliary body may also be obscured from view by abnormalities of the angle wall, such as a narrow angle, the anterior insertion of the iris as in some forms of pigment dispersion syndrome, PAS, a mass or foreign body in the angle, or, as noted, prominent iris processes (Plates 6, 31, 36, and 41).

The anterior chamber angle is thought to be wider inferior and temporal and narrower nasal and superior. This may be related to the fact that the ciliary body is broader in the inferior and temporal quadrants and narrow in the superior and nasal quadrants (7). This alters the insertion of the iris onto the ciliary body face. The narrowness of the superior angle compared to the other quadrants probably accounts for closure occurring first in this quadrant in many cases of angle closure. The thickness of the ciliary body has been implicated as a factor influencing angle closure in some individuals.

The ciliary muscle consists of three groups of fibers: the longitudinal (meridional), the oblique (radial), and the circular. The longitudinal fibers attach to the scleral spur and trabecular meshwork and posteriorly as far as the equator in some eyes. Contracture of these fibers pulls the trabecular meshwork open. Contraction of the circular fibers causes relaxation of the zonules, and thus the crystalline lens changes shape. The oblique fibers are located more internally. The circular fibers run continuous with the oblique fibers and run in a circular direction behind the insertion of the iris root (1). The oblique muscle connects the longitudinal and circular fibers, and their contracture may widen the uveal trabecular spaces in the external portion of the ciliary body (23).

The gonioscopic color of the ciliary body has been described as a gray-white in light eyes and darker—almost a charcoal gray—in eyes with darker pigmented irides. It may also appear reddish-brown, chocolate brown, or reddish-gray. In some blue eyes, it has been described as grayish with an orange hue (23) (Plate 7). In general, in darker eyes with darker pigmented irides, the ciliary body also is darker, and the iris processes are also more pigmented (23). There are, however, numerous exceptions. In some normal darkly pigmented eyes, the ciliary body may have a mottled gray-brown appearance with a mixture of white. This coloration can be easily confused as evidence of a recessed angle (22). This is often observable in deep chambers. The absence of a history of trauma, a similar appearance in the fellow eye, and symmetry to the ciliary body appearance helps rule out angle recession. Changes to the ciliary body from blunt trauma produces variable color, texture, and asymmetry.

Scleral Spur

The scleral spur is a fibrous ring that is attached anteriorly to the trabecular meshwork and posteriorly to the sclera and the longitudinal portion of the ciliary muscle (Table 2.7) (23). The spur is unique to higher primates and is first evident during the fourth month of gestation (1). The size of the scleral spur is not the same in all eyes. The spur forms a complete ring, triangular in shape, with the apex pointing toward the

TABLE 2.7
Scleral Spur

Finding	Condition
Entire spur visible	Angle open
Spur hidden	Iris processes/uveal meshwork
	Excessively narrow angle
	Closed angle
	Synechia
	Inflammatory exudates
Spur unusually prominent and white	Uveal meshwork or iris processes torn
	Ciliary muscle torn
	Cyclodialysis cleft

Adapted from Epstein DL. *Chandler and Grant's Glaucoma*, 3d ed. Philadelphia: Lea & Febiger, 1986.

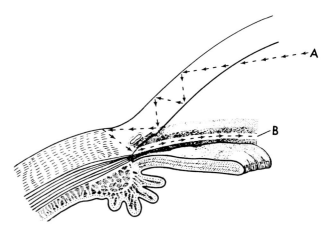

Figure 2.10. Example of retroillumination of the angle. Light is directed from point A on the cornea and is internally reflected within the sclera and cornea. The light can be seen lighting the scleral spur (B). (Reprinted with permission from Hoskins HD Jr. Interpretive gonioscopy in glaucoma. Invest Ophthalmol. *1972;11:97.)*

anterior chamber. The scleral spur represents the posterior ring of the scleral sulcus, and just anterior to it lies Schlemm's canal, which when filled with blood can be visualized with a gonioscopic lens (Plate 5). As a gonioscopic landmark, the scleral spur is of utmost importance; its identification and visualization confirm that the filtering meshwork is not obstructed in the area of observation. The technique of transillumination is helpful in identifying the scleral spur when the angle is heavily pigmented or when there are significant iris processes.

Gonioscopically the scleral spur may appear as an internal projection of the angle wall and is white in color when contrasted with the grayish coloration of a nonpigmented trabecular meshwork. When the trabecular meshwork is pigmented, the white scleral spur is more obvious unless there are significant iris processes hiding the spur from view. The longitudinal fibers of the ciliary body attach to the spur, and some may continue as far anterior as Schwalbe's line as fibers of the corneoscleral trabecula (23).

The iridotrabecular processes (iris processes), when they are dense, may cover the angle wall hindering direct observation of the scleral spur. Use of sclerotic scatter with a gonioscopic lens will cause the scleral spur to light up behind the iris processes. Sclerotic scatter can also be used to localize the spur to contrast the darker trabecular meshwork and ciliary body (Figure 2.10).

This technique was originally described using a Koeppe (25) lens but is also useful with indirect gonioscopy lenses. The technique calls for the light beam to be parallel to Schwalbe's line and decentered so that it lands on the cornea anterior to the angle. The light will be internally reflected within the sclera, and because of sclerotic scatter, the sclera will light up and appear brighter than the trabecular meshwork and ciliary body. In eyes with narrow angles and nonpigmented trabecular meshwork, the sclera may be difficult to observe directly, particularly if the peripheral iris is bowed. In these cases, this technique can be used to highlight and localize the spur (25). If the IOP is elevated and the spur can be identified in its entire circumference, the angle is confirmed as open, and the angle closure is not the reason for the raised IOP.

Trabecular Meshwork

The trabecular meshwork runs from Schwalbe's line to the anterior limit of the cornea, where it inserts into the scleral spur posteriorly (Table 2.8). In cross-section, the trabeculum forms an obtuse angle, with the base in contact with the scleral spur, the anterior face of the ciliary body, and the iris root. The apex terminates at the corneal-scleral boundary, Schwalbe's ring (26). The trabecular meshwork can be divided into two portions. One is the anterior part, which runs from Descemet's membrane to the area anterior to Schlemm's canal. This is considered the nonfiltering portion of the trabecular meshwork because it has no contact with Schlemm's canal. The other portion is the filtering part of the trabecular meshwork. It covers over Schlemm's canal and is made up of three portions: the outermost cribriform layer or juxtacanalicular tissue, the corneoscleral meshwork, which runs from the scleral spur to the cornea, and the innermost uveal meshwork, which borders the anterior chamber and runs from the corneoscleral meshwork posteriorly to the ciliary body and iris root (27).

Gonioscopically, compared to the cornea, which is transparent, and the sclera, which is opaque, the filtering portion of the trabecular meshwork has a gray, translucent appearance. In older patients or in heavily pigmented eyes, the filtering portion of the trabecular meshwork is often pigmented and darker than the remainder of the meshwork (Plate 41). This helps to identify the portion of the meshwork involved in filtration and localization of the canal of Schlemm, which lies internal to the meshwork at this point. The pigment band over Schlemm's canal is slightly wider than the width of the canal. In eyes without pigmentation, the filtering portion can be identified by its known location from the scleral spur and Schwalbe's line, as well as by its gray, granular appearance in comparison to the white scleral spur. With slight gonioscopic pressure against some eyes (Plate 5),

TABLE 2.8
Trabecular Meshwork

Finding	Condition
Normal variables	Covering by iris processes or uveal meshwork
	Pigmentation inferior
	Blood in Schlemm's canal
Characteristic feature	Filtration area finely granular, gray, translucent, with or without pigment
Acquired abnormalities	Excessive pigment 360° or localized
	Inflammatory deposits
	Blood vessels
	Synechia
	Loss of normal texture
	Traumatic rupture
Congenital abnormalities	Posterior embryotoxon
	Iridocorneal malformations

Adapted from Epstein DL. *Chandler and Grant's Glaucoma*, 3d ed. Philadelphia: Lea & Febiger, 1986.

TABLE 2.9
Pigment in the Angle

Pigment in the Angle	Condition
None	Normal in young
Band nasally and inferiorly	Normal in elderly
Faint band, whole circumference	Normal in elderly
Dense band, whole circumference, both eyes	Pigmentary glaucoma
	Pigment dispersion syndrome
Dense band, whole circumference, one eye	Exfoliation
	Malignant melanoma
	Cysts of iris or ciliary body
Scattered, mostly in lower angle	Previous intraocular surgery
	Previous inflammation
	Previous hyphema, melanoma
Patchy band, whole circumference	Occasional in open-angle glaucoma
Black, fine and coarse, balls and granules	Old blood
Dense isolated velvety patch	Nevus/melanoma

Adapted from Epstein DL. *Chandler and Grant's Glaucoma*, 3d ed. Philadelphia: Lea & Febiger, 1986.

blood will reflux back into Schlemm's canal, marking the location of the filtering trabecular meshwork. This will produce a reddish coloration to the filtering meshwork. In youths, the trabecular meshwork has been described as having a bluish-gray coloration (23), as "glistening and translucent like a semi-transparent gelatin with a stippled surface," and as a smooth, glistening, pinkish-white, moist-appearing structure (3).

Trabecular Pigmentation

According to Spaeth (22), it is rare for the trabecular meshwork to be pigmented before puberty, which he suggests may indicate some hormonal control over pigment release. He notes that during pregnancy there is a transient increase of pigmentation to the Krukenberg spindle, which he feels is related to a partial hormonal control over the release of pigment from the posterior pigment epithelium of the iris (22).

In most adult eyes, pigmentation of the trabecular meshwork is a normal finding, and it tends to become denser in the aged (Table 2.9). This is the result of pigment epithelium's becoming free from the iris and ciliary body. Most liberated pigment is phagocytosed, and smaller pieces actually pass through the inner walls of the canal of Schlemm (7). The larger pieces of pigment are trapped on the surface of the trabecula. The normal-appearing angle thus will often have a diffuse dark brown or black pigmented trabecula, particularly in the inferior and nasal angle. The temporal and superior angles often remain free of pigmentation. If there is significant pigmentation of the trabecula, especially in the superior as well as inferior angle, other reasons for the pigmentation, such as exfoliative syndrome, pigment dispersion syndrome, or previous inflammation, should be considered. Pigment in pigment dispersion or exfoliation syndrome lies within the trabecula itself and on the surface, and the angle wall may have a scalloped pigment wave above Schwalbe's line known as *Sampaolesi's line.*

Increased pigmentation is also noted in diabetes, chronic iridocyclitis, malignant melanoma, necrotic nevi, uveal tract

cysts, and iris atrophy (23). Deposition of pigment from these conditions may lie on the surface of the trabecula and lie as high as Schwalbe's line. Spaeth suggests that in some cases of primary chronic angle-closure glaucoma, the posterior trabecula may have an increase in pigmentation similar to the appearance in pigment dispersion syndrome (22). The presence of this appearance in a patient with narrow angles should suggest the possibility of chronic angle closure rather than solely a narrow angle. Irregular pigmentation of the trabecular meshwork may be an indication that the portion without pigment is a nonfunctioning sector and the pigment is collecting only in the areas actively filtering aqueous (20) (Plate 6). In albino eyes, there is a total lack of pigmentation.

The resistance to outflow probably does not occur at the visible trabecular meshwork; it is more likely to occur at the internal wall of the canal of Schlemm (7). Thus, unless the aqueous is blocked from entering the canal, little can be said about the gonioscopically open angle with visible pigmentation and the pigment's effect on outflow.

Schlemm's Canal

Lying within the trabecular meshwork is the canal of Schlemm. Gonioscopically it has been measured to be 0.2 mm to 0.3 mm. This compares to the histological measurement of 0.282 mm (28). The canal of Schlemm connects with the venous system through a system of collector channels anastomosing to form a deep scleral plexus. This plexus drains the aqueous into the anterior ciliary veins and episcleral veins (26). The canal of Schlemm cannot be detected by gonioscopy unless it is filled with blood. The blood will appear as a pinkish band anterior to the scleral spur, thus highlighting Schlemm's canal (25) (Plate 5 and Table 2.10).

Normally there is no visible blood in the canal because the pressure within the canal is lower than the pressure in the

TABLE 2.10
Reasons for Blood in Schlemm's Canal

Excessive external pressure from gonioscopy
Increased episcleral venous pressure
    Severe thyroid ophthalmopathy
    superior vena cava syndrome
    carotid-cavernous fistula
    Orbital varices
    Sturge-Weber syndrome
    Inflammatory lesions at orbital apex
Low intraocular pressure

Adapted from Stewart C. *Clinical practice of glaucoma.* Thorofare, N.J.: Slack Inc, 1990.

anterior chamber. When the normal pressure gradient is altered so that the pressure in the intrascleral circulation is elevated higher than it is in the canal of Schlemm, blood will reflux back in toward the canal. This reversal can occur in a congested, inflamed eye when the anterior chamber pressure is low. Increases in venous pressure or relative hypotony occurs when a patient squeezes against the gonioscopy lens and then relaxes. This action can also cause a reflux of blood into the canal. Most often blood in Schlemm's canal is observed when excessive force is applied against the globe with the gonioscopic lens. The direct mechanical pressure increases the pressure in the intrascleral circulation, resulting in an elevation of the venous pressure. If the external pressure is excessive and prolonged, it is possible to observe minute amounts of blood flow from the canal into the anterior chamber (29). This can be stopped by withdrawing the lens. Blood in Schlemm's canal is rarely observed in eyes with elevated IOP.

Pathological changes causing increased episcleral venous pressure include carotid cavernous fistula, severe thyroid ophthalmopathy, superior vena cava syndrome, orbital varices, and inflammatory lesions at the orbital apex. These conditions do not usually present with blood in Schlemm's canal as an isolated feature (30).

Schwalbe's Line

This structure is the condensation of connective tissue fibers supported by elastic fibers and collagen material (7). It is the region where the corneal scleral meshwork terminates anteriorly and is the anterior limit of the angle wall. Gonioscopically, its appearance is variable. In some eyes, it appears white or as a thin, white, glistening line. In others, it may be thicker and protrude into the chamber. In most eyes, it is barely distinguishable. The angle recess originates from this area, creating a shelflike ledge resulting from the difference in the radii of curvature of the angle recess and the internal cornea. The ledge provides a location for normally liberated pigment to collect, particularly in the inferior angle. This pigment collection can be granular or black and powdery and dense and be mistaken for the pigmented portion of the trabecular meshwork. Sampaolesi's line is a wavy pigmented

granular deposit above Schwalbe's line and has been described in the exfoliation syndrome. It is found in the inferior angle and is located superior to Schwalbe's line and should not be confused with pigmented trabecular meshwork or pigmented Schwalbe's line.

Gonioscopically, the position of Schwalbe's line can be identified by the use of an optic section. The optic section creates the focal lines representing the anterior and posterior cornea. These focal lines merge at the end of the internal cornea and denote the internal limbus. The location of the merging point also marks the location of Schwalbe's line representing the end of the cornea and the anterior limit of the trabecular meshwork. Gonioscopically, the ability to identify Schwalbe's line by use of the optic section prevents the examiner from misinterpreting a pigmented Schwalbe's line as the pigmented trabeculum (Figure 2.11). This is important information when assessing whether an angle is opened or closed. Being able to identify this structure accurately and repeatedly provides a frame of reference that can be used to identify the remainder of the gonioscopic landmarks.

When Schwalbe's line is narrow, it is usually more prominent and can be retractile and glistening compared to the cornea, which is anterior, and the trabecula, which is posterior. In approximately 15% of eyes, Schwalbe's line is anteriorly placed. In these instances, it can be identified on routine slit lamp examination as posterior embryotoxin or as the trabecular zone and a prominent line of Schwalbe (31). In some cases of angle dysgenesis, Schwalbe's line may be more anteriorly placed, with iris strands attached to it. This may be visible on slit lamp examination without a goniolens and is known as *Axenfeld's sign* (Plate 35) (2).

Ciliary Processes

In some conditions, the ciliary processes will be visible by gonioscopic observation (Table 2.11). They are most obvious

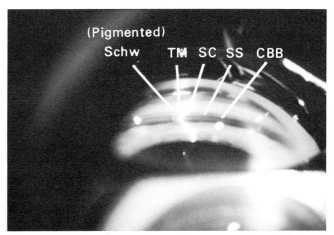

Figure 2.11. Normal-appearing angle, open to ciliary body band. (Courtesy Rodney Gutner, O.D.)

TABLE 2.11
Ciliary Processes

Finding	Condition
Visible gonioscopically	In extreme mydriasis
	With cyst or tumor behind iris
	With dislocated lens
	In surgical coloboma
	In aniridia
Enlargements	Cysts, tumor
Lateral displacement	By epithelial implantation cysts
	By tumors of ciliary body
Gray covering or	Exfoliation
discoloration	Epithelization
	Cyclitic membrane
Shrinkage and pallor	Postinflammatory atrophy
Elongated or sheetlike	Buphthalmos
Anteriorly rotated	Plateau iris, angle closure
	Choroidal effusion
	Malignant glaucoma (ciliary block glaucoma)
	From adherence to limbal scar

Adapted from Epstein DL. *Chandler and Grant's Glaucoma*, 3d ed. Philadelphia: Lea & Febiger, 1986

when examining eyes in which the iris is detached or removed from its insertion, such as in a case of traumatic iridodyalysis or surgical iridectomies (Plate 25). In a widely dilated eye, they may become visible. The ciliary tips may also be evident when a mass or cyst pushes the lens forward or when the lens is dislocated or subluxated (Plate 49). Eyes with exfoliation may have a powdery light-gray deposit on the ciliary processes. They may also be observed to be shrunken and whitish in chronic iridocyclitis (8). Ciliary processes have been observed to be rotated forward, holding the lens forward in cases of plateau iris and in cases of malignant glaucoma.

The Angle in Primary Open-Angle Glaucoma

Gonioscopy greatly aids in the determination of the etiology and classifications of glaucoma. It is generally agreed that the angle in primary open-angle glaucoma is similar to the angle in the normal eye. The depth and width in the normal eye and the glaucomatous eye are similar, with the same distribution of wide intermediate and narrow angles (32). It is the observation of abnormalities along the angle wall and the angle wall iris relationship that provides valuable information regarding the etiology of the glaucoma.

Over the years, there have been attempts to study the angle in cases of primary open-angle glaucoma, looking for gonioscopic differences from the normal angle. This has led some observers to assign importance to such observations as a grayish-white feltlike appearance to the ciliary body, a loss of translucency of the trabecular meshwork, giving it a porcelain-like appearance, increased pigmentation to the trabecular meshwork, and increased iris processes (18,32,33). At one time or another, these have been thought to have been significant findings for identifying open-angle glaucoma.

However, these are findings observed in equal numbers of normal eyes (29).

Evidence of blood in Schlemm's canal and the ease or difficulty with which this can be induced have also been investigated as a means of differentiating a glaucomatous from a nonglaucomatous eye. This has been found to be of little value. It becomes difficult to observe in older eyes, as well as in eyes with ocular tensions above 30 mm Hg (31,32).

Gonioscopy actually provides little information regarding the location of aqueous flow abnormalities in a primary open-angle glaucoma (28). It does provide essential information for differentiating the glaucomas into the secondary forms of open-angle glaucoma or a primary or secondary form of angle-closure glaucoma.

References

1. Tripathi BJ, Tripathi RC. Embryology of the anterior segment of the human eye. In Ritch R et al, eds. *The glaucomas,* vol 1. St Louis: CV Mosby, 1989; Chapter 1.
2. Anderson DR. The development of the trabecular meshwork. *Trans Am Ophthalmic Soc.* 1981;79:458–485.
3. Jerndl T et al. *Goniodysgenesis: A new perspective in glaucoma.* Copenhagen: Scriptor, 1978.
4. Spaeth G. Gonioscopy: Uses old and new. The inheritance of occludable angle ophthalmology. *Ophthalmology.* 1978;85(22):232.
5. Barkan O. Pathogenesis of congenital glaucoma. Gonioscopic and anatomic observation of the angle and anterior chamber in the normal eye and in congenital glaucoma. *Am J Ophthalmol.* 1955;40:1–11.
6. Rodrigues MM et al. In Tasman W, Jaeger EA. *Duane's Foundations of Clinical Ophthalmology,* vol 1. Philadelphia: Lippincott, 1990; Chapter 11.
7. Gorin G. Gonioscopy. In Bellows JG, ed. *Glaucoma: Contemporary international concepts.* New York: Masson Publishing, 1979; Chapter 10.
8. Epstein D. *Chandler and Grant's glaucoma,* 3d ed. Philadelphia: Lea & Febiger, 1986 and Tripathi BJ, Tripathi RC. Functional anatomy of the anterior chamber angle. In Tasman W, Jaeger EA, eds. *Duane's foundations of clinical ophthalmology,* vol 1. Philadelphia: Lippincott, 1990.
9. Fellman RL et al. *Gonioscopy: The ophthalmologist's hidden view.* St Louis: CV Mosby, 1987.
10. Fontana S, Brubacker R. Volume and depth of the anterior chamber. *Arch Ophthalmol.* October 1980;98:1803.
11. Fallman RL et al. Module #7: Gonioscopy: Key to successful management of glaucoma. In *Clinical modules for ophthalmologists.* Focal Points 1984, American Academy of Ophthalmology.
12. Gorin G, Posner A. *Slit lamp gonioscopy,* 3d ed. Baltimore: Williams & Wilkins, 1967.
13. Lowe RF. *Primary angle closure glaucoma.* Singapore: PG Publications, 1989.
14. Henkind P. Angle vessels in normal eyes. *Br J Ophthalmol.* 1964;48:551–557.
15. Shihab ZM, Lee PF. The significance of normal angle vessels. *Ophthal Surg.* June 1985;16(5):382–385.
16. Chatterjee S. Gonio-vessels in normal and abnormal eyes. *Br J Ophthalmol.* 1960;44:347.
17. Spaeth G. The normal development of the human anterior chamber angle: A new system of descriptive grading. *Trans Ophthalmol Soc UK.* 1971;91:709–713.
18. Boyd TAS. Gonioscopic appearance in open angle-glaucoma. *Trans Can Ophthalmol Soc.* 1962;25:206–220 and Lichter P.

Iris processes in 340 eyes. *Am J Ophthalmol.* 1969;68(5):872–878.

19. Barkan O. The structure and function of the angle of the anterior chamber and Schlemm's canal. *Arch Ophthalmol.* 1936;15:101–110.

20. Greenidge KC. Angle-closure glaucoma. *Int Ophthalmol Clin.* 1990;30(3):177–186.

21. Palmberg P. Gonioscopy in the glaucomas. In Ritch R et al, eds. *The glaucomas*, vol 1. St Louis: CV Mosby, 1989.

22. Spaeth GL. Distinguishing between the normally narrow, the suspiciously shallow, and the particularly pathological anterior chamber angle. *Perspectives Ophthalmol.* 1977;1(3):205.

23. Hoskins HD, Kass M. *Becker-Schaffer's diagnosis and therapy of the glaucomas.* St Louis: CV Mosby, 1989.

24. Lichter PR, Shafer RN. Iris processes and glaucoma. *Am J Ophtalmol.* 1970;70:905.

25. Hoskins HD Jr. Interpretive gonioscopy in glaucoma. *Invest Ophthalmol.* 1972;11:97.

26. Newell FW. *Opthalmology principles and concepts.* St Louis: CV Mosby, 1969.

27. Rohen JW, Drecoll EL. Morphology of aqueous outflow pathways in normal and glaucomatous eyes. In Ritch R, Shields MB, Krupin T, eds. *The glaucomas.* St Louis: CV Mosby, 1989.

28. Kronfield PC. Further gonioscopic studies on the canal of Schlemm. *Arch Ophthalmol.* 1949;41:393.

29. Hobbs HE. The trabecula in chronic simple glaucoma with special reference to the gonioscopic appearance of blood in the canal of Schlemm. *Br J Ophthalmol.* 1950;489.

30. Stewart WC. *Clinical practice of glaucoma.* Thorofare, NJ: Slack Inc; 1990.

31. Burian HM et al. Visibility of the ring of Schwalbe and the trabecular zone. *Arch Ophthalmol.* 1955; 53:767–782.

32. François J. Gonioscopy in primary glaucoma. In Duke-Elder S, ed. *Glaucoma: A symposium.* Oxford: Blackwell Scientific Publications, 1955.

33. Gradle HS, Sugar HS. Concerning the chamber angle III. A clinical method of goniometry. *Am J Ophthalmol.* 1940; 23:1135.

34. Smith R. Blood in the canal of Schlemm. *Br J Ophthalmol.* 1956;40:358.

Chapter 3

Uses and Application of Gonioscopy

Evaluation of the anterior chamber provides a means of making a proper diagnosis in many cases of eye and systemic disease and is necessary for the appropriate diagnosis and treatment of the glaucomas (Table 3.1). In practice, gonioscopy is most often limited to a glaucomatous eye or an eye with narrow angles. This limited use prevents an appreciation for the large variation in the appearance of the normal angle (1). Not performing gonioscopy will certainly lead to errors in diagnosis, but not appreciating subtle abnormalities will result in diagnostic errors as well. It is thus incumbent upon examiners to become familiar with the large number of normal and abnormal findings observed with the gonioscopic lens (2). This can be accomplished by implementing this technique as part of the routine assessment for every patient, at least until one becomes comfortable with the variations in normal angle appearance.

Gonioscopy will alter the corneal surface, resulting in changes to refraction. It can lower intraocular pressure (IOP) by forcing aqueous out the anterior chamber. And it may open a narrow or closed angle and lower the IOP. For these reasons, when it is done as part of an initial examination, it should be performed after tonometry as the last technique before dilating the pupil.

Routine Dilation and Angle Closure Risk

In routine patient care, a primary application for gonioscopy involves the evaluation of the anterior chamber angle in the suspected narrow angles before dilating the patient's pupils. The decision to dilate a patient should include the assessment of this risk, which is increasingly minimized by systematically evaluating the anterior chamber angle because narrowness of the anterior chamber angle is a key physical characteristic in angle closure glaucoma.

By identifying an eye at risk for angle closure, the clinician can better predict the likelihood of mydriatically precipitating an angle closure attack and prepare themselves and the patient for the potential consequences for such an occurrence. The patient can then be properly observed after the dilated exam for any signs of angle closure; if any are present, the attack can be aborted early, thus avoiding the possibility of a distressed patient calling hours later with a painful sore eye in angle closure. The earlier in the course the attack is identified and treated, the easier it is to break, because there is less congestion to the eye, and, consequently, damage to the eye is reduced and a cure is more likely (3). The examiner can also discuss with the patient the potential risk and benefits from the dilated examination, with the possibility of an angle closure attack being induced from dilation. Actually it can be considered as a mydriatic provocative test. The patient can then be advised that it is best for this situation to take place in an environment where treatment is available (4).

It is inappropriate to dilate a patient without first evaluating the anterior chamber and assessing the potential risks for a mydriatic-induced angle closure and advising the patient of the potential risk. In clinical practice, there are many instances when dilation may be indicated even in the presence of the risk of inducing an angle closure attack—for example, in a patient with narrow angles but with symptoms suggesting retinal detachment. Often patients with active disease require therapeutic dilation, as in cases of anterior uveitis or corneal abrasions. Failure to recognize the potential of further embarrassment to the eye by inducing a secondary angle closure can lead to serious sequelae. Prior dilation without angle closure is not an assurance that future dilations will be safe.

Clinical Techniques for Assessing Angle Width and the Risk for Angle Closure

A goal of the anterior chamber assessment is to predict which angle, based on the position of the iris in relation to the angle

TABLE 3.1
Indications and Contraindications for Gonioscopy

Indications
  Shallow anterior chambers
  Open but narrow angles
  Corneal edema (localized)
  Intraocular inflammation
    Rule out synechia
    Evaluate for granulomas
  Iris contour changes
    Suspected iris or ciliary body masses
    Intumescent lenses
    Dislocated or subluxated lenses
  Patients at risk for angle neovascularization
    Chronic inflammation
    CRVO
    BRVO
    CRAO
    Diabetes
    Ocular ischemia
  Asymmetric anterior-chamber depths
  History of blunt trauma
    Iris sphincter tears
    Angle recession
  History of sharp trauma
    Retained foreign body
  Intraocular foreign bodies
  Pupil distortion
    Iris synechia
  Pigment dispersion
    Pigment peppering of inferior iris
    Krukenberg's spindle
    Iris transillumination
    Heterochromia
  Iris nevi
  Anterior uveal melanoma
  Exfoliation
  Patients with symptoms or signs of angle closure
    Glaukomflecken
    Intermittent blurred vision
    Frontal pain headaches
    Transient vision loss
    Colored halos
    Iris atrophy
  Classifying glaucoma or glaucoma suspects
  Deciding on the safety of mydriasis
  Family history of angle closure
  Posterior chamber examination
  Examination of corneal endothelium
  Wilson's disease or other copper metabolic disease
  Prior to anterior segment surgery (cataract)
  Laser surgery
    Argon laser trabeculoplasty
    Iridoplasty
    Goniophotocoagulation

Contraindications
  Hyphema
  Compromised corneas
  Lacerated globes
  Perforated globes

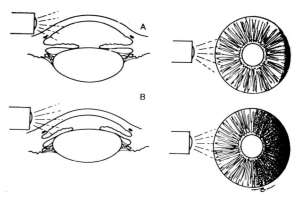

Figure 3.1 Flashlight technique. Oblique flashlight illumination as screening measure for estimating the anterior chamber depth. A. With a deep chamber, nearly the entire iris is illuminated. B. When the iris is bowed forward, only the proximal portion is illuminated, and a shadow is seen in the distal half. (Reprinted with permission from Shields MB. Textbook of glaucoma, 3d ed. Baltimore: Williams & Wilkins, 1992.

and gonioscopy (Figure 3.3) are clinical methods used to provide this information.

The flashlight technique is the crudest. Clinicians using it are unable to view the structures necessary to determine if the angle is actually opened or closed, and they can only infer the iris contour. The van Herick is more reliable. Studies indicate a high correlation between slit lamp angle estimation and gonioscopic angle depth (1,5,6,7,8). If one includes the observation of the anterior chamber axial depth and slit lamp observation of the iris contour, the slit lamp technique becomes that much more informative. Nevertheless, it provides only indirect information regarding the angle recess and the iris angle wall relationship within that recess. Gonioscopy is the only means available that provides a direct view of the iris within the recess and its relation to the wall. In addition, iris contour and anterior chamber depth can be evaluated. The other methods, however, do have clinical value for the status of the angle and chamber, and have been correlated with gonioscopic appearance.

The Flashlight Technique

The flashlight technique uses a light source such as a penlight or transilluminator. The light is held perpendicular to the outer canthi/limbal area at the level of the pupil. The examiner observes whether the light is transmitted across the iris, thus lighting the entire iris, as occurs in a deep-chambered eye. In a shallow-chambered eye, the lens-iris diaphragm is displaced anterior, shallowing the chamber, and thus it prevents the light from passing across the iris, creating a shadow on the nasal portion of the iris (see Figure 3.1). A shadow will be produced when the iris creates an angle of 20 degrees or less with the anterior chamber wall (Shaffer grade 2 to 0) (6). Basically all eyes can be categorized as either open, greater than 20 degrees, or narrow, 20 degrees or less.

This method does not differentiate closed angles from narrow angles or the variations in narrow and open angles.

wall and particularly the trabecular meshwork, is most likely to close when the eye is dilated. The flashlight technique (Figure 3.1), van Herick slit lamp estimation (Figure 3.2),

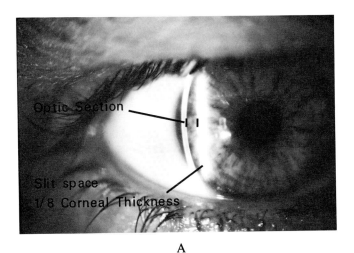

A

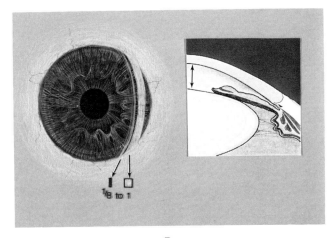

B

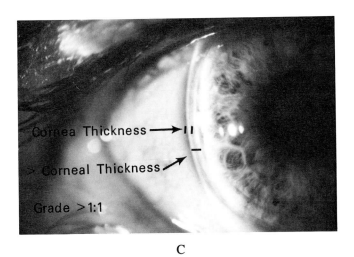

C

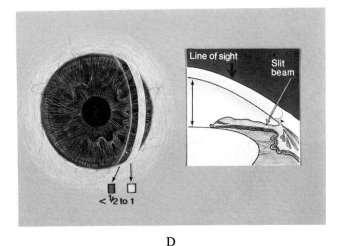

D

Figure 3.2. van Herick Technique. Slit lamp angled 60 degrees. Use optic section. The thickness of the space between the posterior cornea and the iris is judged in relation to the corneal thickness at this location. A. Angle width is slit closed. B. Artist's representation. Note that the central chamber is shallow as well. C. Angle width is open normal appearance > ½:1. D. Artist's representation. Note normal depth of central chamber. (Art courtesy Laurel Cook)

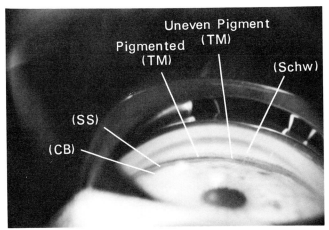

Figure 3.3. Gonioscopic view of open angle. Open to tip of CB. Pigmented trabecula. Pigment scattering along Schwalbe's line. (CB = ciliary body, SS = scleral spur, TM = trabecular meshwork, Schw = Schwalbe's line)

Nevertheless, there may be instances when this is the only means available for estimating the risk for angle closure, and in those cases it is important to understand that there is large variation in anterior chamber configurations. For example, in older patients with enlarged lenses, a slight bowing of the iris centrally with the peripheral iris well away from the meshwork may prevent the iris from lighting up. The erroneous information by the flashlight technique in this instance will lead the examiner away from dilating the eye in a situation where it would be acceptable to do so. Misinterpretation with this technique can also occur in cases of plateau iris, where the iris will fully light up but full dilation may result in angle closure (9). In these instances, the examiner erroneously concludes that the eye is safe to dilate because no shadow is created; however, the angle recess is shortened due to the anterior placement of the iris into the angle wall, and the iris, when dilated, becomes bunched into the recess, closing off the angle.

The reliability of this method can be affected by placement of the light source and the patient's gaze. If the light is placed too far anterior and/or is angled improperly, the entire iris will light up even in the presence of a narrow angle. If the light is placed too posterior, the iris will fail to light up, producing a false-positive test. The patient's gaze will also interfere with accurate assessment; if the eye is rotated nasally, the nasal iris will not be illuminated, yielding a possible false-positive result in an eye with a normal angle.

van Herick Technique

The slit lamp technique of angle grading is often referred to as the van Herick technique (see Figure 3.2). In 1969 van Herick and associates reported on their evaluation of more than 5000 patients using the slit lamp to estimate the angle depth at the extreme nasal and temporal portions of the anterior chamber (5). They concluded that the estimation at these points serves as a reliable average of the angle as a whole. It is particularly valuable as a screening technique to identify patients requiring gonioscopy. It is also valuable for patients with corneal ulcers, corneal abrasions, or uveitis, where gonioscopy may be relatively contraindicated or difficult to perform because of poor patient cooperation because an estimate of the angle is needed to ensure that dilation will not cause secondary problems for the patient by inducing an angle closure.

For this technique, the patient is seated at the slit lamp in a room with reduced illumination to prevent pupil constriction. The patient should fixate straight ahead. The slit lamp magnification should be set at approximately 16×. The illumination arm of the slit lamp and microscope are set at an angle of 45 to 60 degrees, with the narrow (optic section), sharply focused slit beam placed almost perpendicular to the peripheral corneal surface. van Herick and colleagues recommend that the measurement be taken "just before the point of disappearance of the corneal—iris space at the periphery." At this point, the width of the corneal optic section beam is used as the unit for estimating the anterior chamber depth. Giving the optic section width the value of one, the distance from the posterior corneal surface to the iris is graded in terms of the corneal optic section. If the space is equal to the width of the corneal optic section, the angle is estimated to be 1:1. If the space is only one-fourth of the corneal optic section width, the angle is judged to be ¼:1 and correlates to the Shaffer gonioscopic grade 2 (10) (Table 3.2).

Van Herick and associates noted that the slit lamp grading is based on the results of the nasal and temporal judgment. Anatomically, the temporal angle is considered to be the deeper of the lateral angles; however, interestingly with this technique it appears that the temporal angle is the narrower (6). This was also noted by Alsbirk in his study of 505 adult Greenland Eskimos (11). Utilizing the van Herick system, he found that 50% of eyes had a deeper chamber nasally than temporally, however, this asymmetry was not found on gonioscopy. Thus, a narrower slit lamp temporal quadrant did not reveal a narrower temporal quadrant on gonioscopy when comparing the two quadrants. Alsbirk feels this slit lamp

asymmetry is the result of an asymmetry of the corneolimbal portion of the ocular anatomy where the temporal portion of the eye is stretched more than the nasal portion, causing the temporal limbal portion to be closer to the iris insertion. He concluded that the slit lamp temporal aspect evaluation is the more important measurement (11).

The results of this evaluation can also be affected by room illumination and slit lamp light width and intensity, all of which can alter the status of the iris, giving false-positive or -negative test results unless accounted for. For example, in an eye at risk for relative pupillary block with a narrow angle and a bombe iris, the angle may widen when the pupil is fully constricted and narrow when the pupil is mid-dilated. This fluctuation in angle depth, associated with dimming and brightening of the illumination, is also suggestive of an iris anteriorly pushed forward by the lens. Older patients with miotic pupils have a wider van Herick estimation because of the pupil constriction, and patients with a larger pupil than normal may have their iris bunched peripherally more than average, giving a narrow van Herick estimation, particularly if the peripheral iris has a prominent last roll. Eyes with larger than normal lateral scleral overhangs will have deeper van Herick estimations because the iris point of reference is closer to the pupil and farther from the angle recess. Thus, the location of judgment is different from the so-called normal location. Peripheral lesions of the cornea, including scars, pterygiums, and corneal arcus may all interfere with slit creation, decreasing the accuracy of the angle estimation and will also alter corneal thickness.

With this technique, any angle judged to be ¼:1 is considered narrow and capable of closure. Thus, this value is critical. It follows that any eye judged to have a van Herick angle estimation of ¼:1 or less should have gonioscopy performed before dilation to assess the openness of the angle and estimate the risk of inducing a mydriatic angle closure attack. Actually, observation of an angle this narrow on routine examination indicates the need for gonioscopy regardless of whether the patient is to be dilated (12) (Table 3.2).

According to van Herick and colleagues, the gonioscopic appearance of a slit lamp grade 2 angle by this technique will often reveal a Shaffer gonioscopic grade 1 or less superior angle and a grade 2 or 3 inferior angle (5). Rarely was there disagreement between slit lamp evaluation and gonioscopy (only a few in 400 eyes), but when there was a discrepancy, usually the angle was a half to one grade shallower on gonioscopy. The relationship and close association between gonioscopy and slit lamp angle estimation is particulary helpful for neophyte gonioscopists. The slit lamp evaluation provides an excellent reference for beginning gonioscopists to use as a check against the gonioscopic estimation and, helping to prevent misinterpretation, particularly in some anomalous-appearing angles where the structures are pale. If the slit lamp evaluation provides a grade of 1:1, it is unlikely that the angle will be narrow by gonioscopy.

In a group of 2185 unselected patients, van Herick and associates found an incidence of only 1.64% of eyes with a grade 1 or 2; 4.2% of eyes in those age 60 years and over had

van Herick	Central Chamber	Shaffer Grade	% of Population van Herick, Shaffer Schwartz	Risk for Closure	Gonioscopy 1° Gaze 2° Gaze	Dilation Recommendation	Agent
>½:1	6:1	40°	38.6	Not possible	CBB 360° 1° gaze	Yes	Mydriatic/cycloplegic
½:1	≥5:1	30–40°	60	Not possible	CBB 360° 1° gaze	Yes	Mydriatic/cycloplegic
¼:1	≤4:1	20°	1.0	Closure possible but unlikely	If CBB 360° 1° gaze or 2° gaze	Yes	Mydriatic/cycloplegic
					If CBB inferior SS superior 1° gaze or 2° gaze	Yes	Cycloplegic and mydriatic if primary gaze
							Cycloplegic only, if secondary gaze
<¼:1	<4:1	10°	.64	Closure possible	SS inferior Trab. superior If 1° gaze or 2° gaze	Caution one eye each visit	*Use tropicamide* only. Reverse with dapiprazole. Follow in office until dilation resolved and check IOP
				Closure likely	Trab. only. Inf. and Sup. 1° gaze or 2° gaze	No unless for provocative test One eye each visit	Prepare for closure Consider Prophylactic PI
				Closure likely	If secondary gaze	No	Consider prophylactic PI
Plateau Iris Configuration							
≤¼:1	≥5:1	≥20°	?	Possible	If open to SS superior and inferior	Caution	Weak mydriatic or cycloplegic
					If open to CBB	Yes	Reverse quickly with dapiprazole if angle crowded

1° gaze = primary gaze, 2° gaze = secondary gaze. Lens tilted toward angle of observation and patients look into goniomirror. Recommended mydriats 1.0% or 0.5% tropicanide.

an incidence of grade 1 or 2. They also noted a more common association between narrow angles and hyperopia (5,10).

Cockburn's Method

Cockburn (6) used a modified van Herick technique to obtain a slit lamp estimate of the angle. He then correlated that estimate with the gonioscopic evaluation of the superior quadrant of each eye and created a graph to be used as a method for estimating anterior chamber slit lamp appearance to predict gonioscopic angle appearance (Figure 3.4). He found that approximately 7.5% of optometric patients had narrow angles by his slightly modified van Herick estimation (7). He evaluated the left eye of 50 patients in one trial and in a second evaluated the right eye of 1113 patients (9). He judged the anterior chamber depth in decimal units of corneal thickness. For convenience, evaluation was made as close to the temporal limbus only. The nasal angle was not used because there was difficulty in a number of patients obtaining proper placement of the slit lamp due to their prominent noses. van Herick and associates used both lateral angles for their estimates. This may account for the slight difference in their results.

Cockburn commented that the superior and inferior locations are not suitable for estimation (7). The limbus is ovoid, with its shortest diameter superior, so estimation vertically will be made farther from the angle recess resulting in the slit lamp angle appearing deeper vertically than laterally. This would probably have some normal range of values, but no studies have been done to correlate superior and inferior gonioscopy appearance to the superior and inferior slit lamp angle estimation. Since the superior angle is the narrowest angle and tends to close off first in most cases of primary acute angle closure, it may be worth investigating.

For the gonioscopic correlate to the slit lamp estimate, Cockburn limited the evaluation to the superior angle of each patient's left eye using a Zeiss gonioscope lens. He chose this quadrant because of the anatomical narrowness and its proclivity to closure. Thus, the comparison was between the temporal slit lamp estimation of angle width to the superior quadrant's gonioscopic appearance. van Herick and associates did not describe their gonioscopic technique in detail regarding their method; thus, factors of lens type used and quadrants evaluated are unavailable for comparison.

Cockburn manipulated the Zeiss lens to provide the best view possible into the angle recess, with the combined width of the trabecular and scleral spur used as the unit of comparison. If the posterior segment of the scleral spur was visible, the angle was gonioscopically graded as 1.0. If only

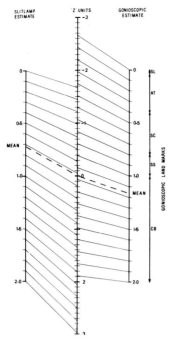

Figure 3.4. Estimates obtained by the slit lamp method and the gonioscopic grading system of the width of the anterior chamber angle. The approximate location and width of the gonioscopic features appear on the right of the figure. An estimate of the probable gonioscopic appearance of an angle may be obtained by following a line from the appropriate slit lamp grade to the z unit axis and then to the gonioscopic grade by the nearest connecting line. SL = Schwalbe's line; AT = anterior trabeculae; SC = Schlemm's canal region of the trabeculae; SS = scleral spur; CB = ciliary body. (Adapted from Cockburn. Predicting visibility of angle structures. Am J Optom & Physiol Optics. 1982; 59:11. The American Academy of Optometry.)

portions of the trabecular were seen in the superior angle, other quadrants were examined as a means of observing to the scleral spur. The superior quadrant was then gauged in terms of the width of the band in the deeper quadrant. Thus, the superior quadrant was graded as a proportion of the entire band (to scleral spur) seen in the superior quadrant or, if not visible in that quadrant, some other quadrant of the eye where it was visible. If the scleral spur was not visible in any quadrant, compression gonioscopy was performed to reveal it, and that distance was used as the reference. When the entire angle was visible to the ciliary body, the width of the visible ciliary body was estimated as a proportion of the trabecular meshwork scleral spur band (Schwalbe's to posterior scleral spur equals 1.0). Thus, an angle with visible ciliary body half the width of the Schwalbe's line to scleral spur would be graded as 1.5 units (6). Cockburn's results indicate that in any angle estimated as 0.3 on slit lamp observation, one should be able to observe only a portion of the trabecular band visible in the superior quadrant with a Zeiss four-mirror lens. This is considered a narrow angle in that quadrant.

When the angle is very narrow, the slit lamp and gonioscopic estimations did not correlate as well. Cockburn related this to a possible prominent iris bowing interfering with the gonioscopic view. It may also be related to the type of lens

chosen for the study—it is more difficult to view the angle recess over a bowed iris with a Zeiss four-mirror lens than with a Goldmann-type lens. As the Zeiss lens is tilted, more artifacts and distortion develop; also, because of the adherence of the Goldmann-type lenses, they can be tilted to more extreme angles, and their larger optic zone offers a larger field of view. Thus, in any of these studies, the type of lens and methods used will alter the results. Cockburn concluded that any angle estimated as 0.2 or less is at risk for angle closure and should have gonioscopy performed. If the angle is 0.3, the risk for angle closure is at threshold; gonioscopy would be advisable, especially if there are other signs and symptoms of angle closure. Cockburn's graph does not correlate with my clinical experience or with van Herick's results. It indicates that a temporal slit lamp angle of 0.50 (van Herick ½:1) correlates to a gonioscopic angle open superiorly only to the mid- to posterior trabecular meshwork. I expect and usually can visualize the scleral spur to ciliary body band superiorly in an eye with a slit lamp estimation of 0.50. The superior angle is normally the most gonioscopically shallow, thus the angle can be expected to be even wider and deeper in the inferior quadrant by as much as a quarter to a half a structure.

Table 3.3 shows the results of a number of other reports on the population distribution of narrow anterior chamber widths. Results vary from a low of 1.64% in the van Herick and associates study to a high of 19.0% in the Kessler study. Most are in the range of 4.6% to 7.5%. The problem is that each study has a different method of angle evaluation population group, and different criteria for narrowness.

Dynamic Anterior Chamber Evaluation

Too often clinicians use the slit lamp technique solely to evaluate the angle, thus failing to observe other valuable signs of an eye at risk for angle closure. The technique described by van Herick and colleagues should be expanded on to include assessment of the central chamber depth and iris contour routinely. Starting at the pupil margin, the optic section should be moved slowly along the iris toward the periphery, noting the contour of the iris and looking for evidence of iris bombe and depth of the anterior chamber centrally, mid-peripherally, and at the lateral extreme. This should be done both nasally and temporally. Estimates of central chamber depth should be done using the central corneal thickness, approximately 0.5 mm, as a reference.

The average adult eye has a chamber depth of 3.15 mm with a range of 2.6 to 4.4 mm, which is normally equal in the two eyes. The chamber shallows 0.01 mm per year of life and is normally deeper in myopes and shallower in hyperopes (13). Tornquist calculated that an eye with a central chamber depth of 1.5 to 2 mm had a risk of developing angle closure 175 times greater than an eye with a chamber depth between 2.0 and 2.5 mm (14). Furthermore 97% of Lowes' patients with angle closure glaucoma had anterior chamber depths of 2.3 mm or less (15). Thus an eye with a chamber depth less than 2.4 mm (16) (five corneal thicknesses or less as compared

TABLE 3.3
Surveys of Narrow, Occludable Anterior Chamber Angles

Author	Method and Criteria	% Narrow Angles	Sample Size	Sample Selection
Spaeth[a]	Gonioscopy 10° or less	6.5	947	Nonophthalmic subjects all ages
Kessler[b]	Gonioscopy (ciliary body not visible)	19.0 or 17.5[f]	400	Ophthalmological practice
van Herick et al.[c] (before 1963)	Slit lamp estimate ≤ 0.25 units	4.6	3251	Ophthalmological practice
van Herick et al.[c] (1963–1968)	Slit lamp estimate ≤ 0.25 units	1.64	2185	Ophthalmological practice
Cockburn[d]	Slit lamp estimate ≤ 0.3 units	7.5	509	Optometric practice (consecutive series of presenting patients)
Cockburn[e]	Gonioscopy (ciliary body not visible)	6.0	300	Optometric practice (consecutive series of presenting patients)

Reprinted with permission from Cockburn DM. Prevalence and significance of narrow anterior chamber angles in optometric practice. *Am J Ophthalmol Physiol Opt.* 1981; 58(2):171–175.
[a] Spaeth GL. The normal development of the human anterior chamber angle: A new system of descriptive grading. *Trans Ophthalmol.* 1971; 91:709–739.
[b] Kessler J. Depth estimate of the peripheral anterior chamber. *Ann Ophthalmol.* 1969–1970; 1:373–374.
[c] van Herick W, Shaffer RN, Schwartz A. Estimation of width of angle of anterior chamber. *Am J Ophthalmol.* 1969; 68(4):626–629.
[d] Cockburn DM. *The reliability and validity of the van Herick test in the assessment of anterior chamber angle width.* Melbourne, Australia: Baillieu Library, University of Melbourne, 1978.
[e] Cockburn DM. Prevalence and significance of narrow anterior chamber angles in optometric practice. *Am J Ophthalmol Physiol Opt.* 1981; 58(2):171–175.
[f] Uncertainty due to absence of label on published table.

to a more normal six corneal thicknesses or greater) is an eye at risk for angle closure and will also be narrow on gonioscopy (9). This emphasizes the need to evaluate the central chamber depth as well as the peripheral angle.

Systematically evaluating the contour of the iris and the entire chamber depth axially, as well as in the extreme periphery, and looking for asymmetry in and between eyes makes recognition of an eye at risk for angle closure by means of relative pupillary block, plateau iris, and malignant glaucoma easier to identify. The expanded van Herick technique, however, is not a replacement for gonioscopy.

The combination of slit lamp estimation and gonioscopy will aid in identifying those eyes at risk for angle closure (Figure 3.5). Although gonioscopy, like other tests, is a subjective evaluation of the angle's narrowness, it is the only technique that allows direct visualization and observation before, during, and after dilation of the openness of the trabecular meshwork.

Configurations at Risk for Angle Closure Requiring Gonioscopy

Pupillary Block

The most common form of angle closure glaucoma is the result of pupillary block. In these cases, slit lamp observation of the anterior chamber will reveal that the axial depth is shallower than usually observed—less than 2.5 mm (five corneal thicknesses or less as compared to six corneal thicknesses or greater)—the iris is bowed forward in the mid-peripheral area, and the estimation by van Herick technique is often ¼:1 or less. The configuration suggests posterior

chamber pressure greater than anterior chamber pressure in an eye with a shallow-anterior chamber. Pharmacologic dilation of these eyes may result in closure of the angle hours after the drops were instilled. This is the result of greater apposition of the iris to the lens when the iris is mid-dilated and somewhat lax. This tends to occur when the iris is recovering from the pharmacologic dilation. With the iris in relative apposition to the lens, the aqueous has difficulty moving from the posterior chamber to the anterior chamber. Pressure builds up in the posterior chamber, forcing the only movable portion of the angle, the iris root, forward against the anterior wall of the angle. Once the iris is in contact with the wall, it may remain in apposition or become attached to the wall. Either event will result in the iris blocking the anterior trabeculum and thus blocking the exit of aqueous from the eye. Although these episodes are uncommon in routine practice, the consequences of loss of vision from angle closure glaucoma are serious enough that each clinician must evaluate the risk-benefit of dilating patients with occludable angles. Any patient suspected at risk based on slit lamp evaluation must have gonioscopy performed prior to dilation for accurate diagnosis (5.12). To avoid bilateral angle closure, each eye should be dilated at separate visits when both eyes have narrow angles.

Plateau Iris

The flashlight technique is particularly problematic in cases of plateau iris. The test results in the erroneous observation of a normal anterior chamber angle in the cases of plateau iris configuration (Figure 3.5). This type of configuration occurs in younger people in an eye with a relatively normal central anterior chamber or axial depth, with a flat iris and a narrow

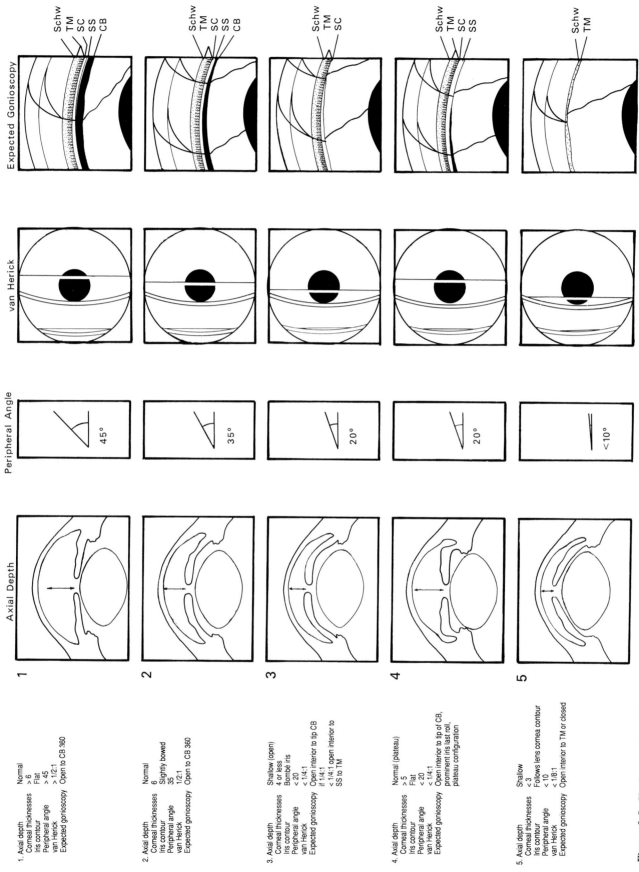

	Axial Depth	Peripheral Angle	van Herick	Expected Gonioscopy
1		45°		Schw TM SC SS CB
2		35°		Schw TM SC SS CB
3		20°		Schw TM SC
4		20°		Schw TM SC SS
5		<10°		Schw TM

BÜTELHÜ

1. Axial depth   Normal
   Corneal thicknesses   >6
   Iris contour   Flat
   Peripheral angle   >45
   van Herick   >1/2:1
   Expected gonioscopy   Open to CB 360

2. Axial depth   Normal
   Corneal thicknesses   6
   Iris contour   Slightly bowed
   Peripheral angle   35
   van Herick   1/2:1
   Expected gonioscopy   Open to CB 360

3. Axial depth   Shallow (open)
   Corneal thicknesses   4 or less
   Iris contour   Bombé iris
   Peripheral angle   <20
   van Herick   <1/4:1
   Expected gonioscopy   Open interior to tip CB
     if 1/4:1
     <1/4:1 open interior to
     SS to TM

4. Axial depth   Normal (plateau)
   Corneal thicknesses   >5
   Iris contour   Flat
   Peripheral angle   <20
   van Herick   <1/4:1
   Expected gonioscopy   Open interior to tip of CB,
     prominent iris last roll,
     plateau configuration

5. Axial depth   Shallow
   Corneal thicknesses   <3
   Iris contour   Follows lens cornea contour
   Peripheral angle   <10
   van Herick   <1/8:1
   Expected gonioscopy   Open interior to TM or closed

Figure 3.5. Slit lamp and gonioscopic correlation. (Schw = Schwalbe's line, TM = trabecular meshowork, SC = Schlemm's canal, SS = scleral spur, CB = ciliary body) (See also Table 3.2).

angle. Slit lamp evaluation in these eyes will result in an abnormal van Herick evaluation because the slit lamp will reveal an angle that is narrow in its extreme periphery. Thus, the van Herick estimation will be much narrower than expected based on the central anterior chamber depth, which is usually of normal depth. The presence of the narrow peripheral angle by van Herick, the flat iris, and the relatively normal axial chamber depth should make the examiner suspicious of plateau iris configuration. Because of the abnormal van Herick observation, the angle should be evaluated with gonioscopy. In plateau iris configuration, the gonioscopy examination will reveal that the peripheral iris is curved posterior just before its wall insertion. The flat iris surface curving backward before its insertion gives the iris a shape of a plateau (17). Gorin has suggested that some of these eyes will have a more anterior insertion of the iris along the angle and will close from posterior to anterior (18). Some have also described this configuration as having a prominent last roll of the iris just before insertion (Figure 3.6) (1).

In plateau iris configuration, full dilation may cause the iris to attach to the angle wall, resulting in an angle closure (Figure 3.7). Thus, in these rare instances when the eye is fully dilated, the risk of angle closure is greatest. Measurement of IOP when the eye is fully dilated or performing gonioscopy at that time will help detect these cases. Gonioscopy on all patients during dilation is not practical as a

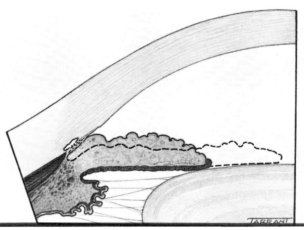

Figure 3.7. Artist's representation of plateau iris closure. Note that the iris physically bunches into the angle recess, iris plane is flat and angle is narrow. (Reprinted with permission from Kanski JJ, McAllister JA. Glaucoma: A colour manual of diagnosis and treatment. London: Butterworth-Heinemann, 1989.)

routine procedure. Postdilation tonometry is more practical; however, observation by slit lamp and predilation gonioscopy of eyes suspected of plateau iris from the slit lamp observation is often sufficient to identify patients at risk. Gonioscopy would reveal a flat iris plane with a prominent last roll of the iris lying abnormally close to the angle wall, a more anterior insertion of the iris than normal, or an iris with its most peripheral portion curved posterior prior to insertion with the bend of the iris close to the angle wall.

When necessary, it is best to dilate these eyes with weaker doses of anticholinergic agents such as ½% tropicamide or an adrenergic agent such as 2.5% phenylephrine HCl. It is best to avoid combining these agents in the eye with plateau iris thereby avoiding iris bunching into the angle.

Cases of plateau iris angle closure are rare. They are often misdiagnosed as narrow open-angle glaucoma or, if advanced, as relative pupillary block angle closure glaucoma. The condition is often diagnosed retrospectively in eyes treated with iridotomies or iridectomies for presumed angle closure from pupillary block. These eyes, however, will experience a significant rise in IOP when dilated in the presence of patent iridotomies. This is the result of the iris continuing to be mechanically (pharmacologically) placed against the angle wall, blocking the trabecular meshwork.

Recent ultrasound biomicroscopy studies in plateau iris syndrome reveal that these eyes have anteriorly positioned ciliary processes when compared to normal eyes or eyes with angle closure from relative pupillary block. This is considered an anatomic variant, and the occludability of such an angle may depend on the size and amount of anterior placement of the ciliary processes and the accompanying iris periphery thickness although there is usually a contribution from pupil block when these angles do occlude (19).

In cases of plateau iris angle closure, the scenario often is as follows. A patient presents with signs and symptoms of angle closure glaucoma. Once the eye is quiet and the acute

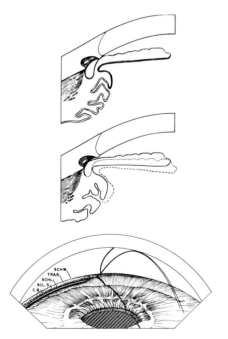

Figure 3.6. Two modes of angle closure. The top represents the usual mode in pupil block—closure from anterior to posterior. The middle represents closure in plateau iris closure, creeping angle closure, or chronic angle closure. In these cases, peripheral anterior synechiae form in the depths of the angle. Anterior third of trabecula remain visible. The bottom represents the progression of PAS from deep in the angle to the anterior angle. (Reprinted with permission from Gorin G, Posner A. Slit lamp gonioscopy, 3d ed. Baltimore: Williams & Wilkins, 1967.

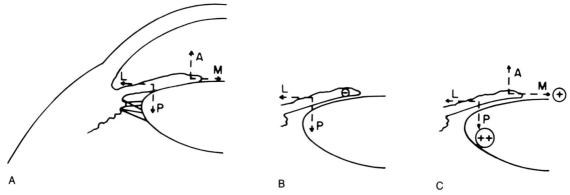

Figure 3.8. Mechanics of pupillary dilation A. Components of iris muscle activity. Anterior component of iris sphincter activity (A), medial component of iris sphincter activity (M), lateral component of iris dilator activity (L), and posterior component of iris dilator activity (P). B. Pupillary dilation with anticholinergic mydriatic. The iris sphincter is inactivated, and the posterior component of the iris dilator acts peripherally. C. Pupillary dilation with adrenergic mydriatic. The iris dilator is stimulated and its posterior component is augmented while the medial component of the iris sphincter persists. (Reprinted with permission from Bartlett JD, Jaanus SD. Clinical ocular pharmacology, 2d ed. Boston: Butterworth–Heinemann, 1989; 404.)

attack is medically broken, laser surgery is performed, resulting in a patent iridotomy or iridectomy and an open angle. When the patient is subsequently dilated, a significant rise in pressure occurs, and the angle is observed to be closed. Gonioscopy at that time will reveal the iris blocking the trabecular meshwork. Thus the pupil blocking component of the angle closure has been resolved by iridotomy, but the angle remains occludable from the plateau configuration because of the anteriorly placed ciliary processes (19). (This assumes that other potential causes, such as significant peripheral anterior synechia, multiple cysts or a mass of the ciliary body or iris, ciliary block glaucoma, effects of topical steroids, or cycloplegic agents, have been ruled out as a potential cause of postlaser iridotomy elevated ocular tension and that the pressure was normalized by the successful iridotomy.)

Treatment for plateau iris angle closure consists of iridoplasty by laser or long-term miotic therapy as a means of keeping the iris from contacting the wall and blocking the trabecular meshwork. Patients on long-term miotic therapy may experience shallowing of the angle so that an iridotomy is probably justified therapy as well in these cases.

Choice of Agents for Dilation in Narrow Angles

The dilator muscle moves the iris peripherally and posteriorly. Its posterior movement is quicker than its peripheral movement, and with its location below the sphincter in the pupil area, it pulls the sphincter posteriorly as well (20) (See Table 3.2). In an eye at risk for pupil block, use of an adrenergic (agonist) stimulating agent such as phenylephrine will force the iris posterior, increasing the pupil block. If the sphincter is still active, it will pull the iris medially against the lens, further increasing pupil block. Thus, in cases where there is real concern for pharmacologically inducing angle closure from routine dilation, one should theoretically avoid the use

of iris dilator stimulating agents because the posterior vector forces of the stimulated dilator muscle and the unopposed action of the sphincter place the eye at great risk when the pupil is mid-dilated (4,20,21) (Figure 3.8).

This was especially true before the availability of dapiprazole (brand name: Rev-Eyes®). Prior to this alpha-adrenergic blocker, pilocarpine was routinely used to reverse dilation. If pilocarpine is used to reverse dilation, when the pupil is mid-dilated, the combination on the iris of the dilator posterior pulling effect from the phenylephrine HCl and the medial pulling forces of the sphincter from the pilocarpine places the pupil blocking forces at their greatest. In addition, pilocarpine causes forward movement of the lens in some eyes and steepening of the anterior lens surface, which can further increase pupil blocking forces. Dapiprazole, unlike pilocarpine, does not act on the sphincter muscle and therefore does not cause a shallowing of the anterior chamber, does not cause ciliary congestion, and does not pull the iris medially against the lens. Thus, dapiprazole is a better choice to reverse the action of adrenergic stimulating dilating agents. In eyes with narrow angles, routine pilocarpine use should be avoided.

Tropicamide, a fast-acting anticholinergic agent, paralyzes the sphincter and allows the dilator to work uninhibited. The dilator muscle is still active but with less force than when a dilator stimulating agent is used; also, the sphincter's medial action is absent. Therefore, it may be a safer drug to use in narrow-angle eyes where there is a concern for mydriatically inducing an angle closure attack, particularly in comparison to other anticholinergics, such as cyclopentolate, which should be avoided in eyes at risk for angle closure glaucoma.

In his study looking at various dilating agents in eyes at risk for angle closure, Mapstone (22) found that cyclopentolate was a slower acting agent than tropicamide, thus placing the eye in a position of pupil block for a longer period of time, and if pressure became elevated, it was more difficult to normalize. In cases where pressure increased with tropicamide, much of the angle was still open and the pressure was easier to normalize.

In general to reverse dilation, the use of a cholinergic stimulating miotic agent is best avoided. Its use is controversial. It is often taught that the use of an agent such as pilocarpine is appropriate because it constricts the pupil and draws the iris away from the trabecular meshwork, thereby reducing the risk for angle closure. However, in some cases, particularly if an adrenergic stimulating agent is used and the pupil is mid-dilated, the pupil blocking forces can be increased by pilocarpine (20,21). The use of parasympathomimetic miotic and an adrenergic stimulating agent is actually the basis of a very potent pharmacologic provocative test. The best theoretical option to break an adrenergic stimulating agent–induced angle closure attack would be to use an alpha-adrenergic blocking agent such as thymoxamine (which is not available in the United States) or dapiprazole (23), which is available.

In cases of plateau configuration, weak dilating agents should be used, and one should avoid placing the iris physically against the angle wall. Use of pilocarpine is not contraindicated in pure cases of plateau iris configuration; however, there is some thought that many cases of plateau iris have some amount of pupil block as well. It is probably best to use the alpha-adrenergic blocking agents for reversal in these cases as well.

Glaucoma Suspects

The evaluation of any glaucoma patient or glaucoma suspect must include the examination of the anterior chamber and angle. Before initiating treatment, proper diagnosis is imperative. This can be ensured only if gonioscopic evaluation has occurred. Observation of the angle will provide vital information. First, it will help answer the most basic question as to whether the angle is opened or closed and further differentiate within these two broad categories. For example, is the angle blocked posteriorly as in plateau iris, syneched or closed by apposition? Treatment will de different in each case. Other abnormalities related to glaucoma can also be readily assessed, such as whether there is evidence of neovascularization of the angle (Plates 20 and 21), angle recession, the presence of exfoliative material on the pupil frill (Plate 26), or the presence of excess pigmentation of the trabecular meshwork. The information gathered will alter the treatment protocol for the patient.

In glaucoma patients, gonioscopic examination should be repeated at least yearly during the course of therapy to enable the examiner to identify any change in the status of the glaucoma mechanism. There is always the possibility that an open-angle glaucoma may become a chronic, intermittent, or acute form of angle closure. The angle is usually considered normal in cases of primary open-angle glaucoma; however, even these eyes may have subtle gonioscopic abnormalities, such as higher insertion of the iris, increased numbers of iris processes (Figure 3.9 and Plates 28 and 29), a fine textural wooly substance, and increased trabecular pigmentation

(Plate 6) that may suggest a secondary form of glaucoma and provide further insight into the etiology of a particular patient's glaucoma (8,24).

Abnormalities of the Angle Wall

On routine slit lamp evaluation, some patients present with abnormalities of the angle wall and anterior chamber that need further examination by gonioscopy. Some examples, such as mesodermal dysgenesis from prominent posterior embryotoxin to Peter's anomaly, require gonioscopic examination. Eyes with irregular contour to the iris may have tumors or cysts of the iris or ciliary body (Plate 49) that may not be observable unless gonioscopy is performed. Patients with Wilson's disease or other abnormal copper metabolizing disease may have a Kayser-Fleischer ring, which can be confirmed and diagnosed by gonioscopic appearance (25). This deposition on the cornea is at the layer of Descemet's and therefore would be expected to be visualized, depositing up to Schwalbe's line. This would help differentiate it from a case of arcus senilis. Eyes that have suffered blunt trauma may have evidence of angle recession. Many of these conditions can be observed, monitored, and photographed through gonioscopic examination. Recognition of these and other abnormalities requires an understanding and recognition of the normal anterior chamber appearance (Figure 3.9).

Laser Treatment

The value of gonioscopy became more fully appreciated at about the time that argon laser trabeculoplasty (Figure 3.9) became a viable therapy for patients with open-angle glaucoma (1). The treatment of narrow angle and closed angle by iridotomies and iridoplasties, as well as goniophotocoagulation for neovascular glaucoma, requires an excellent working knowledge of the anterior chamber and angle appearance by gonioscopy. An understanding of these surgical techniques in the management and treatment of glaucoma allows for appropriate management and follow-up for patients requiring these modes of therapy.

Argon laser trabeculoplasty (ALT) has been a significant adjunct in the therapy for open-angle glaucoma. Laser trabeculoplasty lowers IOP by one of possibly three mechanisms: (1) a mechanical effect secondary to thermal shrinking of the collagenous tissue of the trabecula, which opens the intertrabecular spaces, (2) a cellular response, which removes extracellular material from the trabecular spaces, or (3) a biochemical response caused by the laser damage to the endothelial cells of the trabecula, which causes remaining cells to increase their activity (26). What the laser treatment does *not* do is create a new or direct opening between Schlemm's canal and the anterior chamber.

ALT is most commonly done with an argon blue laser set at $50\mu m$ spot size, 0.1 second duration, and a 600 to 1200 mW power. The laser is aimed at the juncture of the pigmented

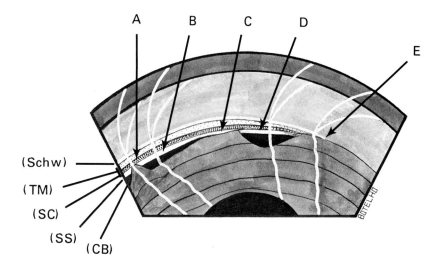

Figure 3.9. Examples of various gonioscopic angle appearances: (A) tenting synechia (PAS) more common in inflammatory conditions; (B) focal lines in normal angle open to the ciliary body band; (C) broad-based synechia seen in chronic angle closure glaucoma, creeping angle closure, or plateau iris angle closure where synechia occurs from posterior to anterior; (D) angle recession where the ciliary body is visible more posterior than normal; and (E) angle closure along Schwalbe's line, seen most typically in primary angle closure from pupil block or in high PAS with ICE syndrome.

and nonpigmented trabecular meshwork. (If the beam is placed too far anterior, it may cause injury to the corneal endothelium. If the burns are placed too far posterior, it may cause pain during the treatment, iritis, postoperative pressure rises, and postoperative peripheral anterior synechia [PAS]) (26). The power should be sufficient to create a blanching effect, pigment dispersion, or a small bubble. It is usually scheduled for two sessions at least one month apart. Approximately 50 burns equally spaced are applied over 180 degrees of the angle at each session (27). The benefits of the surgery tend to diminish over time, with a five-year success rate of about 50% (16,28). Presentation of unusual complications after ALT requires careful gonioscopic examination to detect postoperative PAS or large inflammatory trabecular meshwork precipitates (29).

The degree of pigmentation and the width of the angle may alter accurate laser application. The lack of pigmentation may make it difficult to identify the exact location of the trabecular meshwork. Excess pigmentation may cause a pigmented Schwalbe's line to be confused as the trabecular meshwork, resulting in inaccurate placement of the laser energy. Use of an optic section for localizing Schwalbe's line will help reduce these potential problems. Also, if the trabecular meshwork is heavily pigmented, a lower laser power will be sufficient to treat the trabecula. Patients with pigmentary glaucoma and exfoliation seem to do well with this procedure, but, interestingly, postoperative transient pressure rises seem to be greater in eyes with pigmented trabecular meshwork (30). This could be related to post-surgical pigmentary clogging of the meshwork. Postoperative rises in IOP appear to be well controlled with the use of 1% apraclonidine, an alpha-2 adrenergic agonist given 1 hour before and 1 hour after surgery. Postoperative inflammation

is common and is usually effectively managed with topical steroids—1% prednisilone acetate 4 times a day for 7 days (30). Generally ALT is more successful in primary open-angle glaucoma, pseudoexfoliative glaucoma, and pigmentary glaucoma and somewhat less effective (50–60% relative success) in angle recession glaucoma and postiridectomy treatment. It has poorest success in uveitic glaucoma, juvenile congenital glaucoma, and steroid-induced glaucoma (Table 3.4) (26).

Iridoplasty (gonioplasty or peripheral iris retraction) changes the configuration of the iris by application of a low-energy, long-duration laser burn to the peripheral iris. It is used as a treatment in cases of plateau iris angle closure. The placement of the burns causes the iris to retract from the angle. It is also used as an adjunct before ALT when the trabecula is hidden by a prominent or bowed iris. Shrinking the iris from the wall improves the visibility of the angle wall, ensuring an unobstructed view for proper placement of the ALT burns. The common laser settings are 200 to 500μm spot size, a 0.2 to 0.5 second duration, and a power of 200 to 600 mW (27). Usually anywhere from 20 to 80 spots are delivered to the peripheral iris through a goniolens. Proper placement of the burns, approximately one to two mm from the iris root, will avoid producing synechia by unwanted centrifugal retraction (31). In some cases of recently formed synechia, laser gonioplasty is a valuable treatment. Gonioplasty can also be used to differentiate appositional closure from long-standing synechia. In cases of angle closure glaucoma with significant corneal edema, nanophthalmos, and angle closure secondary to ciliary body edema, iridoplasty may cause sufficient iris retraction from the angle wall to lower the pressure (30). Iridoplasty or pupilloplasty may be employed to treat medically nonresponsive cases of angle

CHAPTER 3. USES AND APPLICATION OF GONIOSCOPY

TABLE 3.4
Anterior Laser Trabeculoplasty

Good success
    Primary open-angle glaucoma
    Pseudoexfoliation
    Pigmentary glaucoma
Intermediate success
    Angle recession
    Postiridectomy
Poor success
    Uveitic glaucoma
    Juvenile glaucoma
    Congenital glaucoma
    Steroid-induced glaucoma

closure. The pressure can be lowered if 100 degrees of the angle is opened. Once the pressure is lowered, the inflammation will resolve sufficiently to allow the eye to undergo a laser peripheral iridotomy within three to ten days (32).

Research Applications

Goniosocpy can be used for analyzing and observing the area of aqueous outflow within the eye. Using suction gonioscopy, Iwata was able to visualize the reflux and efflux of blood from Schlemm's canal. His findings suggest the primary open-angle glaucoma in middle or late stages of the disease showed impaired blood reflux into Schlemm's canal and impaired efflux (delayed clean-up time). He also evaluated this phenomenon in cases of infantile glaucoma and felt the results indicated that the area of compromise in aqueous outflow resides in the lumen of Schlemm's canal and not by a membrane covering the trabecular meshwork or in the meshwork itself (33).

References

1. Fellman RL et al. Gonioscopy: Key to successful management of glacuoma. In *Focal points 1984: Clinical modules for ophthalmologists*. American Academy of Ophthalmology; 1984.
2. Palmberg P. Gonioscopy. In Ritch R et al, eds. *The glaucomas*, vol 1. St. Louis: CV Mosby, 1989.
3. David R et al. Long term outcome of primary acute angle closure glaucoma. *Br J Ophthalmol*. 1985;69:261–262.
4. Bartlett J, Jaanus SD. Dilation of the Pupil. In *Clinical ocular pharmacology*, 2d ed. Boston: Butterworths, 1989.
5. Van Herick W et al. Estimation of width of angle of anterior chamber. *Am J Ophthalmol*. 1969;68:626–629.
6. Cockburn DM. Indications for gonioscopy and assessment of gonioscopic signs in optometric practice. *Am J of Optom Phys Optics*. September 1981;58(9):706–717.
7. Cockburn DM. Prevalence and significance of narrow anterior chamber angles in optometric practice. *Am J Optom Phys Optics*. 1981;58(2):171–175.
8. Kimura R. Gonioscopic differentiation between primary open angle glaucoma and normal subjects over 40. *Am J Ophthalmol*. 1975;80:56.
9. Vargas E, Drance SM. Anterior chamber depth in angle-closure glaucoma. *Arch Ophthalmol*. 1973;90:438–439.
10. Hoskins DH Jr., Kass MA. *Becker-Shaffer's diagnosis and therapy of the glaucomas*, 3d ed. St. Louis: CV Mosby, 1989.
11. Alsbirk PH. Limbal and axial chamber depth variations. *Acta Ophthalmol*. 1986;64:593–600.
12. Clemmesen V. Gonioscopic screenings in Greenland. *Canadian J Ophthalmol*. 1972;8:270–273.
13. Tripathi RC, Tripathi BJ. Functional anatomy of the anterior chamber angle. In Ritch R et al, eds. *The glaucomas*. St Louis: CV Mosby, 1989; vol.1, Chapter 10.
14. Tornquist P. Chamber depth in primary acute glaucoma. *Br J Ophthalmol*. 1956;40:421–429.
15. Lowe R. Aetiology of the anatomical basis for primary angle-closure glaucoma. *Br J Ophthalmol*. 1971;54:161.
16. Lowe RF. Primary creeping angle-closure glaucoma. *Br J Ophthalmol*. 1964;48:544.
17. Tornquist R. Angle-closure glaucoma in an eye with a plateau type of iris. *Acta Ophthalmol*. 1958;419–423.
18. Gorin G. Shortening of the angle of the anterior chamber in angle-closure glaucoma. *Am J Ophthalmol*. 1960;49:141.
19. Pavlin CJ et al. Ultrasound biomicroscopy in plateau iris syndrome. *Am J Ophthalmol*. 1992;113:390–395.
20. Lowe RF. *Primary angle closure glaucoma*. Singapore: PG Publications, 1989.
21. Lowe RF. Primary angle-closure glaucoma. *Br J Ophthalmol*. 1967;51:727.
22. Mapstone R. Dilating dangerous pupils. *Br J Ophthalmol*. 1977;61:517–524.
23. Doro D et al. How safe is safe-mydriases in high risk eyes? *Glaucoma* 1988;10:178–181.
24. Boyd TAS. Gonioscopic abnormalities in open-angle glaucoma. *Tr Can Ophthalmol Soc*. 1962;25:207.
25. Brodland D, Bartley G. Kayser-Fleischer rings in a patient with basal cell carcinoma; fortuitous diagnosis of presymptomatic Wilson's disease. *Mayo Clinic* 1992;67:142–143.
26. Krupin T. *Manual of glaucoma 1988*. New York; Churchill Livingstone, 1988.
27. Higginbotham EJ, Shahbazi MF. Laser therapy in glaucoma: An overview and update. *International Ophthalmol Clinics*. Summer 1990;30:3.
28. Shingleton BJ et al. Long-term efficacy of argon laser trabeculoplasty. *Ophthalmology*. 1987;94:1513–1518.
29. Fiore PM, et al. Trabecular precipitates and elevated intraocular pressure following argon laser trabeculoplasty. *Ophthalmic Surgery*, October 1989;20(10):697–701.
30. Shields MB. *Textbook of glaucoma*, 3d ed. Baltimore: Williams & Wilkins, 1992.
31. Araia F et al. Argon laser techniques for narrow angle glaucoma. *Glaucoma*. 1979;1(2):103.
32. Greenidge KC. Angle-closure glaucoma. *Int Ophthalm Clinics*. 1990;30:177–186 and 1987;9:53–55.
33. Iwata K. Suction Gonioscopy analysis of aqueous pathway. *Glaucoma* 1:103,1979.

Chapter 4

Instrumentation

The anterior chamber wall cannot be directly observed externally because of the limbal overhang; moreover, as the observer moves parallel to the iris surface, the light rays from the chamber angle undergo internal reflection, preventing the light from leaving the eye (see Figure 1.2). In the early 1900s Salzmann laid the foundation for modern gonioscopy when he employed a contact lens made of glass to create a different radius of curvature, thus neutralizing the corneal refractive power and negating the internal reflection. Since that time, two systems have been used clinically to visualize the anterior chamber wall structures. Earlier in this century, the primary gonioscopic method used direct-view lenses of the Koeppe type. This system relies on the refraction of light rays from the anterior chamber angle wall at the steep outside curve of the lens. Now, most clinicians use indirect-view lenses, utilizing mirrors to reflect light, as exemplified by Goldmann-type indirect lenses or the four-mirror-type indirect lenses, such as the Zeiss, Posner, or Sussman designs. In one survey, 60% of clinicians utilized the Goldmann-type lenses and 40% used the Zeiss lens, with a majority of glaucoma specialists preferring the latter (1,2). In another survey, 70% used a Goldmann-type lens, 12% used a four-mirror lens, and 18% used both types (3).

The Direct System

This direct system is frequently referred to as the Koeppe system, after the lens type most frequently employed (Table 4.1). The Koeppe lens design uses simple light refraction (Figure 4.1) to produce an image that is upright, virtual, and magnified. The lens is a 50 diopter concave base curve lens with a convex bubble-shaped outer surface (1). It is made of either glass or plastic and is available in four diameters: 17.0 mm, 18.0 mm, 19.0 mm, and 22.5 mm. If the lens is too large, insertion is difficult. If it is too small, the lens will be difficult to keep centered (4). This can interfere and compromise

the view; therefore, choosing the appropriate diameter is important. Smaller direct-view lenses, such as a Richardson lens, are used with children. The Layden lens is used for premature infant gonioscopy (5). The Koeppe A lens has a dimple in the center to help in the positioning of the lens. The Barkan lens, which has a portion in the dome that is cut out, is used for goniotomy (6). The Swan-Jacob gonioprism and Thorpe surgical gonioscope lens are examples of direct-view lenses used for surgical goniotomy, where direct gonioscopy has its greatest use. These lenses are also used for other surgical procedures, such as trabeculodialysis and goniosynchialysis (1,7).

The lens curvature provides 1.5× magnification, with additional magnification coming from a microscope that is often supported and counterbalanced (traditionally it is suspended on a rope from a pulley mounted to the ceiling) (1). The angle is illuminated by a hand-held focal light source, typically a Barkan focal illuminator, or from a finely focusable fiberoptic light source. A hand-held microscope with an attached illuminating system can also be used; however, without support, slight movements cause the object of observation to move out of focus easily. Zeiss manufactures a hand-held slit lamp with 12× magnification that can be used as the microscope and illuminating source for direct gonioscopy (Figure 4.2). This slit lamp is also useful for performing indirect gonioscopy in patients unable to be placed at the conventional slit lamp. This fixed attached light source and viewing system, however, prevents illumination of the angle by retroillumination or backlighting in the direct system.

TABLE 4.1
Direct-View Koeppe Lens System

Image is upright, virtual, magnified
System uses simple light refraction
Lenses are made of glass or plastic
Diameters vary: 17.0 mm, 18.0 mm, 19.0 mm, 22.5 mm

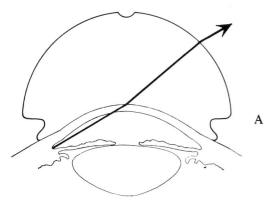

A

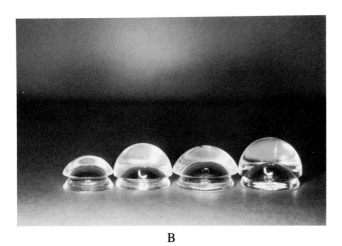

B

Figure 4.1 (A) Koeppe lens design. The light is refracted directly to the observer. When viewing inferior, the inferior angle is being observed. (Reprinted with permission from Hoskins HD, Kass MA Jr. Becker-Shaffer's diagnosis and therapy of the glaucomas, 6th ed. St Louis: CV Mosby, 1989.) (B) Various diameter direct-view lenses.

The Koeppe-type lens allows the examiner to observe the anterior chamber directly from an external observation vantage point. Thus, when the examiner is looking superiorly, the superior angle is under observation. The view

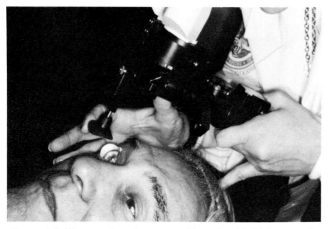

Figure 4.2 The examiner is using a Zeiss hand-held lamp and a Koeppe lens for direct observation of the angle.

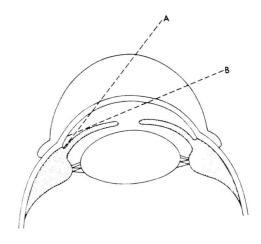

Figure 4.3 The examiner changes position (B to A) to view deeper into the angle. Unlike the indirect system, the lens does not require tilting, and the patient can maintain fixation. (Reprinted with permission from Hoskins HD Jr. Interpretive gonioscopy in glaucoma. Invest Ophthalmol. 1972; 11:97.

provided is more panoramic, providing a larger field of view than that obtained with the indirect lenses. (Figure 4.3).

Technique

Saline is most often used as the fluid to fill the space between the lens and the cornea; however, a more viscous solution, such as commercially available gonioscopy solutions, may be used. Use of the viscous gonioscopy solutions, however, will interfere with corneal integrity, the patient's vision, and the examiner's subsequent evaluation of the eye's surface, as well as direct or indirect ophthalmoscopy of the internal ocular structures. Thus, whenever possible, gonioscopy should be performed after these evaluations. Usually it is performed just after ocular tensions are measured and just prior to dilation.

The patient should be placed in a supine position with head flat, the chin and forehead at the same level. Apply one drop of a topical anesthetic. Hold the lens by the lip located at the edge. (The dome of the lens should be avoided to prevent smudging of this surface.) Without any intervening solution, insert the lower lip of the sterilized lens under the edge of the lower lid; as the patient looks inferior, pull the upper lid over the superior lip of the lens. If a bubble forms, ask the patient to turn his or her head to the opposite side; lift the temporal edge of the lens minimally and introduce the saline solution until there are no air bubbles. If gonioscopic gel is used, the concave surface can be filled with the solution and then the lens placed directly on the eye as described. With the lens in place and the patient looking straight ahead, direct the broad light source toward the angle sector of observation. Using a hand gonioscope or a hand-held slit lamp, move slowly toward the eye until the pupil area is in focus. Then evaluate the iris contour as fixation is shifted toward the angle recess for examination.

Advantages (Table 4.2)

The direct system is flexible in that the light source and the examiner are mobile (8). The lenses rarely need any manipulation after insertion, and the patient is often comfortable in a supine position. The examiner is not required to hold the lens once it is placed on the eye, and because the lens is held in place by the patient's lids, the examiner can place a lens on each eye and more easily and quickly compare the two eyes by rapidly moving back and forth between them. This is particularly beneficial in suspected cases of unilateral angle recession where comparison of the angle depth between the eyes is critical or in examination of an infant (Plates 14 and 21). This type of examination can also be utilized in nonambulatory patients at bedside and for patients who may be unable to be placed conveniently at the slit lamp for indirect gonioscopy.

To see over a bowed iris or into a narrow angle, the examiner needs only to alter the axis of view to a higher position (see Figure 4.3). Patients do not need to move their eyes, and no pressure is exerted onto the eye, causing artifacts. Because of the lens' large diameter and peripheral flange, very little pressure is placed on the limbus, thereby minimizing the possibility of distorting the shape of the angle and providing a more natural view of the anterior chamber (9).

Transillumination of the scleral spur is more dramatic with the Koeppe lens direct view method. This is particularly useful when the angle wall is heavily covered with iris processes. It is also useful in defining the exact location of the scleral spur in anomalous angles or when the examiner is unsure as to whether he or she is seeing the complete trabecula. Visibility of the scleral spur ensures that the functioning portion of the trabecula is not covered with iris tissue. Transillumination is accomplished by directing the illuminating source toward the cornea anterior to the angle wall or by placing the separate light source behind the portion of the angle under observation. The light will then become internally reflected within the sclera. The scleral spur will be lit up internally by sclerotic scatter and will stand out as a bright line, in comparison to the remainder of the wall, thus highlighting the scleral spur. This procedure also makes the iris processes more pronounced as they stand out as darker lines in comparison to the highlighted wall and appear closer to the observer as if they are standing off the wall. This can be accomplished with the indirect system, but the effect may not be as dramatic (see Figure 2.9).

This direct system has application in teaching situations because it provides a panoramic view. Also, familiarity of the angle wall and structures may be easier to grasp as the direct system provides a direct, more natural view of the angle. It is also easy for multiple observers to examine the eye without lens manipulation. The patient is often more comfortable in a supine position, and less ocular surface irritation occurs, particularly if a nonpreserved saline or nonpreserved viscous wetting solutions such as Celluvisc® has been used as an intervening solution (6).

The direct system has very real and practical application in cases where the indirect system provides equivocal views of the lateral angles. For example, the direct system may be very helpful as an adjunct because stereoscopic view is obtainable in the lateral angles. (This is extremely difficult in many cases with the indirect system.) It also provides the examiner with a useful view in eyes with very narrow angles with a convex iris (9) because observation into the angle recess is easier. Some of this may be related to gravity. With the patient supine, the iris may drop posterior by gravitational forces and open or widen the angle. This allows the observer to see deeper into the angle recess, which is helpful in narrow angles as long as one takes into account the effects of gravity; otherwise, this dropping back of the iris may cause interpretation errors.

Disadvantages (Table 4.3)

Use of the direct system requires a large working area so that the examiner can move around the patient in order to view the different portions of the angle. It may be difficult to observe certain quadrants in patients with prominent noses or brows (10). In addition, an assistant is often required to coordinate the use of the separate illumination and viewing system or on occasion to hold the lens in place. The steep outside curve of the lens can create distortion (11).

This method is somewhat inconvenient because it is unwieldy and more time-consuming; therefore, it is used less frequently than other methods for gonioscopy. The major disadvantages, however, are the lack of variable magnification and illumination and the inability to produce an optic section. This prevents exact localization of structures, so the examiner often has to rely on concentric rings of color variation to localize anterior chamber landmarks. Exact identification of Schwalbe's

TABLE 4.2
Advantages of the Direct System

Panoramic view
Patient comfort
Simultaneous lens placement each eye (good for angle recession)
Useful for bedside examination
Narrow angles—good view
Binocularity for lateral angle
Transillumination
Teaching situations
Less chance for lens-induced distortion
Pediatric exam
Goniotomy

TABLE 4.3
Disadvantages of the Direct View System

Time consuming
Requires large working area
Often requires an assistant
Requires separate illumination and magnification systems for best results
Lacks magnification and illumination compared to slit lamp
Cannot create optic section to localize Schwalbe's line
Poor detail

line with this method can be difficult. In some eyes, there is a band of pigment anterior to Schwalbe's line and along Schwalbe's, which can be easily mistaken for trabecular meshwork. The trabecular meshwork could be mistaken for ciliary body band, and a narrow or closed angle could be judged erroneously as an open or wide angle. Also, subtle changes in the anterior chamber wall are difficult, and sometimes impossible, to resolve with the direct system. Early neovascularization, small localized areas of peripheral anterior synechia, or localized pigment spattering (Plate 15) along the angle wall from resolved iris apposition in cases of subacute angle closure glaucoma could easily be missed because of inadequate magnification.

Distortion can be a problem with this system. This can occur if a vacuum suction is created when fluid escapes from under the lens without air becoming aspirated (12). To prevent this and distortion from pressure, the lens should remain centered on the eye with as little force as possible. Unfortunately, with some patients, force against the lens may be needed to keep the lens in place, and the force will distort the view (4). Also, if the lens is not centered, the lens edge away from the limbus on the corneal side will be in a position to create direct pressure on that portion of the angle. This direct pressure will result in the narrowing of that angle portion. The side opposite will be artificially opened by the aqueous forced posterior into that angle section, and that angle portion will be widened (4).

Direct Koeppe-type gonioscopy is a method that is rarely used in routine clinical practice. However, there are times in the course of a busy practice, particularly practices concentrating in the area of glaucoma, where this technique can provide very useful information. It is often easier with the Koeppe system to view the angle recess in a narrow-angle eye with a bowed iris. In situations where stereoscopic observation of the lateral angle is important, this system is superior to the indirect system. When multiple examiners will be observing the angle, patient comfort will be better. The more natural direct panoramic view obtained with this method makes it particularly valuable as an introductory method for identification of anterior chamber landmarks for the student or resident learning gonioscopy.

The Indirect System

The indirect gonioscopy method is more often used than the direct system (Table 4.4). In a busy practice, this method is much more convenient for implementation during the examination. Following tonometry, with the cornea still anesthetized, gonioscopy can be conveniently performed while the patient is seated comfortably at the slit lamp. It rarely requires an assistant, no additional space is needed to perform the examination, and other than the lens itself, no additional microscopes or illumination systems are needed (Figure 4.4).

The system combines lenses with mirrors mounted within them, or silvered prisms, used in conjunction with a slit lamp (Figure 4.5). The angle is observed by reflected light, and the mirror is placed opposite to the section of the angle

TABLE 4.4
The Indirect System

Advantages	Disadvantages
Focal lines for localization of Schwalbe's line	Poor lateral view (stereopsis difficult)
Magnified view	Patient discomfort
Excellent for small details	Difficult for repeated examination
Use for laser treatment	Need for gonioscopic fluid
Easy to implement in examination	Small field of view
	Observation is reversed by mirrors (when mirror is superior, inferior angle is under observation)

being observed. When the mirror is superior, the angle being observed is the inferior angle. The angle under observation is inverted but not reversed laterally. The image will not be rotated around a vertical axis. Thus, with the lens superior, a lesion noted in the lens at 12 o'clock is actually located in the angle at 6 o'clock (13). The image with the indirect system is indirect, virtual, and unmagnified (Figure 4.6).

The mirrored lenses allow the anterior chamber to be observed in a straight-ahead position. The examiner and the patient remain seated upright. Rather than the examiner physically moving to view over a bowed iris or to view into the different angle quadrants, he or she need only rotate or tilt the lens or have the patient rotate the eyes into different fields of gaze. For example, in a case of narrow angles, the angle recess can be easily observed by tilting the lens to the angle of observation and having the patient rotate the eye toward the gonioscopy mirror.

The indirect lenses rely on the slit lamp for illumination and magnification. The clearer the optics and the brighter the illumination from the slit lamp, the greater advantage this system is in detecting discrete changes in the angle wall. Small foreign bodies (Plate 36), areas of posterior synechia (Plate 11), inflammatory debris, exfoliative deposits (Plate 18), and subtle neovascularization (Plate 20) are more easily detectable with the increased magnification and illumination provided by the slit lamp.

One of the most important advantages with this system is the ability to utilize an optic section in order to identify structures and determine the place of attachment of the iris root.

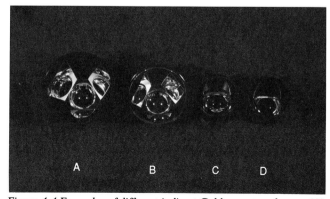

Figure 4.4 Examples of different indirect Goldmann-type lenses: (A) *large three-mirror (gonioscopy mirror inferior),* (B) *small three-mirror (gonioscopy mirror inferior),* (C) *two-mirror, and* (D) *one-mirror (Haag-Streit).*

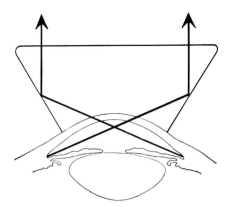

Figure 4.5 Example of light rays being reflected from mirror goniolens. To observe the inferior angle, the examiner looks into the superior mirror. (Reprinted with permission from Hoskins HD, Kass MA Jr. Becker-Shaffer's diagnosis and therapy of the glaucomas, 6th ed. St Louis: CV Mosby, 1989.)

The anterior termination of the angle wall is located at the juncture of the posterior and anterior corneal focal lines. This marks the internal limbus or termination of the cornea internally, and Schwalbe's line is located at this point. Thus, the examiner can locate the anterior limit of the trabecular meshwork (Figure 4.7 and Plate 34).

There are some disadvantages. In cases where the angle is narrow or the iris is bowed, observation of the angle recess can be difficult with the indirect system. Artifacts may be

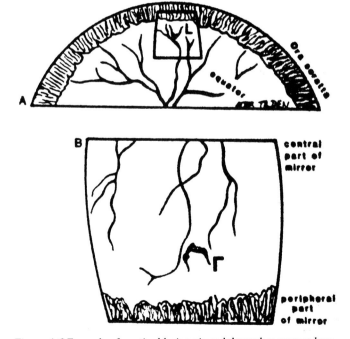

Figure 4.6 Example of a retinal lesion viewed through a contact lens mirror. When viewing into the angle, the same effect takes place. The image is inverted, nor reversed laterally. (A) The upper half of the peripheral fundus. (B) A view of that corresponding part of the fundus showing that a particular lesion (L) is inverted but not reversed laterally as seen by the observer. (Reprinted with permission from Kassin E. Fundus lens biomicroscopy theory and practical methods. Optom Month. August 1984.)

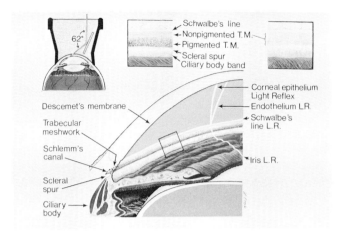

Figure 4.7 An artist's representation of an open angle and focal lines coursing along the iris and angle wall. The optic section terminates along the angle wall at Schwalbe's line. This iris insertion along the angle wall is observed where the focal line along the iris is observed meeting the focal line along the wall. (Drawing by Laurel Cook)

introduced because the lens may require tilting up and down or side to side, and the patient may need to rotate the eyes to allow the examiner to observe the angle recess. This may produce folds of the corneal epithelium and endothelium, thus distorting the view. Unwanted pressure may be produced by this manipulation, which will change the dynamics of the aqueous flow from the posterior chamber to the anterior chamber, creating an unwanted and unpredictable opening of the angle in one quadrant with a narrowing in another quadrant. This can lead to errors in diagnosis. The lateral walls are difficult to observe stereoscopically because the slit lamp viewing axis is horizontal while the mirror axis is vertical. The examination can be uncomfortable for the examiner and the patient if the examination is lengthy. Some patients may be unable to be seated at a slit lamp, although in some of these instances, a hand-held slit lamp can be used, with a small one- or two-mirror Goldmann-type lens. With the larger Goldmann lenses, focusing of the hand-held slit lamp is problematic; the lamp has to be held farther from the patient because of the larger lens cone, and in some cases, this places the slit lamp beyond its fixed focused range.

Lenses

Indirect Lenses (Figure 4.8)

The prototype lens used is the Goldmann lens, manufactured by Haag-Streit. Ocular Instruments also manufactures a series of Goldmann-type indirect lenses and a number of other specialty gonioscopy and laser application lenses. Twomey Corporation manufactures a small-diameter series of indirect gonioscopy lenses.* Generally the lenses are made as a one-mirror lens, a two-mirror lens, and a large and small

*Wherever possible, the discussion is intended to be generic; mention of a Goldmann-type lens means all lenses made in that design and does not suggest, unless specifically noted, that the discussion is about the Haag-Streit lens.

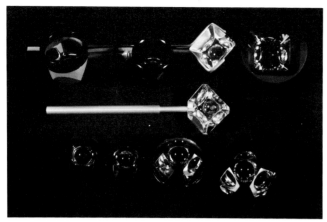

Figure 4.8 Indirect gonioscopy lenses. Read each row from left to right. Top row: Sussman four-mirror lens, Twomey four-mirror lens, Zeiss four-mirror lens with holding fork. Middle row: Posner four-mirror lens. Bottom row: Goldmann type-one mirror, Goldmann type-two mirror, Goldmann type-three mirror (small), Goldmann type-three mirror (large).

TABLE 4.6
Goldmann-Style Three-Mirror Lenses

Parallel view good for detail
Causes less vacuum than smaller lens
Good for beginning gonioscopist
Can use for retina examination
Stable view
Easier to handle

three-mirror lens with one mirror for gonioscopy. The Thorpe four-mirror lens is the exception; it is a large Goldmann-type lens design with four mirrors placed for gonioscopy.

Goldmann-Style Indirect Lenses

The one- and two-mirror lenses are used primarily for gonioscopy, although the central portion of the lens can be used for examining the posterior pole (Table 4.5). The two-mirror lenses have mirrors across from each other, so the lens needs to be rotated only 90 degrees to evaluate the whole angle. Lenses with one gonioscopy mirror must be rotated 270 degrees to evaluate the entire angle. In the Haag-Streit series, the one- and two- mirror lenses are smaller than the three-mirror lens (Table 4.6) and are particularly valuable in patients with small apertures or for patients who are squeezers. The smaller lenses tend to adhere to the eye more because their peripheral curves are steeper than those of the larger lenses. This makes these lenses more practical with patients who are apprehensive and tend to squeeze tightly with the lens on the eye. The tighter adherence of the smaller lenses makes them more difficult for the patient to blink out.

In some instances, the tighter adherence may result in the lens producing a partial vacuum, causing a distortion of the

TABLE 4.5
Goldmann-Style One- and Two-Mirror Lenses

Advantages	Disadvantages
Higher vantage good for narrow angles	Foreshortened view
Applicable with hand-held slit lamp	Cannot use for peripheral retina examination
	Can cause partial vacuum, causing distortion
Useful with:	
Patients with small aperture	
Patients with deep-set eyes	
Patients who squeeze	

cornea; thus degrading the image and also causing a lens-induced deepening of the angle (14). Ocular Instruments manufactures a one-mirror lens described as a bubble-free gonio-lens that, because of a flatter base curve, should not produce lens adherence (15). This lens design does not require methyl-cellulose because there is no vaulting between the lens and the cornea, and therefore air bubbles are not a problem. Tomey Technology also manufactures a small lens but with a four-mirror design. This has the advantage of being small without adhering tightly to the eye. In all of these lenses, the mirrors are inclined at 62 degrees, but placement of the mirrors must vary because the view of the same angle varies with the different lenses. The Haag-Streit lenses provide a higher vantage point than do the other small lens designs.

The gonioscopy mirrors of the Haag-Streit smaller lenses are located closer to the center of the lens and are higher than the mirrors in the three-mirror lens or in the bubble-free Tomey lens. This produces a higher vantage point for observing the angle and is of benefit in eyes with a narrow angle or a bowed iris. The examiner can view the angle recess over the bowed iris—particularly advantageous in cases with narrow angles. For example, say that a patient suspected of having angle closure presents with elevated ocular tension of 30 mm Hg and by slit lamp examination evinces narrow angles, bowed iris, and shallow chamber. If the angle wall is observed to be open on gonioscopy (without compression), the examiner can be reassured that the pressure is not elevated from angle closure. Observation of the entire filtering trabecular meshwork by observing the scleral spur assures the examiner that the angle is open (Figure 4.9). The lens of choice in this situation would be the one that provides the best view over the mounded iris with the least amount of distortion—a lens with a high mirror closer to the center of the lens. The small one- or two-mirror Haag-Streit lenses fit this category.

Comparing Different Goldmann Designs

The view of an angle will be affected by the examiner's choice of lens. In general, a lens designed with higher mirrors, located closer to the center of the lens, and a large angle of inclination will provide a higher vantage point for the observer. The higher mirror allows a view over the iris, and the central location allows visualization across the iris. It is critical for an examiner to be aware that variations in these factors result in different observation points. Sometimes a high observation point is better, as in cases of a narrow angle with a deep angle recess. Sometimes it is important to have a more parallel view—for example, when there is a concern

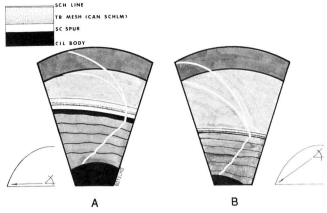

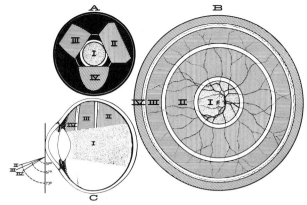

Figure 4.9 Same angle viewed with different lenses. (A) In primary gaze without lens tilting and the patient looking straight ahead: the view of the angle with a large Goldmann-type lens. The vantage point is more parallel to the iris. The examiner's eye is level with the pupil border. (B) Observation with a smaller Haag-Streit lens where the vantage point is higher and oblique to the iris. The observer is looking down into the angle recess. This causes the same angle wall structures to look closer together.

Figure 4.10 Large Goldmann-type lenses can be used to examine the fundus and the vitreous. Mirror IV is used for gonioscopy and far peripheral retina examination. The diagram depicts the mirror required for examining a particular fundus location. (Reprinted with permission from Tolentino FI et al. Vitreoretinal disorders: Diagnosis and management. Philadelphia: WB Saunders, 1976.)

of angle neovascularization. In this instance, the gonioscopy mirror in the large Goldmann-type three-mirror lens will provide a stable, clear, panoramic view of the posterior wall. Small details along the wall will be easier to observe with this lens. The foreshortened view obtained with the smaller lenses may make it more difficult to discern angle wall subtleties because details tend to appear closer together and bunched (Figure 4.9). Again, this is related to mirror height, centration, and inclination. In some patients with deep-set eyes, it is difficult to tilt the larger lenses sufficiently because the orbital rim and brow area prevent it. The angle may be difficult to observe, especially if the iris is bowed. In this instance, the higher view with the smaller Haag-Streit design would be an advantage, because the smaller lenses may provide a deeper view without as much tilting being required.

The larger Haag-Streit lenses have a wider peripheral curve than the smaller lenses, which allows the lens to be rotated freely and rarely produces lens-to-cornea adherence. This reduces the potential for corneal epithelial compromise from the lens. The larger lens, because of its larger diameter and subsequent edge location, also causes less corneal indentation or vacuum than the smaller Goldmann-type lenses. This reduces the potential for distortions because a lens too steep for a particular cornea will have its contour altered by pressure or by the relative vacuum created under the goniolens. This change in corneal curvature translates to an alteration of the aqueous in the anterior chamber, resulting in a change of the iris root and angle wall relationship. Clinically, this vacuum can be detected when a lens placed on the eye does not rotate freely. Distortions can also be minimized by avoiding pressure on the lens and keeping the lens centered over the cornea.

Recommending a particular Goldmann-type lens is difficult because each lens has advantages and disadvantages; however, the three-mirror lens design is an excellent choice for neophyte

gonioscopists. With this lens, the view of the angle is not foreshortened; thus, the wall structures are easier to differentiate because they appear less crowded and bunched together, particularly when compared to the view with the one- and two-mirror lens. This difference in view between the lenses is significant, especially for those learning the technique and becoming familiar with the gonioscopic anatomy. The three-mirror lens also has another benefit: it provides excellent views of the peripheral retina when the eye is dilated. In the Goldmann design, the three mirrors are located around the central lens at 120 degrees from each other and are angled at 59 degrees, 67 degrees, and 73 degrees in relation to the plane parallel to the concave surface of the lens (13). The mirror, set at 59 degrees and shaped like a flat-top bifocal lens, is used for examination of the angle (Figure 4.10). In the dilated eye, the mirror angled at 73 degrees provides a view from the edge of the posterior pole to the equator region. The longer and thinner mirror angled at 67 degrees provides a view from the edge of the equator to the ora. The gonioscopic mirror angle at 59 degrees can be used to view the ora serrata area. The central portion of the lens can be used to examine the posterior pole.

Technique

Goldmann Lenses

Patient Preparation

The gonioscopic procedure should be done at the end of the routine examination after tonometry and just prior to dilation. A slit lamp evaluation should be done prior to the lens insertion to evaluate the corneal integrity. The anterior chamber and angle should be analyzed for depth and iris configuration for comparison to the gonioscopic findings. No additional anesthetic is necessary as the eyes are usually sufficiently anesthetized from the anesthetic used for tonometry.

Explain the examination completely to the patient and prepare him or her for the eyelids to be sensitive to the lens. Some patients may be apprehensive when they see the size of the lens; when they are reassured that only the small concave surface contacts the numbed cornea and that a coupling solution is utilized to cushion the eye, most are quite cooperative. The coupling solution often runs down the cheek of the patient; placing a tissue on the cheek, under the lens, will prevent this.

Seat the patient comfortably in the slit lamp with forehead and chin secure, and caution him or her about moving back away from the slit lamp. The patient's eyes should be parallel to the slit lamp table, with the slit lamp set for the examiner's proper pupillary distance and the illumination placed at a high setting. Initially, the beam of the slit lamp should be a narrow optic section, with the angle of the illumination source set at 0 degrees. Caution the patient against squeezing the eyes and urge him or her to keep both eyes open and the gaze in a straight-ahead position. It is important that the patient gaze where directed, and the examiner should be aware of where the patient is looking. Not paying attention to this detail is a common error for beginning gonioscopists. If a patient looks down while the examiner is evaluating the inferior angle, the quadrant will appear narrower than it actually is.

Examiner Preparation

The examination can sometimes take up to 5 minutes or longer per eye. To avoid examiner fatigue and discomfort, adjust the slit lamp to a comfortable height. Dim the room lights to avoid unwanted reflections off the front lens surface, which can interfere with the view. Once the lens is inserted, it may be held in place. You should be able to rest your elbow on the table top when holding the lens against the patient's eye (Figure 4.11). If the distance is too great and your elbow

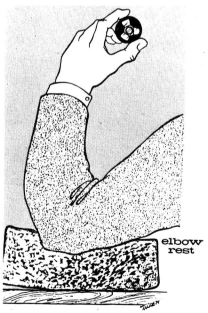

Figure 4.11 An elbow rest allows the examiner's hand to remain vertical (Reprinted with permission from Tolentino FI et al. Vitreoretinal disorders: Diagnosis and management. Philadelphia: WB Saunders, 1976).

not supported, place an elbow rest on the slit lamp table at a height that allows your forearm to remain vertical. This will provide better balance and prevent fatigue and discomfort to your arm, hand, or shoulders. It also prevents you from placing unwanted force against the eye.

Lens Preparation

Because the curvature of the lens portion that contacts the eye is steeper than most corneas, all the Goldmann-type gonioscopy lenses with steep base curves require a somewhat viscous, optically homogenous solution with an index of refraction similar to the cornea. The solution acts as an interface between the lens and the cornea. Because it may interfere with other examinations, such as visual fields, ocular photography, or indirect ophthalmoscopy, gonioscopy with these lenses should be done only after those procedures (7,16). Practically, this problem is dramatically reduced when the gonioscopic fluid is irrigated out of the eye with sterile nonpreserved saline after the lens is removed. When using gonioscopic solution, place the fluid into the concave surface of the lens, filling it with a few drops or to the peripheral curve juncture. Any excess solution will run down the patient's cheek, making him or her uncomfortable during the examination. In some cases, excess solution can be trapped under the lens, creating a partial vacuum and apical compression of the cornea, which will distort the view (17). The solution used should have an index of refraction equal to the cornea; otherwise the image will not be clear. If the solution is not sufficiently viscous, as with normal saline, bubbles will form.

Just prior to insertion, hold the lens up above your head and inspect the solution for air bubbles (Figure 4.12). The air bubbles prevent good lens adherence and also will produce an optical obstacle, interfering with the view. Smaller air bubbles that are present either initially or during the examination can sometimes be eliminated by rocking the lens and by having the patient alter the field of gaze while exerting slight pressure against the cornea with the lens. If this is unsuccessful, remove, rinse, clean, and reinsert the lens. Air bubbles can be avoided by storing the gonioscopic solution upside down,

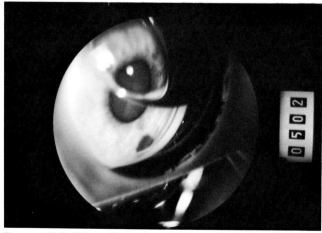

Figure 4.12 Bubbles will interfere with lens adherence and block the view into the angle.

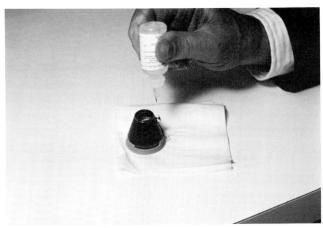

Figure 4.13 To eliminate bubbles, a small stream of goniofluid can be squeezed out while moving the solution onto the concave lens surface.

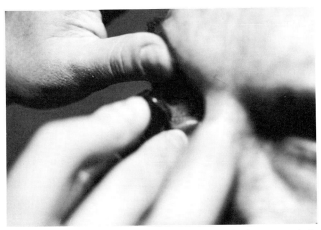

Figure 4.14 Insertion technique. The patient looks up, and the examiner holds the superior lid against the superior orbital rim. The lower edge of the lens is placed against the conjunctiva and is used to hold down the lower lid. The inferior edge of the lens is held against the conjunctiva while the patient fixates straight ahead. The lens is fulcrumed against the globe, and the upper lid is then released.

causing the air to rise to the top, away from the tip of the bottle, and shaking the bottle before applying the solution. It has also been suggested to remove the spout of the bottle and pour the solution onto the lens (18). Releasing the first few drops onto a nearby tissue before applying the solution onto the lens will also help to release any bubbles present. Without releasing pressure on the bottle, thus preventing air into the bottle, the slow stream of solution can be applied to the concave surface of the lens (Figure 4.13).

Some patients may be sensitive to the preservatives in commercially available methylcellulose-based gonioscopy solutions. A nonpreserved wetting agent such as Celluvisc® serves as an adequate binding solution. Adherence is not as great in some eyes, and bubbles will occur more frequently than with the gonioscopic solutions, but usually it serves as an adequate intervening solution for many examination purposes. This type of solution is quite beneficial in teaching situations or when patients require multiple applications of a contact lens. I have found that it reduces patients' complaints of irritation and postgonioscopy epithelial stippling. It should also have a theoretic advantage in cases requiring gonioscopy but where corneal disruption could be promoted by the examination—for example, with a patient with a history of epithelial basement membrane disease or with microcystic edema, or when there is an anticipated need for the patient to have multiple applications of the lens, as in provocative testing.

Some patients may be sensitive to corneal anesthetics as well as the preservatives in the gonioscopy solutions. Disposable soft lenses may be useful in this situation. Semes (19) and Forgacs et al (20) have reported on the use of soft lenses for this purpose. Semes used Acuvue® lenses and concluded that it is a viable option when used with a large three-mirror gonioscopy lens. Nonpreserved saline is used on the goniolens in place of the methylcellulose solution. It tends to run off quickly, and the frequency of bubble formation and soft contact lens displacement tends to make this a technique unnecessarily cumbersome for routine or detailed examination.

It is a viable alternative where there is concern for interference of corneal integrity or in teaching situations.

Lens Insertion

After inspecting the lens for air bubbles or debris, place the gonioscope mirror so that it will be located superior when inserted. Grasp the lens with the thumb and first finger of your dominant hand. With the patient looking superiorly, place the bottom edge of the concave surface of the lens against the inferior conjunctiva, slightly above the lower lid (Figure 4.14). In this position, the lens can be utilized to keep the lower lid in place. Grasp the upper lid simultaneously with the free hand and hold it against the orbital rim. At this point, the patient should look straight ahead. Tilt the lens up at the same time, keeping in contact with the globe. Once the patient is looking straight ahead, release the upper lid. Only gentle pressure, if any, is needed to hold the lens against the globe because a suction cup effect is created when the lens is against the eye. A patient who squeezes will blink the lens out, and you will have to place more force against the cornea with the lens in this instance. This will prevent the patient from squeezing the lens out.

Observation

Once the lens is on the eye, balance your arm and move the slit lamp forward, focusing the slit lamp light in the gonioscope mirror, which is located superior. With the mirror superior, you will be viewing the inferior angle, normally the deepest quadrant. (The superior angle is normally the narrowest.) This increased visibility of the inferior angle compared to the superior angle may be related to this method of gonioscopy (21). At most, this normal difference may result in a half-structure variance in visibility. For example, if you can see to the tip of the ciliary body in the inferior angle, the

TABLE 4.7
Normal Variation in Angle Depth, Widest to Shallowest

Widest	Inferior—best for focal lines
	Temporal
	Nasal
Shallowest	Superior—focal lines
	possible

scleral spur should be easily visible in the superior angle. In an eye where the ciliary body is visible in the inferior angle (superior mirror) and only the trabecular meshwork or Schwalbe's line is visible in the superior angle (inferior mirror), the lens may be inadvertently tilted away from the angle of observation, the patient may not be looking straight ahead or may be looking away from the mirror, or in fact the angle is abnormally shallow in the superior quadrant, which is reason for concern. It is important to understand the normal anatomic variation that results in the lower angle's being the widest and the upper angle's being the narrowest to prevent errors in interpretation (Table 4.7). The lateral angles are intermediate in their visibility when compared to the vertical quadrants.

With the lens in place, start the examination at the pupil border, looking for any abnormalities, such as neovascularization or exfoliative material (Plates 20, 26, and 46). Then move along the iris surface, note its contour, the angle created between the iris and cornea, and the location of the iris insertion. The observed image obtained with the reflecting surface goniolenses is vertically inverted upside down but not laterally reversed; thus, a lesion located to the right of 6 o'clock in the inferior angle will be observed to the right in the mirror, but it will not be reversed anterior to posterior.

Focal Line Technique

Identification of anterior chamber wall landmarks should follow by utilizing the focal line technique. The creation of an optic section with indirect gonioscopy is critical for localization of the anterior chamber wall landmarks and is one of the major advantages of this system. This can be accomplished with any modern slit lamp (Plate 34).

Anatomically the focal lines are easiest to create and observe in the inferior angle because it is the widest quadrant. Thus, place the gonioscopy mirror superiorly, set the slit lamp illumination at high, and place the light source perpendicular to the slit lamp viewing oculars. Magnification should be approximately 16×. Once the slit beam is set at narrow to create an optic section and clearly focused, rotate the slit lamp light housing slowly 5 to 10 degrees nasally and temporally. While rotating the light source, notice the light beam falling along the angle wall split into an optic section, with two focal lines or a V. The line farthest from you represents the anterior cornea, and the other represents the posterior cornea. Where the focal lines join together, at the point of the V, represents and locates Schwalbe's line or the end of Descemet's membrane (See Figure 4.7 and Plates 7 and 9). Locating Schwalbe's line provides a reference point for identifying the other chamber wall structures and prevents the possibility of errors in angle assessment when using pigment bands as a means for locating angle wall structures. Errors occur when you confuse a pigmented Schwalbe's line as pigmented trabecular meshwork.

The trabecular meshwork inserts into Schwalbe's line. The functioning portion is located in the posterior section of the meshwork. Both Schwalbe's and the filtering trabecular are often pigmented, especially in older individuals and particularly in the inferior angle. Therefore, by utilizing pigmentation to locate the functioning trabecular meshwork, you may easily mistake pigmented Schwalbe's as the pigmented functioning trabecular meshwork. In a case where the angle was actually open only to the pigmented trabecular meshwork, you could erroneously assume that the lighter area under the pigmented Schwalbe's was scleral spur rather than the nonfiltering trabecular meshwork and could assume the pigmented trabecular tissue was the ciliary body band. In this case, a narrow angle opened only to trabecular meshwork would be incorrectly identified as being open to the ciliary body band. Localizing Schwalbe's by an optic section prevents this error and the possibility of mistakenly evaluating a closed or narrow angle as open and/or deep.

The focal lines can also be used to locate the point of iris attachment to the angle wall, as well as to judge the width of the angle. Estimate the width and depth of the angle by evaluating the length of the beam of light from Schwalbe's line to its intersection of the narrow beam of light traveling along the iris surface. Remember that this apparent length will vary depending on the gonioscopy lens used: The distance will appear longer with a Goldmann-type large lens and shorter with a Goldmann-type small lens. The location where the focal line running along the iris surface joins the focal line running along the angle wall marks the place where the iris root attaches to the angle wall. Evidence of angle closure is provided when the focal beam along the iris and the focal beam along the angle wall meet above the filtering portion of the trabecular meshwork, without any displacement of the two beams. This is an indication that the iris is attached to the wall at that location. With the light beam in the same position, scan the angle to determine to what extent the angle is closed (Figure 4.15A and Plates 9, 10, and 37).

When the focal line along the iris is displaced from the focal line along the wall, so that the two beams are not exactly continuous, you are not visualizing the location of the iris attachment (Figure 4.15B). This parallactic displacement is evidence that the angle is open wider than observed and that your vantage point is too low. It may be too low for a number of reasons (Table 4.8):

- The iris may be bowed and you cannot see over it, as in cases of a narrow angle with relative pupillary block or because the iris has a prominent last roll, preventing a view of the iris recess.
- Poor technique may contribute to this situation. The patient may be looking superior when the superior angle is being examined, or you may inadvertently tilt the lens inferior when observing the superior angle.
- Perhaps you do not have a high enough vantage because of the type of lens being used.

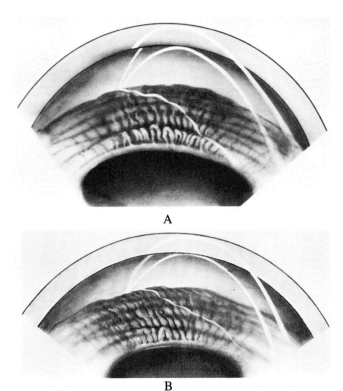

A

B

Figure 4.15 Focal line along the iris meets the focal line along the angle wall above the filtering trabecular meshwork—Scwalbe's line (A). The angle is closed at that location. (B) When the focal line does not meet the focal line along the wall, there is parallax. This indicates that the examiner is not observing the location of iris insertion. The angle is narrow, or the vantage point is too low. (Reprinted with permission from Gorin G, Posner A. Slit lamp gonioscopy, *3d ed. Baltimore: Williams & Wilkins, 1967.)*

To see into the angle recess in these cases, the patient should rotate the eye toward the mirror while you tilt the lens toward the angle under observation (Figure 4.16). This must be accomplished without exerting undo pressure against the cornea; otherwise, the view will be distorted and/or the natural state of the chamber depth will be altered. With the larger, steeper lenses, the cornea is usually vaulted and pressure is on the sclera and this latter problem is averted. When the lens curvature is not steep enough, the cornea will become flattened, and this can result in aqueous being forced back into the anterior chamber and causing a widening of the angle. Sometimes when the lens edge produces pressure against the globe in the area of Schwalbe's line, the angle will become narrower in that region (Figure 4.16B). For example, when viewing the inferior angle, the mirror is superior. If the

TABLE 4.8
Focal Line Parallax

Angle appears narrow but focal lines are not meeting
Vantage point too low
Narrow angle
Lens tilted incorrectly toward angle under observation
Patient is looking away from angle observed

iris is bowed, you will need to tilt the lens inferior to see over the iris. If the inferior edge presses against the globe with too much force at the inferior limbus, the inferior angle will become narrowed. In addition, because of the lens-induced indentation, the aqueous may be forced into the superior angle, causing this quadrant to widen artificially. Then, when the lens is rotated to observe the superior angle, it will appear wider than it actually is. Practically this is not a major problem with the larger, indirect lenses because the edge of the lens is located beyond the limbus. With smaller lenses with outer diameters in the 15 mm range, this is more problematic (12).

When you observe the presence of endothelial or epithelial folds during gonioscopy, it is evidence of excessive pressure (4). Epithelial folds can be recognized as concentric lines that follow the limbus. The endothelial folds, caused by an indentation of the entire thickness of the cornea by the edge of the lens, are branched irregularly, running in different directions (21). The relationship between the cornea and the goniolens is rarely considered by clinicians; however, eyes may vary in corneal diameter and corneal curvature, and yet we expect the gonioscopy lens to act the same on each eye. Consider that the type and size of lens chosen may alter the corneal curvature, and thus the appearance of the angle. The lens you choose should be the one that provides the most accurate view of the angle without causing unwanted alterations in the view. This varies with the eye being examined.

After observing the inferior angle by focal line technique and localizing the anatomic landmarks, widen the beam and study the angle in detail, slowly rotating the lens while observing the angle through the slit lamp. Maintain your fixation on the most posterior visible structure while rotating and tilting the lens, and then scan along the wall at each interval. This can usually be accomplished with one hand on the lens and the other on the slit lamp.

The focal line technique can be used most easily in the inferior quadrant, in the widest quadrant, and also in wide angles in the superior quadrant. It is difficult to obtain in the lateral segments unless the inclination of the light source is altered vertically to produce an optic section. This can be obtained with slit lamps of the Haag-Streit design by rotating the illuminating beam horizontally or using the rotary prism in the Zeiss slit lamp (2). However, it is difficult to obtain and maintain a stereoscopic view laterally. In general, it is more difficult to examine the nasal and temporal quadrants because of this. Posner (21) recommends reducing the angle between the light source and the microscope to a minimum and directing the light into the middle of the mirror. This brings into view the opposite lateral angle. Often it is necessary to have the patient look toward the mirror to the right or left as needed and to tilt the lens toward the angle under observation. Maintain observation of the angle while continuously rotating and tilting the lens.

Lens Removal

Once all quadrants are satisfactorily observed, remove the lens. This can be accomplished by having the patient forcefully

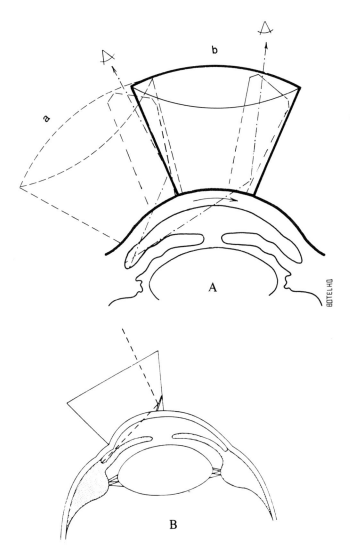

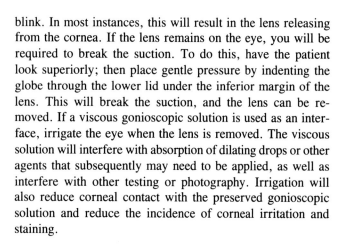

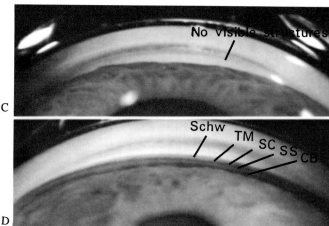

Figure 4.16 With a centered goniolens (a), the observation point does not provide a view into the angle recess. This will occur in a narrow-angle, plateau iris configuration, with prominent bowing to iris, or in malignant glaucoma. The examiner will need to tilt the lens toward the angle segment of observation, and the patient will need to rotate the eye toward the gonioscope mirror (b). This will maximize the view into the angle recess. Pressure against the cornea should be avoided. (B) Pressure against the globe should be avoided, especially with the smaller-diameter lens, as this may narrow the angle under observation and widen the opposite quadrant by forcing aqueous into it. (Reprinted with permission from Hoskins HD Jr. Interpretative gonioscopy in glaucoma. Invest Ophthalmol. 1972;11:97–102.) (C) Poor technique: The angle appears closed. The patient is looking away from the mirror, and the examiner is tilting the lens away from the angle. (D) The patient now looks straight and the examiner holds the lens straight. The same angle will now be observed correctly as open. (Schw = Schwalbe's line, TM = trabecular meshwork, SC = Schlemm's canal, SS = scleral spur, CB = ciliary body) (Reprinted with permission from van Buskirk EM. Clinical atlas of glaucoma. Philadelphia: WB Saunders, 1986.)

blink. In most instances, this will result in the lens releasing from the cornea. If the lens remains on the eye, you will be required to break the suction. To do this, have the patient look superiorly; then place gentle pressure by indenting the globe through the lower lid under the inferior margin of the lens. This will break the suction, and the lens can be removed. If a viscous gonioscopic solution is used as an interface, irrigate the eye when the lens is removed. The viscous solution will interfere with absorption of dilating drops or other agents that subsequently may need to be applied, as well as interfere with other testing or photography. Irrigation will also reduce corneal contact with the preserved gonioscopic solution and reduce the incidence of corneal irritation and staining.

Care of Lenses

Proper care for gonioscopy lenses consists of cleaning the lens to reduce physical damage to it by any residual hardened solution or tear debris and disinfecting it to prevent the potential for disease transmission. Disinfection procedures tend to be highly variable even in hospitals (22).

Gonioscopy lenses fit into the category of semicritical items by the guidelines established by the Association for Practitioners in Infection Control (23). These include items that come into contact with mucous membranes. Most of the studies concerning cleaning and disinfection of semicritical items in eye care have been done using tonometer tips. As with tonometers, which contact the eye, gonioscopy lenses also present a potential vehicle for transmitting infections including viruses such as adenovirus (epidemic keratoconjunctivitis [EKC]), herpes simplex, hepatitis B, and the HTLV-III virus. According to the Association for Practitioners in Infection Control, semicritical items should be free of all microorganisms except bacterial spores and require high-level disinfection with the use of chemical germicides, agents that destroy all microorganisms. Proper procedure calls for cleaning the lens with tepid tap water with a ten-second rinse. This has been found effective for removing hepatitis B surface antigens from tonometer tips (24), and it removes the potential contaminated tear debris and any solution on the lens. Proper cleaning eliminates and reduces any organic load on the lens, as well as the level of microbial contamination. Since the efficacy of the disinfection is effected by the prior cleaning of the lens, this step is important and should not be left out. The lens portion that contacts the eye should then be soaked for five to ten minutes in a disinfecting solution. After disinfection, the lens should be rinsed with sterile water, air-dried, and stored in a dry case. A method of cleaning and disinfection recommended by one of the manufacturers (25) is to clean and wash the lens in water below 110 °F and mild soap, rinse the lens, dry it with a lint-free soft tissue, and store it in a dry case. Avoid rubbing the coated flat surface to prevent scratching. To disinfect the lens, soak it for 20 minutes in glutaraldehyde, rinse with sterile water, and store it dry. To sterilize the lens, oxide gas not greater than 125 °F without maximum aeration is recommended. There is potential for problems with glutaraldehyde as it can be irritating to the eyes and nasal passages especially if there are elevated vapor levels in a poorly ventilated room as well as a cause of allergic contact dermatitis (23,26). There is also concern with this agent getting into the eye (27).

Chlorine and chlorine compounds or 3 percent hydrogen peroxide are acceptable as disinfecting agents; however, manufacturers recommend against the use of hydrogen peroxide, alcohol, and acetone. Isopropyl alcohol is often used in practice, but it is not considered a high-level disinfecting agent, and in one report it was found to be ineffective in EKC (28). In another report using isopropyl alcohol, the human immunodeficiency virus was left firmly embedded in a layer of dessicated protein 20 μ thick, also pointing out the importance of cleaning prior to disinfection (29).

Based upon this information, chlorine, in the form of Dakin's solution, is the most appropriate agent for disinfection. Household bleach contains 5.25% sodium hypochlorite, or 52,500 ppm. Cutting the strength to 1:10 (5000 ppm) is the recommended concentration by Centers for Disease Control guidelines if it is used within 24 hours. In an open or closed polyethylene container, the solution will lose 40% to 50% of its concentration in one month. Therefore, if the solution is mixed and is to be stored in an opaque plastic container, it should be mixed 1 part bleach to 4 parts water; the solution from that bottle can be used for up to 30 days. If it is stored in a closed brown bottle, there will be no decompensation (23). It is important that the solution be washed off the lens surface before it contacts the eye because the bleach can cause corneal defects (although no studies have been performed to evaluate whether the bleach will be harmful to the gonioscopy lens over long periods of time) (Table 4.9).

TABLE 4.9
Lens Care After Use

Rinse with tap water for 10 seconds.
Wipe dry with lint-free tissue.
Disinfect with 1/10 5.25% sodium hypochlorite for 5–10 minutes. (change daily)
Rinse with sterile water.
Air dry.
Store/dry in case.

TABLE 4.10
Four-Mirror Flat-Base-Curve Lenses

Advantages	Disadvantages
No goniosolution required	Requires excellent manual dexterity
Good for screening examination	Patients more aware of lens
Easy to implement into examination procedure	Corneal folds easily induced
	Inadvertent deepening of angle
No lens rotation required	Difficult to see over bowed iris
Used for compression gonioscopy	Cannot use for peripheral retina examination
Difficult-to-handle-lens	Unstable view

Four-Mirror Flat-Base-Curve Lenses (Table 4.10)

The Posner lens, the Zeiss lens, and the Sussman lens are commonly used flat-base-curve small-diameter, four-mirror lenses. They are designed to be used without an intervening viscous gonioscopy fluid, which can irritate the cornea or compromise visual fields or ocular photographs that may be required after gonioscopy (Figure 4.17).

The original Zeiss lens was designed for attachment to the slit lamp and positioned against the eye. That design was replaced by a handle with an Unger grooved holding fork for the prism lens to fit directly into (4). One of the problems with the holding fork design is the tendency for debris from the tears to collect around the edges and in the recesses of the holding fork. This requires the lens to be removed frequently, cleaned, and reinserted back into the holding fork. This maneuver often results in the mirrored surface's flaking, peeling, and becoming irregular, causing poor or altered images. The manufacturer of the lenses does not resilver the lenses, and the frequent replacement required is costly. This is not a problem with the Posner lens because the aluminum handle is embedded into the lens.

A new Zeiss lens design recently available eliminates this problem. It is designed similar to the Sussman lens in that it is hand-held and placed directly against the cornea in the same manner as the Goldmann-type lenses, which the manufacturer

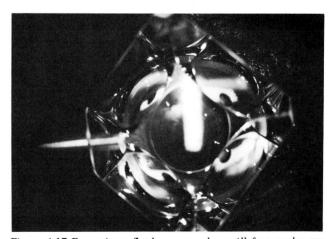

Figure 4.17 Four-mirror flat-base curve lens. All four angles are in view.

suggests makes the lens more natural for delicate maneuvers (14). Because of its small size, the newer Zeiss lens and the Sussman lens may be more difficult for examiners with large hands to hold for any length of time; however, the direct application of this lens without a handle provides the examiner with a greater sense of proprioception, to prevent unwanted pressure exerted against the cornea.

With the four-mirror lenses, all four quadrants of the anterior chamber can be viewed without rotation of the lens. The angle can be observed in its entirety with only minimal movement of the slit lamp. This makes these lenses extremely valuable for quick screening examinations of the anterior chamber. The other most frequently cited advantage is that the four-mirror lenses have a flatter radius of curvature than most corneas, so they do not require a coupling solution. These advantages make gonioscopy with this lens type easier to implement during the course of a routine eye examination.

Technique

The patient, examiner, and slit lamp preparation with these lenses is much the same as for the Goldmann-type lenses. The lens surface that contacts the eye should be clean and disinfected. The four-mirror lenses can be placed directly against the cornea without the use of an intervening methylcellulose solution; therefore, there is only a capillary layer of precorneal tear fluid between the lens and the cornea. However, rigid contact lenses are not generally placed on the eye without the use of a wetting solution, and in the case of these lenses, a drop of nonpreserved saline solution should be used on the concave surface before it contacts the cornea. The excess solution is allowed to run off. Any solution thicker or more viscous will create a fluid-filled chamber and cause undesired corneal compression (5).

Instruct the patient to fixate straight ahead, and focus the slit lamp on the patient's cornea. Then place the lens in front of the cornea, with the concave curve facing the patient's eye. At this point, you should be viewing through the slit lamp binoculars. Move the concave portion of the lens slowly, and center it onto the cornea, attempting to avoid any pressure against the cornea. The lens surface, when close to the cornea, will be attracted onto the cornea by capillary attraction, and a fogging of the lens may be noted immediately before contact. Stabilize the lens by resting the hand with the lens against the patient's cheek, or use your small finger to rest against the side of the slit lamp (Figure 4.18). Unlike the Goldmann lenses, there is little or no suction cup effect, so you must have a steady hand to keep the lens in contact with the cornea without exerting any unwanted pressure against the eye. Orient the lens as either a square or a diamond when placed on the eye. The square position with the Posner or Zeiss lenses surface offers more comfort to the patient because the flat lens rather than the edge of the lens contacts the lids. It s also more awkward to hold the lenses in the diamond position because the wrist has to be in a supinated position rather than straight (1).

Be sure your hand is well supported and balanced to prevent any unwanted pressure against the cornea with these lenses. The lens should barely contact the cornea. Once the light source is placed into the superior mirror, follow the same procedure detailed for the Goldmann-type lenses, including the use of the focal lines. The four quadrants can be examined by simply moving the slit lamp illumination microscope into the different mirrors; the lens requires no rotation. As with the Goldmann-type lenses, this is an indirect system; thus, the view in the superior mirror is actually the inferior angle, and objects are reversed up and down but not laterally. In general, as with all the other indirect systems, the lateral walls are more difficult to view. With the Zeiss or Posner lens, the holding fork or lens stick may need to be rotated superior or inferior to place the mirror in the correct position.

Patients should be advised that they may feel the lens with their lids, and they should refrain from blinking. In some cases, the lids may need to be held apart—the superior lid by the lens and the inferior lid by your free fingers on the hand holding the lens or, more rarely, by your free hand. If the patient squeezes hard, you will have to use more force against the globe, causing the cornea to flatten, the angle to widen, and the recess to deepen.

If a lens is too steep for a particular cornea, the lens will be unable to contact the cornea completely without inducing compression. In other instances with this lens design, the iris is too bowed to view over. In either case, avoid compressing the cornea as a method to view into the angle recess (see Figure 6.18). Instead, rock or tilt the lens (Figure 4.18). This will place the mirror at a more favorable location, providing a view into the angle recess. In order to view the inferior angle, tilt the lens inferior with slight inferior excursion of the lens and the patient gazing slightly superior. To observe the superior angle, have the patient look inferior, and rock or tilt the lens superior with slight superior excursion of the lens. Observation into the lateral angles can also be enhanced by this technique. Actually, this method is frequently required to prevent estimating an angle as being falsely narrow (30). It is important that you place no unwanted pressure against the cornea during this procedure as it will cause distortion of the view and unwanted angle widening. The central cornea is used as the fulcrum point for the rocking. This maneuvre provides a higher, less parallel view over the iris.

The manufacturer of the Sussman lens notes that the lens can be used to perform bedside gonioscopy in a supine position with the aid of a direct ophthalmoscope. Setting the ophthalmoscope at high plus +25 diopters and then moving within ¼ inch of the gonioscope will produce a monocular small but adequate view of the angle. Actually this type of gonioscopy can be performed with any type of gonioprism, and a 20 or 30 diopter lens with an indirect ophthalmoscope can be used as well (31).

Disadvantages

This lens type requires excellent manual dexterity. You must be very delicate when placing the lens against the cornea. Accurate evaluation can occur only when there is no distortion induced by the lens. Even minimal pressure exerted against the corneal surface will alter the aqueous dynamics,

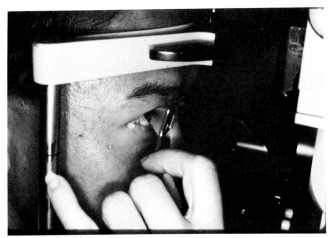

Figure 4.18 Lens tilting. When the iris is bowed and the examiner wishes to avoid unwanted compression, the lens should be tilted or rocked toward the angle quadrant under observation, and the patient should look into the mirror being used. Note the hand is balanced by resting the finger against the side piece.

resulting in the aqueous being forced into the angle recess and artificially opening the angle. Clinically, this can be identified by the observation of corneal endothelial folding and a volcano-like appearance to the iris (Plate 30). (The iris will drop back in the recess and the pupil margin will remain in its position.) In most eyes it takes very little force to create this picture. The endothelial folds result in interference with the clarity of the image, making observation more difficult. The posterior movement of the iris causes the angle to appear deeper than it actually is, causing misinformation of the angle status. In some patients, this is difficult to avoid because the lens used may be either too flat causing compression or too steep for a particular cornea. When the cornea is too steep, the lens will produce too much flattening before the cornea can be completely contacted. In these instances it is better to tilt the lens for observation of each quadrant rather than attempting full contact with the cornea. Screening of eyes with narrow angles is difficult with the four-mirror lenses due to the mirror placements too far from the center of the lens. The lenses often require significant tilting to see over the iris, and if the patient is not extremely cooperative and the examiner extremely delicate, distortions will result. Applying fluorescein prior to lens insertion provides a means for evaluating the lens cornea relationship and identifying corneal flattening before it becomes excessive. This can be conveniently applied by using Fluress® as an anaesthetic, which contains fluorescein with benoxinate. Benoxinate seems to reduce the incidence of corneal irritation, such as epithelial sloughing and conjunctival hyperemia associated with proparacaine (32). When repeated lens applications are anticipated, this may have potential benefit.

Inhibiting patient blinking can be a problem with these lenses because patient awareness of the lens edge may stimulate the normal blink reflex. (This is not as great a problem with the Goldmann-type lenses.) In addition, a strong blinker

can force the lens away from the eye. In either instance, for the lens to remain against the cornea, the examiner will need to exert an equal amount of pressure against the patient's eye with the lens. This will result in undesired corneal compression. Controlling this can be particularly difficult for novice gonioscopists. One method to reduce this problem is to use the upper edge of the lens to keep the lid opened. This must be accomplished without pressing the cornea. It requires a very gentle technique. The ease of inducing endothelial folding and deepening of the angle and difficulty in inhibiting patients' blinking makes mastering gonioscopy more difficult with this design. In essence, it requires a very cooperative patient and an examiner with good manual dexterity. The four-mirror lenses are primarily used for gonioscopy and are of little value for peripheral retina examination, although the central portion of the lens can be utilized for examining the posterior pole of the eye.

Diagnostic Compression Gonioscopy

The mirrors in the Zeiss, Posner, and Sussman lenses are inclined at 64 degrees. The Zeiss lens mirrors are placed 5 mm from the center of the lens, with a height of 12 mm. The mirror height and location for the Sussman and Posner lenses are unavailable from the manufacturer; however, the mirrors for these lenses may be placed differently from the Zeiss lens because they provide different views of the same angle. The base curves are also different. The Zeiss four-mirror lens has a contact surface with a radius of curvature of 7.85 mm (43.00 D). The Sussman and Posner lenses have a radius of curvature of 41.50 diopters. Thus, the Sussman and Posner lenses will compress against a greater range of corneas. During routine gonioscopic examination, this can be undesirable for the reasons noted and should be avoided, or at least accounted for. However, in some situations, the induced compression with these lens designs is desirable and can be a major advantage. It is known as a form of dynamic gonioscopy termed *compression gonioscopy*. Most practitioners utilize the Zeiss, Sussman, or Posner lens for this technique; however, a direct Koeppe-style lens can be used for the same purpose, and Posner has described a similar technique with the Goldmann-type lenses.

Forbes described compression gonioscopy using a Zeiss four-mirror lens in 1966 as a means to distinguish between appositional closure and synechial closure (3). When pressure is exerted against the cornea, aqueous is pushed into the recess of the angle, causing the iris to move posterior at its insertion. Compression with the four-mirror lenses will ascertain whether the synechia is apparent or real. If the angle is closed by apposition, the iris will move posterior and away from the wall, providing a deeper view of the angle recess and enabling observation of the area of actual iris attachment. If the iris is observed to remain against the wall, then synechia is likely present.

Sometimes the iris is noted to be tented against the wall in a few areas, providing an indication of previous angle closure.

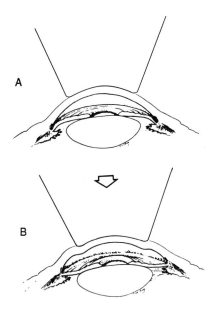

Figure 4.19 Compression gonioscopy. Pressing against the cornea with the small-diameter flat-base curve goniolens will force the peripheral iris posterior and deepen and widen the angle. (A) Without compression. (B) With compression. The pupil border stays in place while the peripheral iris drops posterior, creating a volcano appearance to the iris at the pupil border. (Reprinted with permission from Hoskins HD Jr, Kass MA. Becker-Shaffer's diagnosis and therapy of the glaucomas, *6th ed. St Louis: CV Mosby, 1982.*

This is particularly valuable information for suspected cases of primary intermittent angle closure where the angle would otherwise appear gonioscopically normal (Figure 4.19 and Plate 30).

The cornea is indented by taking the flat-base-curve four-mirror lens and pressing the lens directly against the cornea. The pressure against the eye may cause the globe to move slightly posterior, requiring the slit lamp to be moved slightly toward the patient to keep the view in focus. Observation of corneal folding is an indication that the cornea has been adequately depressed. Forbes noted that areas of appositional closure are easily opened, and in his experience the post-operative gonioscopic appearance agreed with the preoperative evaluation of synechia in eyes with angle closure (33).

In order to increase the posterior movement of the iris and increase the view into a particular quadrant, the lens should be moved slightly from the centered position in the direction of the mirror being used. Pressure is then applied to the cornea. This will displace the aqueous into the quadrant under observation, widening that quadrant to the maximum.

Flattening of the cornea that results in deepening of the angle is also helpful in eyes where the angle wall appears somewhat anomalous. This may occur in cases of significant iris processes and poor cleavage where it is difficult to tell whether you are observing the angle recess and in cases where the angle wall is clear, particularly in eyes with light irides or in young adults, without characteristic wall pigmentation. Here the exact location of the trabecular meshwork may not be easily discernible, and the exact location of the iris attachment is not easily visible. In these situations you

may be uncertain about the depth of the angle or the actual location of the iris insertion. The action of flattening the cornea with the four-mirror lens will cause the aqueous to move posterior into the angle recess and force the iris posterior, widening the angle to its maximum and providing you with the location of actual iris insertion. Comparing the angle view before and after compression provides confirmation for beginning gonioscopists that they were actually observing the point of iris attachment.

The technique of compression gonioscopy is also of great benefit in cases of narrow angles, especially when there is a significantly bowed iris and observation with a Goldmann-type lens is inadequate. Direct corneal compression with the small-diameter flat-base-curve four-mirror lenses will force the iris recess posterior and provide an otherwise unavailable view of the iris insertion.

In his report, Forbes (30) noted that indentation gonioscopy generally provides an accurate assessment of the amount of synechial closure in angle closure, although there may be a tendency to overestimate the amount of closure, particularly when the intraocular pressure is high (33). Palmberg suggests that the mechanism for the deepening of the peripheral angle is the result of a stretching of the limbal ring of the sclera, resulting in a straightening of the corneoscleral angle and a posterior rotation of the iris and ciliary body, and when the intraocular pressure is above 40 mm Hg, there is little more expansion of the limbal ring, and thus indentation gonioscopy is not effective (1), which may explain Forbes's observation.

The information provided by compression gonioscopy is helpful in determining the appropriate method for surgical intervention in cases of angle closure glaucoma. In cases of angle closure where significant synechia is present, the operation of choice is a filtering procedure because there is little functioning trabecular meshwork available. If it can be determined that the closure is mostly appositional, then a laser iridotomy would be effective (1). Laser iridotomy is the preferred treatment for pupillary block, with surgical iridectomy reserved for unusual cases, such as where there has been repeated closing of a laser iridotomy or in cases where there is inflammation (9). In the early 1980s, argon laser was the procedure of choice, but more recently neodymium (Nd:YAG) has been used, particularly in eyes with dark or light irides.

Anderson (34) described compression gonioscopy as a therapeutic technique for relieving an attack of acute angle-closure glaucoma. In one patient, he used several cycles of 30-second compression while instilling pilocarpine to break the attack. He equated the cycles of compression gonioscopy to utilizing a hyperosmotic agent. When the compression opened the angle, it caused removal of fluid from the eye by forcing aqueous out of the anterior chamber. When the compression was relieved, it caused movement of aqueous from the posterior chamber to the anterior chamber. This may not work when significant synechia is present because aqueous will not have an avenue for egress.

Gorin (35) has described a method using Goldmann one- or two-mirror lenses to improve visibility of the angle in narrow angles. The technique, which he called *manipulative gonioscopy*, consists of having the patient look toward the gonioscopic mirror while the examiner applies pressure against the globe with the edge of the lens adjacent to the goniomirror. This results in the goniolens' forcing aqueous into the angle opposite the mirror and widening that quadrant. The pressure will cause the aqueous in the posterior chamber to move into the anterior chamber and thus reduce the iris bombé; the iris will drop posterior and further deepen the chamber. Gorin recommends that the examiner slide the lens toward the angle under observation, bringing the center of the mirror closer to the angle under observation and thus making it easier to see over the iris bombé (35). The opening of the angle with the small-diameter flat-base-curve four-mirror lenses is usually much easier to produce, more predictable, and much more obvious than the effect produced with the Goldmann-type lenses.

Ocular Instruments manufactures a modified domed-shaped Koeppe direct gonioscopy lens, the Kitazawa pressure gonioscopy lens, which can be used outside the slit lamp for direct compression gonioscopy (36). This lens is designed with a cylindrical rod attached to the center of it to aid in manipulation of the lens, and approximately one-fourth of the lens has been cut away, creating a vertical section angled at 135 degrees. The radius of curvature of the contact surface is 7.8 mm, with a diameter of 9.2 mm. The lens is inserted as a conventional Koeppe lens, with only saline needed to moisten the contact surface. To perform compression gonioscopy, the central rod is tilted toward the examiner at the same time that gentle pressure is applied against the cornea. This forces aqueous from the posterior chamber to move into the anterior chamber, widening the angle. Excessive pressure against the cornea will cause endothelial folds, which will distort the view. The vertical plane of the lens should face the angle segment under observation.

Lens Choice

Becker (17) designed a series of lenses in an attempt to avoid corneal contact and its associated distortions, as well as to find the best centration and height for the mirrors. He concluded that for a four-mirror prism, the best view of the angle was obtained when the mirror was placed 3.5 mm from the center. In a single-mirror lens, the best view was obtained with the lens at the center. With the lenses located in these positions, angle recess in most narrow angles could be observed without manipulation of the lens. He then designed a series of lenses with heights at 20 mm and mirrors angled at 65 degrees, with various base curves to avoid corneal distortion. Problems still existed with these lenses, however; corneal contact with the lens still created corneal deformation, and a number of gonioprisms were required, making this impractical (4).

Of all the various lens types and designs available, the Goldmann three-mirror lens provides the most flexibility. It can be used for retina examinations as well as gonioscopy. It provides a more panoramic parallel view of the angle wall than the small Goldmann lenses and four-mirror lenses. It causes less cornea-lens adherence than the small Goldmann-type

lenses. The stability of the view is greater than with the Sussman, Zeiss, or Posner four-mirror lens types. Maintaining stability with the four-mirror compression type goniolenses is difficult, and thus the optical clarity with these lenses is inferior to the large Goldmann-type lenses. This degrades the view in some cases, minimizing the value of this lens type for detailed angle examination.

After one has gained experience with the technique and gonioscopic appearance with the large Goldmann-type lens, the four-mirror lenses become easier to use; however, the flat-base-curve small-diameter four-mirror lens designs all provide different views. If one were to evaluate the same eye with the Zeiss, Posner, and Sussman lenses, the differences in vantage points for each lens would be evident. The four-mirror lens is extremely valuable for quick screenings and compression gonioscopy, but for detailed angle observation, the large Goldmann-type lens is preferable. Knowledge of and familiarity with all the methods and lenses is important, however, because each has a particular value of its own.

Laser Lenses

A number of lenses are available for laser surgery of the anterior chamber; the choice depends on which structure is to receive the laser energy and which type of laser is used. A contact lens with a high plus add, such as the Abraham lens, is used for laser iridotomies. It consists of a modified fundus lens with a $+66$ diopter plano convex lens bonded onto the anterior surface (37). For laser trabeculoplasties, there are a variety of antireflective goniolenses. The Ritch trabeculoplasty laser lens has four highly polished mirrors in opposite pairs. Two mirrors are inclined at 59 degrees, which provide a more parallel view of the inferior angle, and two mirrors are angled at 64 degrees for a more parallel view of the superior angle. One of each of the mirrors is superimposed with a planoconvex button of 1.4 magnification. This decreases the laser spot size from 50 to 35 microns and increases the laser energy by a factor of two with the focal point of the lens calculated so that it is focused at the pigmented band of the trabecular meshwork. This lens is considered helpful in eyes that have light trabecular pigmentation, narrow angles, or anterior iris insertions (38).

Recording Findings

Records of gonioscopic appearance are important for standardization, characterization, classification, reproduction, and documentation of the angle. Records offer a means for determining change over time and for communicating between practitioners. Any system should be simple and descriptive and have the same meaning for all observers. A number of grading systems have been proposed as a means to simplify recording of gonioscopic findings. In one system, grade 1 denotes a narrow angle, and in another system grade 1 denotes a deep, open angle. This obviously can cause confusion when two examiners using different systems attempt to communicate.

TABLE 4.11
Gorin's System

Wide	CBB	45°
Intermediate	Strip CBB	25°–45°
Narrow	Trabecular visible	<25°

TABLE 4.12
Shaffer's system

Grade 3–4	30°–40°	No closure
Grade 2	20°	Possible closure
Grade 1	10°	Eventual closure
Grade S	<10°	Portion closed
Grade 0	0°	Closed

In most cases, the examination of the angle is done in order to determine whether the angle is opened, narrow, or closed, and recording a numerical value signifying this factor actually tells only a small part of the important information provided by the gonioscopic examination. Recording other observations is equally important. Solely grading the angle in terms of its openness does not provide an adequate picture. Categorizing an angle into broad groupings is a simple approach but does not account for the enormous normal variation, from eye to eye. It would be more meaningful for the examiner to record the anatomical structures seen in each segment of the chamber angle, noting the contour of the iris, its location of insertion, the appearance of the wall landmarks, the presence or absence of iris processes, synechia, abnormal pigmentation, and the presence or absence of normal or abnormal vessels.

Grading Methods

Gorin and Posner's Categories

Gorin and Posner (2) categorized angles as wide, intermediate, and narrow (Table 4.11). A *wide angle* is one where the observer is able to visualize the iris insertion onto the ciliary body, with the entire ciliary body being visible. This is correlated with a corresponding angle of 45 degrees created by the iris root and the angle wall. The *intermediate angle* occurs when the entire angle wall is visible along with a strip of the ciliary body but not to the extent of the wide angle. The angle created by the iris root and the angle wall is approximately 25 degrees. These angles are considered open. In a *narrow angle*, the iris lens diaphragm is more anterior than normal. The angle may be slit-like, with only portions of the trabecular meshwork visible. In some cases, with rotation of the patient's eye and/or tilting of the lens, the ciliary body may be visible. This system is based on the visibility of the most posterior wall structure; thus, it is a determination of the angle recess depth with some correlation to angle width. It allows for manipulation of the lens to see into the recess but does not differentiate eyes where that is necessary from eyes where it is not.

Schaffer's System

The most common system used in for classification is the Shaffer system. It is based on the angle created by an imaginary line tangential to the peripheral iris (approximately one-third the distance from the peripheral iris) (39) and the corneoscleral wall at the trabecular meshwork (Table 4.12). An angle of 30 to 40 degrees is considered to be impossible to close and is usually found in eyes that have a deep chamber and a flat iris. In general, as the chamber shallows, the angle

becomes smaller, and when the angle is 20 degrees or less, closure becomes possible. The grades are as follows:

Grade 0: No angle visible.
Grade S: A slit angle less than 10 degrees.
Grade 1: An extremely narrow angle of 10 degrees, with a likelihood of eventual closure.
Grade 2: Twenty degrees, with closure possible.
Grade 3–4: An angle of 30 to 40 degrees or greater, with closure impossible.

This system can be compared with the van Herick system, in which any angle judged as ¼:1 would be equivalent to a Shaffer grade 2 and capable of closure. Shaffer grade 1 or less is at great risk for closure. Grade 2 angles may become more shallow in the future and could also close (1). There is good correlation with the Shaffer system of gonioscopy grading and the slit lamp method of chamber grading (39).

In this system, there actually is no standard or defined location for the iris frame of reference that is used for determining angle width. In Shaffer's text (9), it is diagrammed and appears to be located one-third the distance from the angle wall. Others have defined it as the iris location adjacent to the iris recess. Thus, one observer may not use the same iris location for judging angle width as another. As the iris is more bowed forward, the iris frame of reference moves more centrally. The type of lens used may also alter the angle estimate in this system. With the large Goldmann lens, the view to the angle wall is more parallel than with a Zeiss four-mirror or small one- or two-mirror Goldmann lenses. These different vantage points will influence angle estimation.

This system is primarily concerned with the width of the angle and makes little comment about the depth and the angle of the angle recess. It assumes that these observations are entirely influenced by the angle width. Spaeth contends that the curvature of the iris makes it difficult to describe the width of the angle recess, as this will vary depending on the location of the iris chosen. The Shaffer system does not account separately for plateau iris configuration.

Scheie's System

The Scheie system (40) is used for grading the width of the angle based on the amount of angle structure visible (Table 4.13). This is more informative about the angle recess than the Shaffer system and similar to the Posner method. It has five categories:

TABLE 4.13
Schie's System

Grade 0	Ciliary bodies (CBB)	No angle closure
Grade I	CBB but narrow band	No angle closure
Grade II	Cannot see CBB SS visible	Rare for angle closure
Grade III	Cannot see posterior trabecular meshwork	Closure likely
Grade IV	Gonioscopically closed	Closure likely

Grade 0: The apex of the angle and entire ciliary body is seen.

Grade I narrow: An open but slightly narrowed angle where the ciliary body is visible with effort to see over the iris. Thus, the lens must be tilted or the patient's eye rotated (secondary gaze).

Grade II narrow: The ciliary body cannot be seen.

Grade III: The posterior trabecular is not visible.

Grade IV: The angle is gonioscopically closed, and no angle detail beyond Schwalbe's line can be seen.

According to Scheie, angles graded III and IV have the greater incidence of angle closure and positive mydriatic provocative tests. Eyes with grade II rarely suffer acute attacks of angle closure and usually have normal mydriatic provocative tests. Eyes with grade 0 or I do not suffer acute angle closure. The problem with this system is that the visibility of the wall structures will vary with the amount of lens tilting or eye rotation, and the system does not consider the iris contour, which may interfere with the visibility of the wall structures.

Becker's System

Becker developed a grading system that could be used with his fluid bridge gonioprism. With this lens, the mirror remained centered over the eye, and to view hidden structures, the point of observation along the mirror was raised. The "climb" on the gonioprism was measured by a reticule incorporated on the gonioprism. The narrower the approach, the greater this figure, which he felt reflected the true anatomic configuration of the angle. His grading system was based on two factors for providing an accurate evaluation of the angle: one based on the width of the trabecular meshwork from Schwalbe's line to the scleral spur and the other based on the distance from the iris insertion along the wall to the scleral spur (4). Unfortunately the fluid bridge lens was never commercially available.

Spaeth's System

Spaeth (41) felt that the Schie and Shaffer systems were neither elaborate nor precise enough to characterize the angle structures (Figure 4.20 and Table 4.14). The Schie system was too limited, he thought, in that it describes only the angle recess and does not differentiate between a closed and narrow angle. His concern with the Shaffer system was that the iris contour is variable, and thus there is uncertainty when choosing a reference point in determining the angular value. The Shaffer system does not clearly state the location of the iris to be used for this estimate. Some have inferred that it is the portion adjacent to the trabecular meshwork or the angle recess. Spaeth, however, defines the location more specifically. His system accounts separately for the width of the angle recess or depth of the recess and the angle width. In his

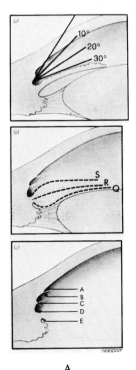

A

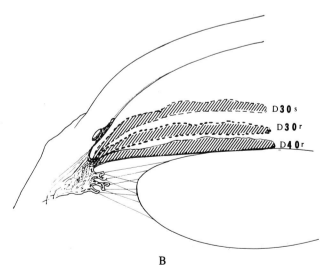

B

Figure 4.20 The Spaeth system. (A) Top: grade of the angle. Middle: grade of the contour most peripheral iris. Bottom: grade of location of iris insertion. (Reprinted with permission from Kanski JJ, McAllister JA. Glaucoma. London: Butterworth–Heinemann, 1989. (B) Schematic representation of the angle. Numbers and figures are grading symbols for iris insertion, angle approach, and peripheral iris contour. They provide an adequate description of the anterior chamber angle for three examples. See table 4.14 for definition of numbers and figures. (Reprinted with permission from Spaeth G. The normal development of the human anterior chamber angle: A new system of descriptive grading. Trans Ophthalm Soc UK. 1971;91:709–739.

TABLE 4.14
Spaeth's System

Iris Insertion
A: Iris inserts onto cornea.
B: Behind Schwalbe's at level of trabecula.
C: Scleral spur.
D: Ciliary body visible.
E: Deep ciliary body.

A and B are considered pathological; these grades usually correlate to angle recess. If compression gonioscopy is required to visualize the insertion, the letter is bracketed—[ ].

Angle
40 Degrees
30 Degrees
20 Degrees
10 Degrees

Contour Most Peripheral Iris	
r:	Regular no forward bowing, no backward arching	Normal
q:	Queer, iris is concave from root	May occur in congenital glaucoma; some cases of pigment dispersion.
s:	Steep, iris rises from root steeply, convex	Narrow approach

Iris Processes
U: Processes seen in brown eyes along the angle recess.
V: Line wall up to posterior trabecula.
W: Line wall up to Schwalbe's line.

Pigmentation: 12:00 o'clock position of posterior trabeculum
O: No visible pigment.
1+: Just perceptible pigment.
2+: More definite pigment but mild.
3+: A moderately dense band.
4+: A dense blackening.

system, the angle created by a line drawn tangentially to the inner surface of the trabecular meshwork and a line drawn tangentially to the anterior iris surface one-third the distance from the most peripheral portion of the iris is the angle width. This does not necessarily define the angle of the iris recess, although they usually correlate. He describes the angle recess as the distance separating the inner portion of the trabecular meshwork from the adjacent anterior surface of the iris. He feels most angles can be adequately described by noting at least three characteristics, each with a variable grade: (1) the location of the iris insertion along the angle wall, (2) the configuration or slope of the peripheral iris, and (3) the angular approach to the iris recess or the width of the recess. He believes this system adequately describes and defines the angle recess as well, but in cases in which the angle recess is atypical and does not fit into one of the categories, then the configuration of the angle recess is the important feature. Grading of iris processes and pigmentation of the posterior trabecular meshwork is also included.

The iris insertion is graded by the location of its insertion along the angle wall where *A* and *B* are considered pathological. *A* indicates insertion onto the cornea; *B*, insertion

at Schwalbe's line or at the level of the trabeculum; *C*, insertion at the scleral spur; *D*, insertion into the anterior ciliary body; and *E*, insertion into the deep ciliary body. The location of the iris insertion usually correlates with the angle recess. If compression gonioscopy is required, it is recorded and noted by placing a bracket around the letter ([ ]) (Figure 4.21). The angle is recorded in degrees in increments of 10° from 10° to 40°. The contour of the most peripheral portion of the iris is recorded as *r* for regular where there is no forward or backward bowing. A peripheral concave iris from the root is labeled *q* for queer, and an iris that rises steeply from the root and is convex is labeled *s* for steep. Iris processes are labeled *U* for processes seen along the angle recess, *V* for processes lining the angle wall up to the posterior trabeculum, and *W* if they line the wall up to Schwalbe's line. Pigmentation is graded in the 12:00 position of the posterior trabeculum where *O* indicates no visible pigment; *1+*, just perceptible pigment; *2+*, more definite pigment but mild; *3+*, a moderate dense band; and *4+*, a dense blackening. Other abnormalities such as peripheral anterior synechiae are also recorded. This system is excellent in that it accounts for not only the angle width but also the angle and depth of the recess and the iris configuration, which are all important aspects in describing the angle and predicting the potential for angle closure. The system, however, has not been generally accepted in the ophthalmic community as it seems to be too cumbersome for most practitioners.

Cockburn's System

Cockburn (3) reported on a group of 300 patients where he used gonioscopy to define the narrow angle (41). His method of categorization involved the gonioscopic evaluation of the superior angle in the left eye of consecutive patients. He used a Zeiss four-mirror lens and manipulated it as necessary in order to see into the angle recess. His definition of a *narrow angle* was an eye in which some portion of the trabecular meshwork was obscured. When only the anterior half of the trabecula was visible, he called this a *critically narrow angle*. He found 6% of the patients had narrow angles and 2% had critically narrow angles. This correlated to his slit lamp estimate of narrow angles in his other study.

Cockburn's method is viable as a quick screening method by using the results to infer the status of the remaining angle. An eye with an open and normal-appearing superior angle is likely to have open angle in the remaining 270 degrees. This relates to the normal quadrant variation where the superior angle is normally the narrowest in an eye. According to Gorin, this may be due to true anatomical differences or due to apparent differences caused by the patient's being seated. The shorter vertical meridian secondary to a greater scleral overhang in this region may also account for this discrepancy. The difference between the superior angle and the inferior angle should not be more than half a gonioscopically visible structure. As a rough guidline, van Herick notes that the slit lamp grade 2 should correlate with a Shaffer gonioscopic grade 1 superior and grade 2-3 inferior. Laterally, the temporal angle is wider than the nasal angle, although on

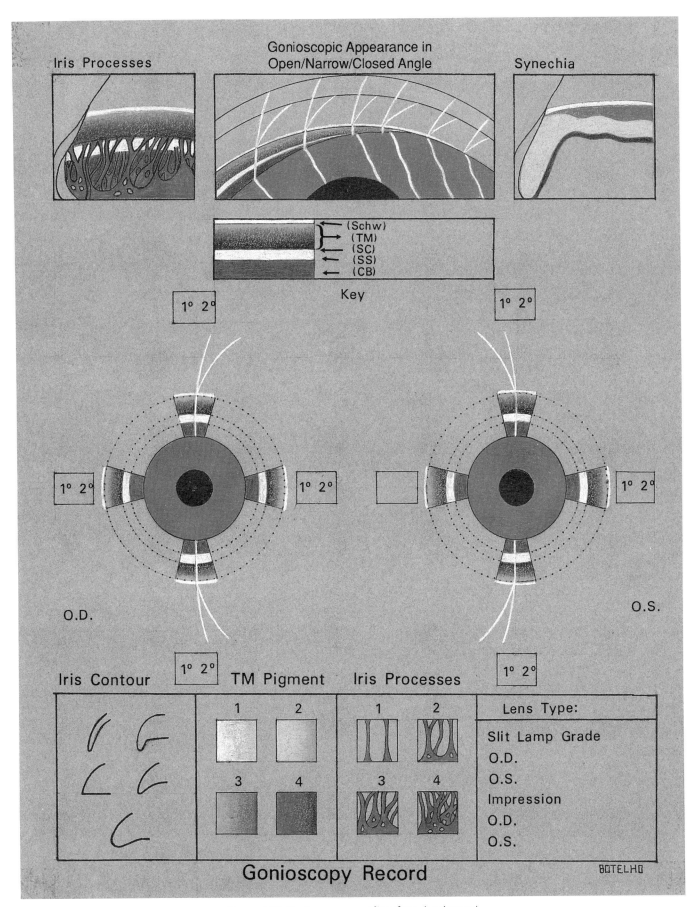

Figure 4.21 Gonioscopy recording form (goniogram).

slit lamp observation, the opposite is seen. Generally angles that are narrow 360 degrees are more at risk for acute angle closure attacks. Eyes narrow in only one or two quadrants are more at risk for partial angle closure of the chronic angle closure variety. Observation of a narrow superior quadrant suggests the need for the entire angle to be examined. Gonioscopy is important in these cases as many may be without symptoms of angle closure. Meticulous examination for smudges of iris pigment on or above the trabecular meshwork and evidence of peripheral anterior synechia are indications of previous intermittent closure and may be missed unless the entire angle is evaluated.

Comparison of Systems

Any record of gonioscopy should include the important features delineated by Schie, Shaffer, Becker, Cockburn, Gorin, and Spaeth. Overall the classification of an angle with any method is subjective. In order to provide more consistency and increase our ability to portray an angle, we need to have a simple yet descriptive method of recording. We should not restrict records to a simple notation of whether an angle was opened or narrow or closable, nor should we designate an angle by certain value in degrees. Classifying an angle as wide or 40 degrees does not provide enough information. Where along the iris was the estimation made? What about a plateau iris configuration or an angle where the iris bows posterior and then sweeps anterior just prior to insertion and attaches at the trabecula or scleral spur? And should we limit inspection to just one quadrant?

Records should also include the method of examination and the type of lens that was used since both can alter the view of a particular angle. It should be noted whether the examination was done with the patient looking straight ahead or whether the examiner needed to tilt the lens or have the patient look in the direction of the mirror (primary position of gaze or secondary position). Seeing the ciliary body in an eye requiring these maneuvers is not the same as being able to view the ciliary body in an eye not requiring this type of manipulation. The record should note whether compression was necessary to observe the angle wall depth.

Spaeth has reported on the importance of the iris contour and configuration, and any system needs to incorporate that information. Gorin has shown the importance of using the focal lines for determining structure location and real or apparent location of iris insertion onto the wall. Any record of the gonioscopic angle appearance would be enhanced and easily communicated to another examiner by graphically reproducing this type of information. Becker's system is intriguing as it is based somewhat on the average lengths of the angle wall and distances between the various landmarks and an attempt to remove subjectivity (4). However, the lens he used for this is unavailable.

Gonioscopically the Shaffer system grades the angle depth. It has been shown that the correlation between the Shaffer system and the slit lamp system is excellent. It is also understood that there is a strong correlation between angle closure and shallow anterior chambers and narrow angles. Since it is easier to use the slit lamp to grade the depths of the central chamber and the peripheral chamber rather than the gonioscope, the slit lamp is recommended for this evaluation, and this information should be included in any record of gonioscopy.

Gorin has described the configurations of the anterior chamber likely to be present in some forms of angle closure glaucoma. This provides useful information if graphically recorded as a comparison to the gonioscopic appearance. This provides a guide for the expected gonioscopic appearance and would be helpful even for experienced gonioscopists. For this reason, the beginning gonioscopist should use Figure 3.5 as a guide.

Any recording system should also include comments about angle wall abnormalities or anomalies, including notations of any synechiae—their type and location. Pigmentation of the angle and presence or absence of iris processes may provide information as to the etiology of a particular type of glaucoma and should be noted in any record. Presence or absence of neovascularization or visibility of normal vessels should be included in the description. To include all this information is cumbersome, and it can be argued that not all of it is always necessary. However, for the beginning gonioscopist, it provides a checklist of important items and an excellent check-and-balance system for correlating gonioscopic and slit lamp appearance.

For recording this information the clinician can use a gonioscopy recording form as in Figure 4.21. The upper left demonstrates an artist representation of iris processes. The middle diagram represents the spectrum of open to narrow to closed gonioscopic angle appearance. The top right represents the appearance of peripheral anterior synechiae. In the boxes the examiner should note whether the angle segment was viewed in primary or secondary gaze. The two circles with dotted lines can be used for recording the most posterior structure observable in the angle circumference as well as noting the height and location of any peripheral anterior synechiae, angle neovascularization, iris processes, or other abnormalities such as angle recession, exfoliation, foreign bodies, or pigment clumping. One can also note the presence and degree of parallax present between the focal line along the iris surface and along the angle wall.

The bottom left key represents the normal and abnormal peripheral iris configurations. The top left configuration is seen in cases of extremely shallow anterior chambers and extremely narrow angles encountered in cases of malignant or ciliary block glaucoma. The top right represents the plateau iris configuration. The middle left represents the configuration in a normal deep angle. The middle right represents a normal but narrow (greater than 20 degrees) configuration. The bottom represents a concave peripheral iris configuration sometimes observed in aphakia or pigments dispersion syndrome. The other keys can be used for reference in grading trabecular meshwork pigmentation as well as iris processes. The bottom right box should be used to note the lens type used for the examination, the slit lamp and chamber depth estimations. The clinician should also record whether compression was necessary and other comments regarding the gonioscopic examination.

References

1. Palmberg P. *Gonioscopy.* In Ritch R et al. *The glaucomas*, vol 1. St Louis: CV Mosby, 1989; Chapter 18.
2. Schwartz B. *Slit lamp gonioscopy.*
3. Author's survey, unpublished.
4. Becker S. *Clinical gonioscopy: A text and stereoscopic atlas.* St Louis: CV Mosby, 1972.
5. Shields M. *Textbook of glaucoma*, 3d ed. Baltimore: Williams & Wilkins, 1992.
6. Fellman RL et al. *Module 7 gonioscopy: Key to successful management of glaucoma.* Focal Points 1984: Clinical Modules for Ophthalmologists, American Academy of Ophthalmology.
7. Kanski JJ, McAllister JA. *Glaucoma.* London: Butterworth-Heinemann, 1989.
8. Hoskins HD Jr. Interpretive gonioscopy in glaucoma. *Invest Ophthalmol.* 1972;11:97–102.
9. Hoskins HD Jr, Kass MA. *Becker-Shaffer's diagnosis and therapy of the glaucomas.* 6th ed. St Louis: CV Mosby, 1989.
10. Gray LA. Fundamentals of gonioscopy, part 1. *Rev Optom.* 1977;114(10):51–60.
11. Richmond PP, Saladin JJ. Gonioscopy using the Brandeth-Saladin goniochamber. *J Am Optom Assoc.* 1978;49(7):761–765.
12. Schirmer KE. Gonioscopy and artifacts. *Brit J Ophthalmol.* 1967;51:50.
13. Kassin E. Fundus lens biomicroscopy: Theory and practice. *Optom Month.* August 1984.
14. Becker S. Critique of gonioscopy. *Curr Concepts Ophthalmol.* 1969;2:195.
15. Kapetansky FM, A bubble-free goniolens. *Ophthalm Surg.* 1988;19(6):414–416.
16. Fellman RL et al. Gonioscopy; The ophthalmologist's hidden view. *Clin Signs in Ophthalmol.* 1987;9(1).
17. Becker S. Unrecognized errors induced by present-day gonio-prisms and a proposal for their elimination. *Arch Ophthalmol.* 1969;82:160–168.
18. Miller JM, Shin DH. A letter on the handling of gonioscopic solutions. *Am J Ophthalmol.* 1984;97(2):252–253.
19. Semes L. An alternative gonioscopy and fundus contact lens protocol. *J Am Optom Assoc.* 1990;61:619–622.
20. Forgacs LS et al. Gonioscopy without the use of corneal anesthetics. *J Am Optom Assoc.* 1974;45(3):258–261.
21. Gorin G, Posner A. *Slit lamp gonioscopy*, 3d ed. Baltimore: Williams & Wilkens, 1967.
22. Rutala WA et al. Disinfection practices for endoscopes and other semicritical items. *Infect Control Hosp Epidemiol.* 1991; 12(5):282–288.
23. Rutala W. APIC guidelines for infection control practice. *Am J Infec Control.* 1990;18(2):99–117.
24. Moniz E, et al. Removal of hepatitis B surface antigen from a contaminated applanation tonometer. *Am J Ophthalmol.* 1981; 91:522–525.
25. Weatherby T, Director of Marketing, Ocular Instruments, Bellevue, WA, product information.
26. Lyon TC. Allergic contact dermatitis due to cidex. *Oral Surg.* December 1971;32:6.
27. Chambers R. West Roxbury (MA), Brockton/West Roxbury VA Medical Center, Infectious Disease Section, personal communication.
28. Koo D et al. Epidemic keratoconjunctivitis in a university medical center etc. *Infect Control Hosp Epidemiol.* 1989; 10(12):547–552.
29. Hanson PJV et al. Chemical inactivation of HIV on surfaces. *Br Med J.* 1989;298:862–864.
30. Forbes M. Gonioscopy with corneal indentation. *Arch Ophthalmol.* 1966;76:488–492.
31. Sussman W. Ophthalmoscopic gonioscopy. *Am J Ophthalmol.* 1968;66:549.
32. Thurschwell L. How to perform gonioscopy and peripheral retina examination with a Goldmann three-mirror contact lens. *South J Optom.* 1983;1(1):18–24.
33. Forbes M. Indentation gonioscopy and efficacy of iridectomy in angle closure glaucoma. *Trans Am Ophthalmol Soc.* 1974; 74:488–515.
34. Anderson DR. Corneal indentation. *Am J Ophthalmol.* 1979; 88:1091–1093.
35. Gorin G. *Clinical Glaucoma.* New York: Marcel Dekker; 1977.
36. Nakamura Y, Kitazawa Y. A new goniolens for corneal indentation gonioscopy. *Acta Ophthalmol.* 1971;49:964–970.
37. Krupin T. *Manual of Glaucoma.* New York: Churchill Livingstone, 1988.
38. Ritch R. A new lens for argon trabeculoplasty. *Ophthalm Surg.* May 1985;16(5):331.
39. Chan R et al. Anterior segment configuration correlated with Shaffer's grading of anterior chamber angle. *Arch Ophthalmol.* January 1981;99.
40. Schie H. Width and pigmentation of the angle of the anterior chamber: A system of grading by gonioscopy. *Arch Ophthalmol.* 1957;58:510–512.
41. Spaeth G. The normal development of the human anterior chamber angle: A new system of descriptive grading. *Trans Ophthalm Soc UK.* 1971;91:709–739.
42. Cockburn DM. Prevalence and significance of narrow anterior chamber angles in optometric practice. *Am J Opt Phys Optics.* 1981;58(2);171–175.

Chapter 5

Primary Angle Closure Glaucoma

In open-angle glaucoma, the aqueous always has access to the trabecular meshwork, and the disruption of aqueous flow is located somewhere along the outflow channel from the trabecular meshwork to the venous blood. Angle closure glaucoma is a condition of the eye whereby the intraocular pressure (IOP) becomes elevated as a result of the iris blocking the aqueous entrance to the filtering portion of the trabecular meshwork. The actual restriction of the outflow occurs in the anterior chamber, before the aqueous reaches the meshwork. Thus, the filtering portion of the trabecular meshwork is made unavailable for the exiting aqueous.

Angle closure glaucoma can be classified as primary with or without pupil block (Table 5.1). It may be acute, subacute (intermittent), or chronic. It may also occur secondarily with or without pupil block. In this chapter, we will discuss primary angle closure, the most common form of angle closure glaucoma. Although it is rare, occurring in 0.6% of the general population and 0.2% per 1000 people in the over-50 age group, it is considered a true ocular emergency because a delay in recognition and treatment can lead to loss of vision (1,2).

Slit Lamp Appearance of the At-Risk Eye

Primary acute angle closure can result from a variety of causes and generally takes place in an anatomically predisposed eye. Traditionally, it is taught that the most common etiology of this form of angle closure glaucoma is from relative pupillary block, a term used to describe the presence of abnormal resistance to aqueous flow, from the posterior chamber through the lens-iris-pupil area to the anterior chamber (Figure 5.1) (2). Normally, the iris contacts the lens in the pupil border area. In an eye with a shallow anterior chamber, the iris may contact the lens to a greater extent than normal, creating greater relative resistance for the aqueous flow (thus

the term relative pupillary block). This increased resistance causes the pressure in the posterior chamber to become elevated in comparison to that in the anterior chamber. The increased pressure in the posterior chamber, in turn, causes the iris to bow or bulge forward in the area free from lens contact at the iris root. This places the iris closer to the angle wall, narrows the angle, and places the iris in position to block the trabecular meshwork trabecula, putting the eye at risk for subsequent angle closure (4). Execution of one of the many triggering mechanisms will set into further motion changes necessary to induce the attack of angle closure glaucoma.

The routine slit lamp examination often detects the physical characteristics that place an eye at risk for this type of primary angle closure glaucoma (Figure 5.2 and see Figure 3.5). These include the observation of a shallow chamber axially (centrally) and peripherally, with the addition of a bowed or bombé iris. Evidence of these findings requires gonioscopic evaluation of the angle recess for changes suggestive of previous attacks or for a configuration that suggests the likelihood of a future attack. This would include a bowed iris causing difficulty seeing into the angle recess in primary or secondary gaze (Plate 9), evidence of peripheral anterior synechia (PAS), a narrow angle recess with the iris close to the angle wall, or pigment dispersion or spattering along the angle wall (5) (Plates 9, 11, and 15).

Classifications

Plateau Iris Angle Closure: Primary Angle Closure without Pupillary Block

A relatively rare etiology of primary angle closure glaucoma is plateau iris angle closure. This is more often a problem in younger patients in comparison to angle closure from pupillary

TABLE 5.1

Classification of Angle Closure Glaucoma

Primary Angle Closure	Mechanism
With pupil block	Relative pupillary block
Without pupil block	Plateau iris configuration
Acute (congestive)	
Intermittent (subacute, subclinical)	
Chronic (creeping angle closure, shortening of the angle)	
Mixed mechanism	Open angle glaucoma with narrow angle component

Secondary Angle Closure	Mechanisms
With pupil block	Miotics, inflammation, phacomorphic, subluxated lens
Without pupil block	ICE syndrome, neovascular, glaucoma, malignant glaucoma, inflammation, nanophthalmos, angle, tumors, or cysts

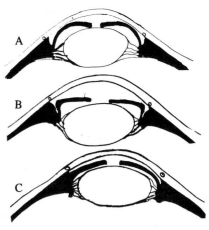

Figure 5.2 Drawing of anterior chamber configurations at risk for angle closure. (A) Closure from increased pupil block. Pressure and volume are increased in the posterior chamber, which pushes the peripheral iris forward and places the iris closer to the angle wall and in position to contact the angle wall at Schwalbe's line. The chamber is shallower peripherally than centrally; however, the central chamber is shallower than normal. (B) Closure by plateau iris or creeping angle closure. The central chamber is of normal depth; the periphery is shallow at the entrance to the angle. Closure occurs from posterior to anterior as the iris contacts the wall from below up to Schwalbe's line. There is little or no evidence of iris bombé, as pupil block may have no role here. (C) Closure from malignant glaucoma. The entire chamber is flat or shallow. The iris contour is parallel to the lens. This is usually a unilateral secondary presentation. (Diagram from Gorin G. Clinical glaucoma. New York: Marcel Dekker, 1977.)

block. The slit lamp configuration in these eyes is characterized by the appearance of a deep or normal axial anterior chamber depth with a shallow angle or peripheral chamber. The presence of a van Herick estimation of less than 1/4:1 with a normal or deep central chamber and a flat iris contour, without iris bombe, should make one suspicious of this configuration. Gonioscopic examination will confirm the presence of this condition by revealing a flat iris plane that makes a sharp angle, dropping posterior just before insertion along the angle wall. This produces an appearance of a plateau; thus, the name. Gorin has noted in some cases that the iris inserts more anterior than normal—possibly higher along the ciliary

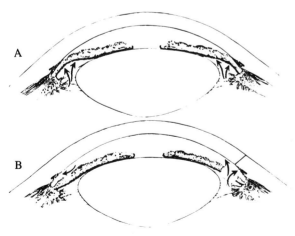

Figure 5.1 (A) Flow of aqueous from posterior chamber to anterior chamber is blocked at the pupil border. The iris is bowed against the angle wall, and the trabecular meshwork is closed off. (B) An iridotomy creates a new pathway for aqueous flow. The posterior chamber pressure decreases. If the iris is not syneched, it will drop posterior in the periphery. (Reprinted with permission from Hoskins HD Jr, Kass, MA. Becker-Shaffer's diagnosis and therapy of the glaucomas, 6th ed. St Louis: CV Mosby, 1989.)

body or even at the scleral spur (6). Barkin (11) has described the condition with the iris having a prominent last roll before insertion. Tornquist had suspected forward rotation of the ciliary body as an etiology of this configuration, but this more likely produces a form of ciliary block glaucoma or malignant glaucoma (4,7). Epstein noted that, in some of his cases, he observed the ciliary processes rotated forward in contact with the posterior portion of the lens, thereby appearing to hold the lens forward (Plate 43) (8). Thus different observers have provided differing descriptions of the same entity. Recent reports, using ultrasound biomicroscopy, have revealed that eyes with plateau iris syndrome display an anatomic variation such that the ciliary processes are in fact located anteriorly when they are compared to either the normal eye or eyes with pupillary block glaucoma (9).

Plateau iris angle closure glaucoma may be precipitated when a predisposed eye is widely dilated. The angle will close off because the short, anteriorly placed iris root folds against the wall, physically blocking the trabecular meshwork.

According to Tornquist, peripheral iridectomy is usually not an effective therapy because pupillary block does not play a significant role, and there is no widening of the angle after the iridectomy (7). Some observers, however, believe that these eyes have some component of pupillary block as well (10). Barkan noted that 20% of noncongestive angle closure cases were found in eyes with normal axial depths but with redundant folds of the peripheral iris (11). The angle in these eyes appeared to close from posterior to anterior rather than the more typical progression of closure, which occurs in relative pupillary block, from Schwalbe's line posterior. He was likely describing a plateau iris configuration. He did comment that the eyes had minimal ballooning in the periphery and responded well to peripheral iridectomy, suggesting that pupillary block had some role in his cases.

Lowe believes that plateau iris configuration is more common in younger people and that when an older person with this configuration suffers an angle closure attack, pupil block plays a role. He notes that because of the anatomical situation created by the iris being so close to the wall in these eyes, less aqueous resistance from relative pupillary block is needed to close the angle. Therefore, there will be less evidence of axial shallowing in these eyes and less evidence of iris bombe (12). One may conclude that the predisposition in plateau iris is not the shallowing of the chamber but rather the peculiar relationship of the iris to the angle wall within the recess created by the anteriorly situated ciliary processes.

Wand et al. suggest differentiating plateau iris angle closure into a preoperative plateau iris configuration and a postoperative condition of plateau iris syndrome (13). Plateau iris configuration is defined as an eye with a normal anterior chamber depth centrally, with a flat iris plane on slit lamp observation but an extremely narrow or closed angle by gonioscopy. They did not comment on the slit lamp appearance of the periphery of the chamber, but it seems probable that eyes with extremely narrow van Herick evaluations, flat iris planes, and normal depth to the central chamber are more likely to have plateau iris configuration. When this configuration is observed on routine slit lamp examination, gonioscopy should be performed to confirm the diagnosis.

They describe plateau iris syndrome as a postoperative condition in which the eye has a normal anterior chamber depth centrally, a flat iris plane, a patent iridectomy, and an angle that will be gonioscopically closed when dilated (13). This situation is rare but does explain the rise in pressure and the angle closure that may occur in eyes dilated in the presence of patent iridectomies. One must rule out other etiologies of pressure increase in this scenario. First the patency of the iris opening should be confirmed by the direct observation of the lens capsule through the opening. Anticholinergic and or mydriatic agents are known to cause elevations of IOP in eyes with open angles, particularly if they have been previously treated with miotic agents (14,15,16). Thus angle closure must be confirmed by gonioscopy in any dilation-induced pressure elevation (Table 5.2). Release of pigment, especially from adrenergic dilating agents or pigment dispersion, can also cause a pressure rise, but the angle again would be open gonioscopically, and the pigment would be visible in the anterior chamber. Another possibility is the presence of malignant glaucoma; this can often by ruled out, however, by the absence of an extremely shallow chamber conforming to the appearance of the lens and the absence of this configuration in the other eye. In addition, the failure of a patent iridotomy to result in angle deepening should make one

TABLE 5.2
Elevated IOP with Dilation after Iridotomy

Mechanism	Differentiation
Peripheral iridotomy not patent	Unable to observe lens capsule
Response to dilating agent	Open angle by gonioscopy
Pigment dispersion from dilating agent or dilation	Open angle by gonioscopy, pigment in anterior chamber (AC)
Malignant glaucoma	Flat anterior chamber, iris contour parallel to cornea, fellow eye without this configuration
Plateau iris	Angle gonioscopically closed, compression gonioscopy moves midperipheral iris posterior not peripheral iris.

suspicious of plateau iris syndrome or malignant glaucoma.

Gorin described a similar anterior chamber configuration of a relatively normal anterior chamber depth in combination with a shallow peripheral chamber, which he called a shortening of the angle (17). In these cases, gonioscopically the iris can be seen to be attached to the angle wall from the bottom of the angle recess slowly moving up to the line of Schwalbe. This is similar to Barkan's description of eyes with noncongestive angle closure and to a chronic form of angle closure described by Lowe as "creeping angle closure" glaucoma. Lowe did note, however, the presence of iris bombe and a shallow chamber depth in his patients (18). Gorin believes that many of the shortening of the angle cases result in long-term noncongestive form of angle closure often mistaken for chronic simple open-angle glaucoma. This misdiagnosis occurs because the eye is not congested and the anterior portion of the trabecular is visible. Therefore the angle is erroneously assumed to be open. Perhaps this accounts for the large number of plateau iris configurations seen clinically but the rare occurrences of plateau angle closure cases. Conceivably they are not recognized as forms of chronic angle closure, are treated as an open-angle glaucoma with narrow approaches, and are placed on weak miotic therapy. The miotic agent pulls the iris away from the wall and prevents PAS. Because there is no, or very little, pupillary block, the weak miotic agent will not cause any secondary chamber shallowing. The cases that eventually do close off are possibly those with some low amount of relative pupillary block, not easily clinically detected as Lowe contends, but enough to force the already anteriorly placed iris against the wall. Future ultrasound biomicroscopy studies of eyes with chronic angle closure glaucoma may answer this question.

It is important to identify plateau iris syndrome angle preoperatively because the treatment may or may not include peripheral iridotomy. Keeping the iris away from the angle wall with miotic agents or laser pupilloplasty or iridoplasty is more appropriate, particularly if there is no pupil block component present. Compression gonioscopy may provide a clue to a potential plateau iris syndrome. In plateau iris configuration, compression gonioscopy will result in the midperipheral iris being bowed posteriorly rather than the peripheral iris. The peripheral iris is the location for posterior iris movement in eyes with pupil block (9).

Acute, Intermittent (Subacute), and Chronic Angle Closure

Primary angle closure glaucoma may be further classified as acute, intermittent, and chronic angle closure glaucoma. The level of signs and symptoms are generally greater for an acute attack and less or absent for a chronic form, with the intermittent attacks manifesting signs and symptoms between the two. In primary pupillary block angle closure glaucoma, the trigger mechanisms that precipitate an attack in an at-risk eye are not well defined. Often they are situations that place the pupillary block forces at their maximum by placing the iris and lens in greater apposition. This can be the result of mid-dilation, normal forward movement of the lens, or from ciliary body swelling. The trigger mechanism may be illness, which can cause ciliary body swelling, emotional stress, pharmacologic pupillary dilation, prolonged near work, causing forward movement of the iris root, or prolonged periods in a dimly lighted environment, resulting in mid-dilation. Most attacks tend to occur in the evening and during the winter; however, direct correlation to meteorological factors is not clear, and Hillman and Turner suggest it may have more to do with the changes in behavior during the winter months (19). There is also evidence of a diurnal variation to the anterior chamber depth, which could account for time-of-day onset (20).

An eye at risk may be moved into angle closure by more than one trigger mechanism (Table 5.3) (10,21). In acute attacks, systemic changes may trigger the onset of an attack. Lowe notes that viral illness is the most common of these, followed by body or face trauma; sudden, severe anxiety; changes in weather; and iatrogenic pupil dilation. Television or movie watching are rarely implicated in acute angle-closure attacks. They are more often cited with subacute attacks (12). Anticholinergic or adrenergic agents taken for systemic conditions may also precipitate an attack in a predisposed eye. This is borne out by a recent report of five cases of angle closure glaucoma in patients treated with nebulized ipratropium bromide, an anticholinergic agent, and salbutamol, a beta-2 agonist (22). Spinal or general anes-

thesia has also been reported to provoke an attack, possibly related to the use of anticholinergic agents prior to surgery, use of ephedrine during surgery, the use of succinylchloride during anesthesia induction, which can cause simultaneous contraction of the extraocular muscles, resulting in a secondary forward movement of the iris lens diaphragm, or psychological stress related to the surgery. Preoperative pilocarpine was not effective in preventing two reported cases (23).

In intermittent angle closure, the attacks continue to resolve spontaneously, but there is a risk of developing an acute attack of angle closure glaucoma, or the intermittent case can turn into a chronic form. Approximately 30% of acute closure attacks are preceded by intermittent angle closure attacks (18). According to Lowe, the clinical presentation of this form of angle closure can present differently in different ethnic groups. In Caucasians, the attacks never last overnight, usually break without synechia, and most often are in one eye. In blacks and Chinese, the intermittent attacks are accompanied by symptoms of short duration, with synechia formation and progression with each attack, even without evidence of obvious inflammation (12).

Chronic angle closure is characterized by the presence of PAS along portions of the angle wall (Plates 4 and 11), the by-product of prolonged appositional closure or frequent, prolonged, intermittent angle closure attacks. Some of these eyes can develop an acute attack of angle closure when pupillary block results in the angle acutely closing off; however, many of them do not and will present with an elevated pressure, with glaucomatous optic nerve damage, but without symptoms of angle closure. These cases will remain unidentified unless careful gonioscopy is performed to detect the presence of PAS (10). They can be mistaken for chronic open angle glaucoma with narrow angles unless the examiner has a high index of suspicion and carefully observes the angle. Use of an alpha-adrenergic blocker such as dapriparzole or thymoxamine can be useful in differentiating an angle closure component in an eye with a narrow angle, elevated IOP, and optic nerve cupping and/or glaucomatous visual field loss. After one or two drops is applied, evidence of a significant IOP drop, along with gonioscopic evidence of angle widening, is suggestive of the presence of a closed-angle component.

Lowe and Ritch have suggested that "creeping angle closure" glaucoma is a form of chronic angle closure glaucoma where the eye develops a quiet and progressive angle closure without evidence of ocular congestion (10). This occurs in patients with thick, darker irides, is more common in Asian and black patients, and uncommon in Caucasions. The iris adheres relatively evenly in all quadrants in a circular fashion, starting deep in the angle and working its way up the wall. Eventually, an acute attack may occur, or the patient may present asymptomatically but with elevated IOP and evidence of glaucomatous nerve damage and field loss. The chamber depths in these eyes are not as shallow as eyes suffering angle closure glaucoma but nevertheless are shallower than normal. These eyes often need additional medical treatment or surgery other than an iridotomy to keep the IOP controlled, possibly the result of chronic trabecular damage from the

TABLE 5.3
Trigger Mechanism for Primary Angle Closure Attack

Viral illness
Trauma (face, body)
Prolonged near work
Anxiety/emotional stress
Long periods in dimly lighted environments
Changes in weather
Iatrogenic pupil dilation
Anticholinergic or adrenergic systemic agents
Systemic surgery

Adapted from Lowe RF. *Primary angle closure glaucoma.* Singapore: PG Publications, 1989.

synechia/apposition. Some of these eyes may actually be suffering from plateau iris syndrome.

Another category has been used to describe eyes in which the IOP is elevated in the presence of a narrow or closed angle and pressure remains elevated even after the angle is open and appears normal: combined mechanism glaucoma or mixed glaucoma (25).

Signs and Symptoms

In population studies only 20% of patients with angle closure glaucoma give histories of experiencing an acute attack (25). This emphasizes the need for careful gonioscopic examination in the at-risk eye, looking for the evidence of previous intermittent closure, listening to patient complaints, and looking carefully for the other signs of angle closure.

Depending on the degree and speed of the elevation of the pressure (acute, chronic, or intermittent), the patient may experience symptoms such as ocular pain or headaches from V nerve stimulation. The pain accompanying an angle closure attack may be significant enough to cause the patient to become nauseous and to vomit from autonomic stimulation (26). Patients have been known to report to an emergency room with symptoms of nausea and vomiting and obtain gastrointestinal consultation before the attack of angle closure is identified as the etiology of the symptoms or to be admitted to medicine or neurology services (27). One recent report describes a patient with eye pain and substernal chest pain, both of which were relieved after an angle closure attack was broken. The symptoms were attributed to trigeminal stimulation and reflex vagal discharge, resulting in esophageal and gastric dysfunction causing noncardiac chest pain (28). Colored halos around lights and blurred vision from corneal edema are classically described as symptoms of acute angle closure glaucoma. Transient vision loss mistaken for ophthalmic migraine or amaurosis fugax has also been reported in cases of intermittent (subacute) angle closure (29).

The congestion of the eye occurs as a secondary complication from the closure. Inflammatory signs may include ciliary injection and cell and flare in the anterior chamber. There may be profuse lacrimation and swelling to the lid and conjunctival chemosis (12). The pain and systemic changes noted may be secondary to iris infarction, corneal epithelial breakdown that exposes the epithelium, and severe anterior uveitis, though not as much from elevated ocular pressure (6). Posner evaluated 410 consecutive cases of primary angle closure in his practice and found only 16% presented in the acute congested phase (30). Pain may actually be an uncommon warning sign in angle closure glaucoma; a complaint of intermittent visual disturbances may be more common, possibly related to the stretching of the globe and disturbance of the corneal lamellae (12,31).

In chronic cases, the patient may remain asymptomatic until vision is severely compromised from optic nerve damage (Table 5.4). When the pressure is significantly elevated in a short period of time (acute), the optic disc will tend to be more pale than cupped. In chronic or intermittent cases, the disc may be significantly cupped (25,32). In severe cases of experimentally induced acute angle closure glaucoma in owl monkeys, Zimmerman noted the presence of severe cupping within 2 weeks. He concluded that cavernous degeneration of the optic nerve was an unusual form of ischemic necrosis in these cases (33). Clinically in the early stages, the disc may have hemorrhages and become edematous secondary to ischemia, and central retinal vein occlusion may occur (34). The final status of the disc is variable and depends on such factors as the length and the severity of the attack. In some instances, the nerve suffers no apparent damage after an acute attack (32).

The cornea may become significantly edematous, preventing an adequate gonioscopic view. The deeper layers of the epithelium are usually involved. The elevated IOP forces aqueous into the cornea, and the endothelial pump is not able to clear the cornea, resulting in a fine, bullous keratopathy (35). Patients with corneal edema may experience colored halos while looking at lights. The inner portion of the halo is blue and the outer red, separated by a green ring. Colored halos are a nonspecific symptom that can occur with any cause of corneal edema (36). To clear the cornea, it may be necessary to apply a few drops of glycerine (75–100%) in the cul de sac after applying a topical anesthetic. The glycerin should be allowed to flow across the whole corneal surface. Clearing usually takes 20 to 30 seconds and lasts for only several minutes. It works as a hypertonic solution, drawing fluid from the corneal epithelium. It has little effect on formed corneal bullae or stromal edema (37). The glycerin may make the epithelium fragile, so the examiner must be cautious to prevent corneal erosions (38). Delicate application of a Zeiss or comparable four-mirror lens may be more forgiving to the epithelium and avoid potential lens-cornea adherence with the Goldmann lens. Also, once the pressure is lowered, the cornea will clear sufficiently to allow an adequate gonioscopic view. If examination is not possible, evaluation of the opposite eye will be extremely helpful. Most cases of primary angle closure glaucoma eventually are bilateral, so evidence of a narrow angle, a shallow chamber and a bombé iris in the quiet eye, suggests primary angle closure in the involved eye. If the quiet eye has a deep normal chamber, the involved eye is more likely to be suffering a secondary form of angle closure (Table 5.5).

Permanent corneal endothelial cell density decreases occur when there is a sustained or sudden increase of IOP (39). The

TABLE 5.4
Symptoms of Angle Closure

Ocular pain/dull ache
Blurred vision
Headache
Nausea
Vomiting
Colored halos
Transient vision loss (intermittent attacks)
Intermittent blurry vision (intermittent attacks)

TABLE 5.5
Signs of Angle Closure

Ciliary injection
Lid swelling
Conjunctival chemosis
Cell and flare in AC
Corneal edema
Fine bullous keratopathy
Endothelial folds
Optic nerve pallor
Optic nerve edema
CRVO
Cupping in chronic cases
Late decreased corneal sensitivity
Pupil dilated vertically oval
Iris atrophy
Glaukomflecken
Cataract
IOP elevated (usually)
Gonioscopically closed angle
Synechia

amount of cell loss correlates to the length of the attack, being as high as 77% in attacks lasting 4 to 8 days (40). However, severe corneal edema will resolve quickly once the IOP is normalized even in cases in which 50% of the corneal endothelium has been lost (12). Clearing usually occurs at the periphery first, but evidence of corneal edema and folds in Descemet's membrane will be evident for a few days after until the corneal endothelium can recover. In severe cases, permanent endothelial damage occurs, with chronic edema remaining, and in some cases, corneal decompensation is severe enough to require later penetrating keratoplasties (12,41). Corneal sensitivity can be permanently decreased, leaving the eye exposed to neurotrophic disease (42).

In acute angle closure glaucoma, the pupil often becomes dilated in a vertically oval form. The dilation occurs early during the attack and progresses, the result of insult to the sphincter muscle secondary to an acute ischemia to the peripheral loops of the minor arterial circle. Observation of this may indicate an iris that will not respond to miotics until the IOP is lowered to the range of 40 mm Hg (1,43). In addition, the iris vessels become dilated, and the iris stroma becomes edematous, adding to an inflammatory response that may promote the formation of posterior and peripheral anterior synechia.

In attacks lasting more than 12 hours, iris atrophy may occur. The longer the attack is, the greater the atrophy will be. The lighter the iris is, the earlier the changes may be detected. They consist of a slight dilation and irregularity of the pupil and a thinning of the sphincter muscle initially localized to one segment. The radial stromal fibers become displaced in the area of the damaged sphincter. In a dark iris, the pupil will be distorted along with a marked depigmentation of the anterior iris. In a very dark iris, the pigment dispersion may be so great that pigment may collect in the anterior chamber, causing a pigment meniscus similar to a hypopion with an evident iris transillumination secondary to the loss of pigment (44). After the attack has subsided, the affected atrophied areas of the pigment epithelium may seem to transilluminate

(12). Evidence of pigment on the posterior cornea located where the iris contacted the cornea may be visible, as well as a line of pigment on the peripheral iris, indicating the extent and location of previous closure (12,25).

It is possible that the iris atrophy will allow passage of aqueous from the posterior to the anterior chamber, thus functioning as an iridotomy and breaking the attack (10). Careful slit lamp examination may provide evidence of the filtration site as a thinned iris where the pigment epithelium is visible because of destroyed iris stroma. According to Gorin and Posner, evidence of a distorted pupil, iris atrophy, and pigment on the posterior cornea is pathognomonic of postcongestive angle closure (38).

Characteristic lens changes known as *glaukomflecken*, first reported in 1930 by Vogt, may occur during acute attacks of angle closure glaucoma (Plate 19). They have also been reported in cases of contusion, chemical burns, and flat postoperative anterior chambers of a few days' duration (12). However, they are associated primarily with events of severe rises in ocular tension. Glaukomflecken appear initially in the first few days as an anterior subcapsular small gray-white discoloration, which can be mistaken for a fibrinous exudate. Once the IOP lowers, they appear more hardened, with variations in their density, and they look like an irregular white net. As time passes, they become more discreet and appear as small blue-white dots or plaques (12). The opacities are permanent but eventually become covered over with new lens fibers. It may be possible to predict when an attack occurred by the depth of the opacification (6). It has been stated that 2 years after an attack they will be located a quarter of the way toward the adult nucleus (45). Glaukomflecken occur because of metabolic disruption of the anterior lens cells from pressure necrosis or toxicity from the necrotic products stagnated in the aqueous (46). The lens may also develop nuclear sclerosis and cortical changes, and in severe cases they may become shrunken and dislocate (12). A slight iridodonesis has been noted in older patients' eyes that have suffered acute angle closure glaucoma.

IOP is most often severely elevated in angle closure glaucoma, but this may vary depending on the amount of angle obstructed and the efficiency of the portion of the angle still open. In general, the more inflamed the eye is, the greater is the tendency toward synechia (4). It is questionable whether synechia develop without inflammation. In some cases, the amount of aqueous produced may decrease, secondary to inflammation, and thus the pressure elevation may not appear consistent with the amount of angle obstructed and may be weeks before the ciliary body rebounds and the pressure becomes elevated.

In cases of intermittent angle closure, the symptoms are more transient in nature (Table 5.7). They occur during the attacks and are relieved when the attack is spontaneously relieved. The intermittent attacks may occur for years before identification or change into either an acute angle closure glaucoma or chronic angle closure. Patients may identify the conditions that precipitate an attack, such as prolonged reading, and, not being aware of the significance of the symptoms, may avoid the precipitating activity. Thus, a scenario whereby a patient complaining of mildly blurred vision with a dull ache in or around an eye while reading notes that the symptoms are relieved by sleep may be indicating that he or she is breaking the intermittent attacks by sleep-induced miosis and does not need a change in reading glasses. Or the patient who complains of blurred vision with a dull ache in or around the eye while at a movie or watching television in a dimly lighted environment, may not need a change in distance glasses but may be experiencing intermittent attacks of angle closure glaucoma.

Most cases of primary closure glaucoma respond to lowering of IOP by medical means, including the use of beta-blockers, hyperosmotic agents, carbonic anhydrase inhibitors, and cholinergic drops. Apraclonodine (Iopodine), an alpha-2 agonist, has also been reported to help in breaking an attack (47). Once the eye is quieted, surgical treatment is most often indicated, with laser iridotomy the preferred treatment.

Angle closure glaucoma may be a secondary disease resulting from changes such as synechia from a neovascular fibrovascular membrane (Plate 25), inflammatory synechia (Plate 13), a subluxated lens, or malignant glaucoma. In these cases, treatment is different than it is in primary angle closure glaucoma because the use of a miotic agent is contraindicated. In one report of patients presenting to an emergency room, almost 40% had a secondary form of angle closure, which would have worsened if miotic therapy were undertaken (48). Gonioscopic evaluation is mandatory in any case of angle closure glaucoma to recognize these secondary causes before therapy is initiated.

Synechia versus Appositional Closure: The Role of Gonioscopy

The choice of therapy in angle closure will vary depending on whether the angle is closed by apposition or by synechia. The degree of angle circumference and height of synechia may also influence therapeutic decisions (Plate 37). If an angle is closed by apposition, medical therapy is more likely to lower the IOP, and the angle is more likely to remain open after an iridotomy. If a significant circumferential area is closed by synechia, lowering the IOP may not open the angle sufficiently, and an iridotomy will most likely not solve the problem so that gonioplasty, goniosynechialysis, or a filtering procedure may eventually be required.

The type of an attack of angle closure may influence the location of the initial synechia or iris apposition. In secondary angle closure from inflammation, the inferior angle may attach first (Plate 13), although there are instances where the lateral angles suffer synechia first. In creeping angle closure glaucoma, the angle tends to close superiorly first, although I have observed several black patients where the angle closed inferiorly first.

In primary angle closure, both apposition and synechia are thought to occur more commonly in the superior angle (Plates 37 and 38). This may be the result of the eyelid's causing greater peripheral flattening of the superior cornea rather

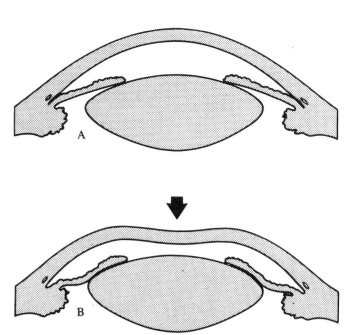

Figure 5.3 Compression gonioscopy in appositional closure: (A) closed angle. (B) Compression gonioscopy. (Left side: With compression, the portion of the iris free from the lens will move posterior. Right side: In plateau iris configuration, the most peripheral iris will recede less than is normal because it is held in place by the anterior-situated ciliary processes. The midperipheral iris, free from the lens and free from the ciliary processes, will recede.) (Reprinted with permission from Kansler JJ, McAllister JA, eds. Glaucoma. A color manual of diagnosis and treatment. London: Butterworth–Heinemann, 1989.

than any other anatomical variation, thus predisposing this area to earlier iris wall attachment (49). Another reason proposed is the variation in the anterior chamber volume, which is greater inferior than superior. Also, the iris surface tends to protrude more superiorly (50). In terms of the lateral angles, the nasal quadrant tends to be narrower because of the nasal crystalline lens decentration; interestingly, it is thought there is a greater tendency for synechia to occur temporarily (49). Once an acute attack is broken, synechia may remain only in the inferior angle. This may be the result of settled pigment and inflammatory debris brought on by the congestive attack (12).

The technique of compression gonioscopy using a Sussman, Zeiss, or Posner four-mirror goniolens is extremely valuable for determining whether the angle is closed from apposition or synechia (Figure 5.3). The flatter base curve and the smaller diameter of contact area with these lenses allow them to flatten the cornea. This indentation forces the anterior chamber aqueous into the angle recesses, pushing the iris root posterior. If the angle is closed by apposition, the posterior movement of the iris will pull the iris away from the wall, exposing the angle wall structures. The portion of the angle wall closed by synechia will remain covered by iris tissue. As noted, however, at times, the cornea is so edematous or the iris so bowed that even compression gonioscopy will not provide this information (51).

TABLE 5.6
Optical Closure versus Actual Closure

Actual Closure	Gonioscopy
Focal lines meet above the filtering meshwork	Use large Goldmann-style lens for diagnosis. Use compression gonioscopy to differentiate apposition versus synechia.

Optical Closure	Gonioscopy
Cannot visualize meeting of focal lines Parallax exists	Require higher vantage. 1. With large Goldmann-type lens, tilt lens toward angle under observation. Have patient gaze toward the gonioscopy mirror. Avoid compression. 2. Use Goldmann style 1- or 2-mirror lens. 3. Use Koeppe system. 4. Use Dapriprazole to open angle and measure IOP. If angle opens and IOP lowers by more than 3 mm Hg, closed-angle component is present.*

*Bonomi L et al. Effects of topical dapiprazole on the intraocular pressure in humans: A controlled study. *Glaucoma*. 1988;10:8–10.

The Goldmann type of three-mirror lens does not adequately or predictably compress the central cornea. However, to determine whether an angle is closed or opened, the Goldmann-type lenses are almost as effective as the Koeppe lens, which is generally accepted as the most error-free way of determining whether an angle is open or closed. The Goldmann lenses cause less artifactual opening of the angle as compared to the four-mirror lenses and allow a better view over a bowed iris (51). Thus, if an angle closure is suspected, Koeppe lenses are the lenses of choice. Of the indirect systems, the Goldmann-type lenses are best to determine whether the angle is closed or opened; subsequently, four-mirror gonioscopy can be performed to determine the type of closure—synechial or appositional. It has even been suggested that compression gonioscopy is a means to break an attack of angle closure. Lateral angles are easier to view with the direct-view Koeppe lens system; thus, in suspected cases of appositional or synechial closure, where the indirect system is inadequate for viewing the lateral walls, use of a Koeppe lens will provide valuable information.

Lowe describes a technique to open the angle with a Goldmann-type lens. This can be used to determine if the angle is closed by synechia or apposition when no flat-base-curve four-mirror lens is available (12). The lens can be tipped and pressed up and back in the direction of the mirror as the patient looks away and then toward the mirror. This will push the aqueous beneath the mirror across to the opposite side and deepen the angle under observation. If this does

not work, the lens can be rotated slowly, with the lens tipped and pressed against the eye while the angle is being viewed. Rotating the lens 360 degrees in this manner may eventually open the angle enough to establish the presence or absence of synechia. This has proved successful in some instances when the angle was unable to be opened with a flat-base-curve, four-mirror lens.

In typical forms of acute angle closure glaucoma, the angle will be totally closed. To determine the actual location of the iris attachment to the angle wall, the use of the focal lines running along the iris surface and angle wall is extremely helpful. Direct observation of the meeting of these two lines assures the observer that he or she is actually seeing the place of iris contact not observing only optical closure (Table 5.6 and Plate 10). If there is separation of the two beams and the posterior trabecular meshwork is not visible, attempts to view into the angle recess are mandatory to confirm actual closure (Figure 5.4). The examiner should rotate the lens toward the angle quadrant under observation, being sure not to put pressure against the eye, and the patient should shift the gaze toward the gonioscopy mirror. Undue pressure against the eye with a Goldmann-type lens produces inconsistent and difficult-to-interpret artifacts. If the posterior trabecular meshwork is still not visible but there is still parallax (separation) between the lines, the site of iris wall attachment is not being observed. A small one- or two-mirror Goldmann-type lens can be used to provide a higher vantage. If this is still unsuccessful, compression gonioscopy can be used to observe into the angle recess. If uncertainty still exists as to whether the angle is closed and the IOP is elevated due to closure, use of an alpha-adrenergic blocking agent will pull the iris away from the wall. If gonioscopically the angle is opened and the

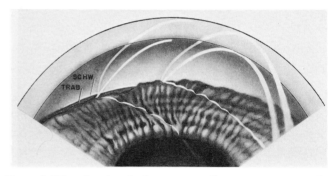

Figure 5.4 Two situations in the same eye. Observation is in secondary gaze where the observer has tilted the lens and the patient is gazing into the mirror. The focal lines to the left indicate a narrow angle; only the trabecular meshwork (TRAB) is visible, but parallax indicates that the angle is deeper than can be observed. The focal lines to the right indicate an area of closure, as the focal lines meet slightly above Schwalbe's line (SCHW), indicated by the fact that the posterior termination of the corneal optic section is not visible. Compression gonioscopy will deepen the angle to the left to provide a view of the location of the actual iris insertion by pushing the iris away from the wall. On the right, if closure is by apposition, the iris will be pulled away from the wall. If synechia is present, the iris will remain against the wall. (Reprinted with permission from Gorin G, Posner A. Slit lamp gonioscopy, 3d ed. Baltimore: Williams & Wilkins, 1967.

TABLE 5.7
Characteristics of Intermittent Angle Closure

Bombe iris
Narrow angle
Shallow central chamber
Pigment peppering along trabecular meshwork (scattered)
PAS (most predictive of future closure)
Iris atrophy
Glaukomflecken
Sporadic recurrent blurred vision with dull ache around eye

pressure is decreased, then the likely diagnosis is elevated IOP secondary to angle closure. If the angle opens but IOP remains elevated, an open angle glaucoma component is confirmed (52).

If the iris focal line and angle wall focal line are observed meeting above the posterior filtering portion of the trabecular meshwork, the angle is closed. A four-mirror lens with a flat-base curve (Zeiss, Sussmann, or Posner) should then be used for compression gonioscopy. This will deepen the angle. If the iris moves easily away from the wall and observation of the entire angle wall is possible, appositional closure is likely. If the iris remains against the wall even partially, synechia is present. If the IOP is very high and compression gonioscopy cannot be performed, it should be done once the pressure is lowered medically.

The best clinical means available to determine whether a particular eye has an open pathway to the trabecular meshwork is by direct observation of the anterior chamber wall via gonioscopy. In the normal angle, 180 degrees of synechia is usually required for elevation of the IOP (4). In the presence of a primary acute attack of glaucoma, the gonioscopic examination will reveal that the trabecular meshwork is blocked by the iris, usually in its entire circumference. During remission in intermittent angle closure, the angle may appear relatively normal although careful examination may reveal signs of a previous attack that may include PAS or a peppering of blotchy or scattered pigment sitting on the surface of the angle wall trabecular meshwork without localization to the Schlemm's canal portion of the filtering meshwork (Plate 13). Additional signs of previous attacks may include pigment on the iris close to the angle, iris atrophy in one or two sectors, or, if the attacks were severe, a dilated pupil, and Glaukomflecken (12). If these findings are associated with an eye with a narrow angle and a bowed peripheral iris, it is even more incriminating because any and all of these findings in some combination provide strong evidence of a previous attack. In addition to these physical findings, patient symptoms of sporadic, recurrent and spontaneous blurred vision or an achy dull feeling, in or around the eye in question, should make the examiner suspicious of previous attacks. This is especially true if the patient can identify a particular activity that precipitates the symptoms and it is consistent with an activity that would increase relative pupillary block (Table 5.7).

Characteristics of an Eye at Risk for Primary Angle Closure

Classification of the glaucomas is attributed to Barkan who introduced the term *narrow-angle glaucomas* (25). Based on his observation of the angle wall with the Koeppe gonioscope, he was able to differentiate what he called the two different forms of glaucoma: narrow angle (iris block) glaucoma and open (or wide) angle glaucoma (11). Earlier investigators had embraced the idea that the narrowing and closure of the angle was a secondary event to the increased IOP. Now it is understood that in primary angle closure, increased IOP is secondary, the result of blockage of the trabecular meshwork by the iris, and that the shallow anterior chamber predisposes the eye to angle closure (53).

Biometric Characteristics

Primary angle closure glaucoma is influenced by the factors that determine the anterior chamber depth, and these have a genetic predisposition. For example, an eye with a shallow chamber and a large lens is considered anatomically predisposed to angle closure. Age is also a factor; generally older hyperopic eyes or eyes with low myopia have shallow chambers with large lenses. With normal aging, the lens tends to thicken and decrease the chamber depth further. In fact, the age of onset of most angle closure attacks is in patients between 50 and 65 years of age (25). Epidemiologically, the risk for angle closure glaucoma increases as the axial anterior chamber depth decreases. Epidemiological association is not as strong with other ocular dimensions, such as corneal diameters or relative lens positions (54).

The physical characteristics of the normal human eye have a Gaussian frequency distribution. They are usually correlated and not randomly combined, thus resulting in a tendency toward emmetropia. This is not always the case; some features may predominate, possibly the result of genetic influence, resulting in refractive errors (12). The human eye dimensions are usually stabilized by 14 years of age. The forward position of the crystalline lens results in a clinically detectable shallow chamber and is correlated to a narrow angle, one feature that predisposes the eye to angle closure. This occurs as a bilateral phenomenon in most people.

Ordinarily as people age, the crystalline lens continues to grow, and this causes the anterior chamber to become more shallow. There is evidence that the anterior chamber depth decreases even during periods when the lens does not appear to be increasing in thickness; thus, the shallowing of the anterior chamber may not be due solely to lens thickening. It has been proposed that the zonule attachments may loosen, allowing the lens to move anteriorly (55). The forward position of the lens also correlates with a larger ciliary body. It has been suggested that the ciliary body thickens by the laying down of connective tissue and by breakdown of hyaline material (56) and that this may contribute to shallowing of the chamber. More rarely a normal chamber may be shallowed by a pathologically swollen lens.

TABLE 5.8
Biometric Values in the Mean Angle Closure Glaucoma Eye

Small corneal diameter
Steep anterior cornea (small radius of curvature)
Steep posterior cornea radius
Shallow anterior chamber (1.8 mm critical value)
Thick lens
Steep anterior lens
Lens positioned anteriorly
Short axial length

From Lowe RF. *Primary angle closure glaucoma.* Singapore: PG Publications, 1989.

Generally eyes with shallow anterior chambers have a large lens, with a steep anterior lens curvature and a lens positioned anterior. The cornea has a steep radius of curvature and a smaller diameter (53). The eye will have a short axial length and a decreased anterior chamber volume (12,57). Lowe describes these characteristics as the biometric values in the "mean angle closure glaucoma eye" (Table 5.8) (15).

The trigger mechanisms that eventually precipitate the iris to come into contact with the trabeculum are not completely understood; however, the anterior chamber depth is considered the most important and measurable feature in the development of angle closure glaucoma because it provides indirect information as to whether the peripheral portion of the angle is open (54). In a number of studies, no patient with angle closure glaucoma was found to have an anterior chamber depth above 2.5 mm (54). Lowe (12) notes that the mean anterior chamber depth in an angle closure glaucoma subject is 1.8 mm, and in a normal subject, it is 2.8 mm. On the slit lamp examination, this equates to axial depths of 3–4/1 and 5–6/1 anterior chamber depth/corneal thickness, respectively. By combining the slit lamp appearance of the anterior chamber configuration with the gonioscopic appearance of the angle, the examiner will have an excellent means of identifying eyes at risk for angle closure. According to Lowe, the anterior chamber depth of 2.5 mm is the threshold depth for pupil block angle closure glaucoma. Lens position and thickness are genetically determined. As we age, the lens normally thickens approximately 0.75 mm to 1.1 mm in the span of 50 years. Half that value is the amount of normal anterior lens surface forward movement, or about 0.4 mm to 0.6 mm. Therefore, an anterior chamber depth of 2.4 mm in early adulthood has the potential to reach the critical value of 1.8 mm, and eyes with chamber depths of 3.1 will potentially shallow to the threshold value of 2.5 mm (12,58). Recent biometric studies of the eye have revealed that the lens thickness/ocular axial length ratio may be useful in predicting which at-risk eyes are more likely to go on to develop an angle closure attack. It has been suggested that angle closure can be predicted by noting the lens thickness in relation to the axial length (59).

Panek and associates (57) studied the biometric variables in 56 patients determined to have occludable angles on clinical examination. Of these patients, 34% eventually required a peripheral iridotomy after a mean duration of 16 months. The only variable measured with predictive results was the ratio of increasing lens thickness to ocular axial length; it was 2.27 compared to the value in normals of 1.91 (57). The conclusion was that this ratio may be a useful predictor for eyes requiring iridectomy. Other investigators have suggested that these values can be used for diagnosing and grading the severity of angle closure glaucoma (59). Volume measurements have also been evaluated; there is a large overlap, however, in the the volume measurement among eyes considered clinically normal and those appearing clinically at risk for angle closure (60,61). In summary, the best clinical methods currently available include the gonioscopic inspection of the entire angle (62).

When evaluating an eye gonioscopically for the risks of primary angle closure, Spaeth suggests that three characteristics of the angle need evaluation on inspection (Table 5.9): the angular approach, the peripheral curvature of the iris, and the point of insertion of the iris onto the angle wall (5). When the iris inserts into the area of the scleral spur, it is by definition an anterior iris insertion. A narrow approach is an approach of the iris that creates an angle between the iris and the cornea less than 20 degrees (Shaffer 0 or Shaffer 1). An anterior peripheral convexity of the iris is a pronounced anterior convexity of the iris at its far periphery so as to obstruct the visualization of the deeper recess. Any and all place an eye at risk for angle closure. According to Spaeth, the characteristic with the most correlation to angle closure is the degree of anterior convexity of the peripheral iris (5).

In his study of the heritable characteristics of the anterior chamber angle configuration, Spaeth evaluated the angles of a group of people with normal eyes, a group of relatives of people with angle closure, and 10 patients with angle closure. In comparing the normal eyes with those that had suffered angle closure, anterior insertion was seen 4 times more frequently, narrow approach 9 times more frequently, and marked peripheral anterior convexity 11 times more frequently in narrow angle eyes. Spaeth concluded that the three characteristics are inherited independently and that there is a hereditary tendency for primary angle closure (63).

Other investigators have also noted the polygenetic dimensions of the anterior chamber associated with angle closure glaucoma (53). Lowe suggests that the anterior lens surface forward position is the partial result of the inherited forward position of the lens and the inherited above-average thickness of the lens, resulting in the familial incidence of shallow chambers (13,58). The conclusion appears to be that "inheritence is not simply wide, narrow, or closed" but some combination of factors that result in an eye at risk for angle closure (5). The anatomic predisposition to angle closure appears to be inherited, yet the familial incidence of angle closure is low (1).

TABLE 5.9
Gonioscopic Risk for Angle Closure

Angle Characteristics
Narrow angular approach
Convex peripheral iris curvature
Anterior point of iris insertion

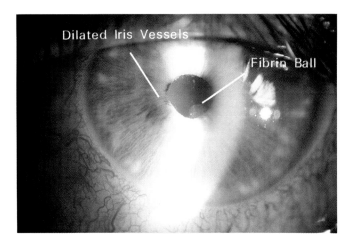

Plate 1 Inflammation. Notice the dilated iris vessels, which could be confused with neovascular vessels. Once inflammation resolves, the vessels return to their normal appearance.

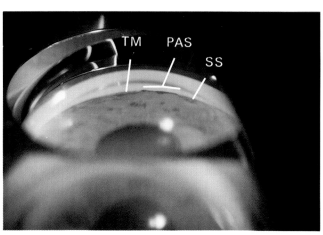

Plate 4 Peripheral anterior synechia (PAS). This was taken six months after a PI in an eye with chronic angle closure glaucoma from pupil block.

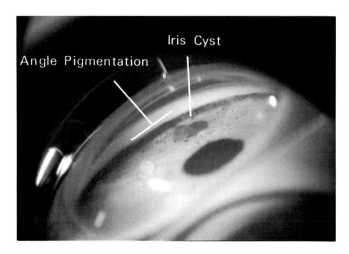

Plate 2 Iris cyst. A free-floating iris cyst located on the iris surface. Notice related heavy pigmentation of the angle wall. (Photo courtesy R. Gutner, O.D.)

Plate 5 Blood in Schlemm's canal. Angle recession from prior blunt trauma. The trabecular meshwork is not pigmented, and the blood in Schlemm's canal localizes the filtering portion of the trabecular meshwork. (Photo courtesy M. Garston, O.D.)

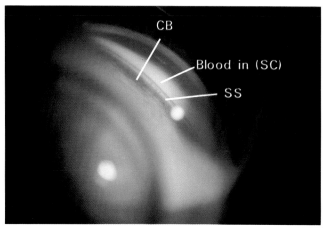

Plate 3 Traumatic angle recession. Remnants of blood in the angle appear as a heavy pigmented ball. (Photo courtesy G. Selvin, O.D.)

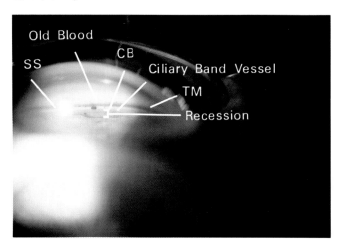

Note: Throughout this color section, the following abbreviations will be used:

CB	=	ciliary body
PAS	=	peripheral anterior synechia
SC	=	Schemm's canal
Schw	=	Schwalbe's line
SS	=	scleral spur
TM	=	trebecular meshwork

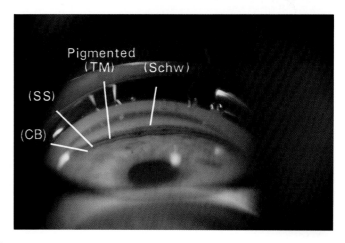

Plate 6   Pigmented trabeculum. Pigment peppering along the angle wall and in the trabecular meshwork. The meshwork has uneven pigment granules on its surface. Pigment may be lightest where little outflow occurs and heaviest where there is normal outflow. Schwalbe's line is also pigmented.

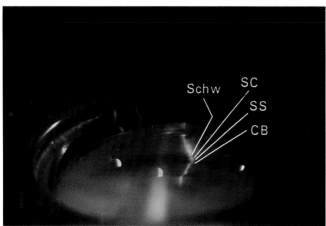

Plate 7   Open angle to the ciliary body. The focal lines meet at Schwalbe's line. Schwalbe's line and the filtering trabecular meshwork are pigmented.

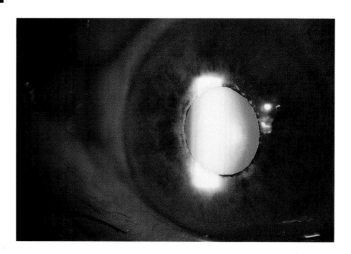

Plate 8   Iris transillumination in the exfoliation syndrome. Transillumination defects typically are located at the pupil border in exfoliation syndrome.

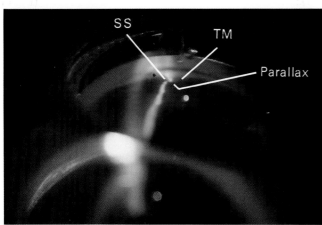

Plate 9   Focal lines in narrow, but open line. Iris is bowed just prior to insertion. The patient is looking into the gonioscopy mirror, and the lens is maximally tilted toward the angle segment under observation. The top of the scleral spur is just detectable, and because the focal lines are not seen meeting (parallax), the angle recess is probably deeper than it appears.

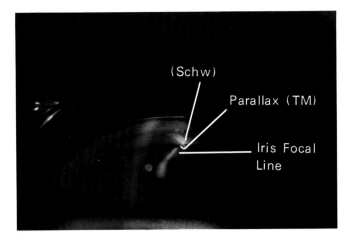

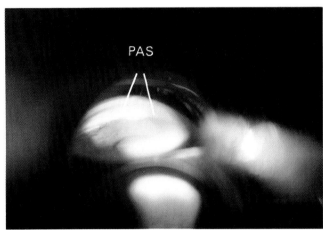

Plate 10 *Narrow open angle. The iris is bowed forward at the recess. The meeting point of the iris light beam and the angle wall light beam is not apparent; therefore the angle recess is deeper than it is visualized. To obtain a view into the angle recess, the patient should look toward the gonioscopy mirror, and the examiner should tilt the lens toward the angle segment under observation.*

Plate 11 *Peripheral anterior synechia (PAS). A large area of iris tissue is attached above Schwalbe's line. (Photo courtesy G. Selvin, O.D.)*

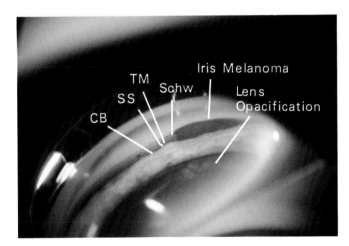

Plate 12 *Iris melanoma. An iris melanoma has invaded into the angle wall. Notice the lens opacification under the pigmented mass. (Photo courtesy R. Gutner, O.D.)*

Plate 13 *Synechia (PAS). Basal (low) synechia tenting to the anterior ciliary body in an eye with active anterior uveitis.*

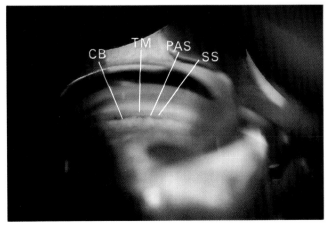

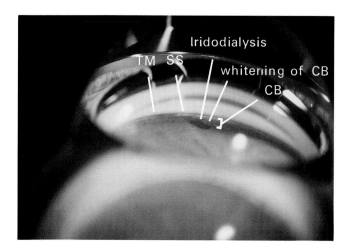

Plate 14   Angle recession. Notice the widening of the angle, the whitening of the scleral spur, and the gray appearance over the ciliary body. The dark area ia a localized iridodialysis. (Photo courtesy R. Gutner, O.D.)

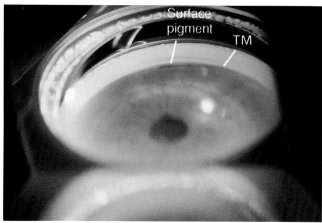

Plate 15   Angle wall pigment peppering. The patient has intermittent chronic angle closure. Peppering of pigment or spattering is an indication of previous iris attachment in this area. Notice the variability of the angle width. This photograph was taken in extreme secondary gaze.

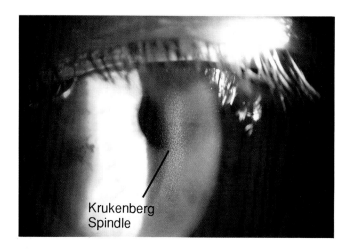

Plate 16   Krukenburg's spindle. Dense spindle in an eye with pigment dispersion syndrome. (Photo courtesy R. Gutner, O.D.)

Plate 17   Iris transillumination in pigment dispersion. Midperipheral-to-peripheral spokelike defects are characteristic locations for iris transillumination in eyes with pigment dispersion syndrome. (Photo courtesy R. Gutner, O.D.)

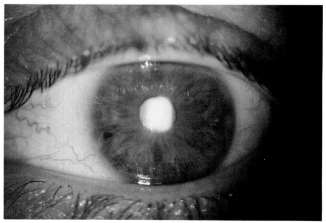

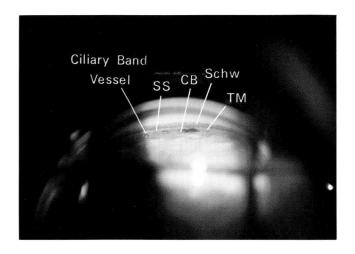

Plate 18   Exfoliation located in the angle recess. A normal cicular *ciliary band is evident. A dense patch of pigment secondary to old anterior uveitis is located on the surface of the ciliary body. Similar pigment patches can be observed in eyes with exfoliation syndrome without uveitis.*

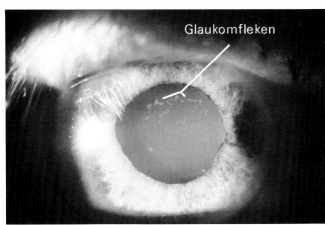

Plate 19   Glaukomfleken documented during an attack of angle closure. Also notice the iris atrophy. (Photo courtesy R. Gutner, O.D.)

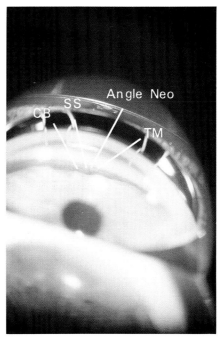

Plate 20   Neovascularization of the angle. Notice the fine branching neovascular vessels spreading along the trabecular meshwork. (Photo courtesy R. Gutner, O.D.)

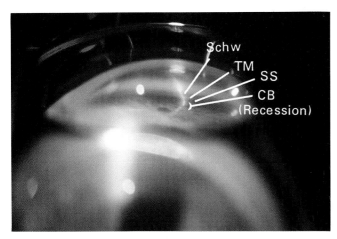

Plate 21   Angle recession. The width of the ciliary body is twice that of the trabecular meshwork.

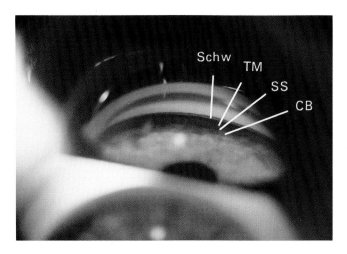

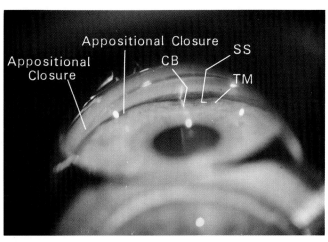

Plate 22   Pigmented trabecular meshwork (TM). Heavy pigmentation of the TM in a 26-year-old patient with pigmentary glaucoma. The iris attaches to the angle wall at the base of the TM. The scleral spur is not visible.

Plate 24   Pigment peppering along the angle wall secondary to anterior uveitis. Appositional closure is also visible secondary to multiple peripheral iris cysts.

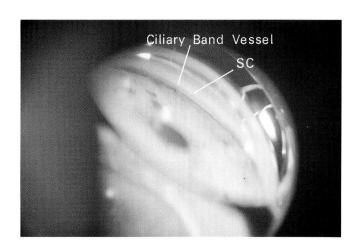

Plate 25   Blood in Schlemm's canal localizes the filtering trabecular meshwork, which is not pigmented. A normal ciliary band vessel is evident.

Plate 26   Pupil frill exfoliation. Exfoliation material is deposited along the pupil margin. This can be observed along the medial aspect of the pupil margin by gonioscopy.

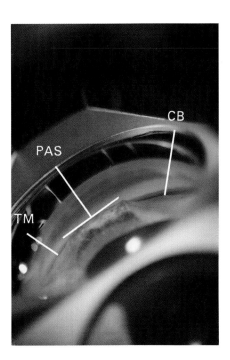

Plate 23   PAS in ICE syndrome. A high broad band of PAS. There is iris atrophy in the area of the synechia. (Photo courtesy R. Gutner, O.D.)

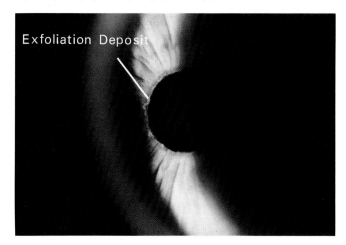

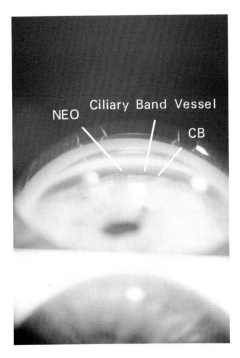

Plate 27 Normal angle blood vessels. Normal circular ciliary band vessels in an eye with neovascular angle vessels. (Photo courtesy R. Gutner, O.D.)

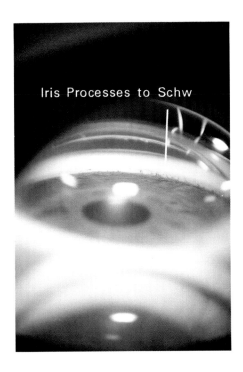

Plate 28 Iris processes. Fine individual iris processes along the angle wall. (Photo courtesy R. Gutner, O.D.)

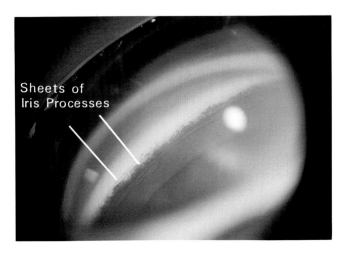

Plate 29 Iris processes. A dense network of iris processes. Notice the lacy appearance. (Photo courtesy R. Gutner, O.D.)

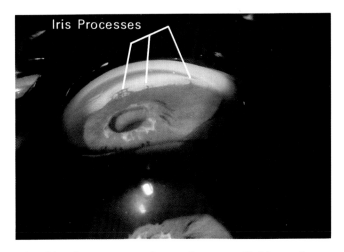

Plate 30 Compression gonioscopy in an eye with iris attachments to the angle wall (Axenfeld's anomaly). The iris attachments are to the level of Schwalbe's line. Notice the volcano appearance to the iris at the pupil border. This volcano appearance is characteristic for compression gonioscopy with a flat-base-curve, four-mirror lens. (Photo courtesy M. Garston, O.D.)

Plate 31 Peripheral anterior synechia (PAS). Small areas of synechia on the left side of the photo. Notice the variability of the width of the scleral spur.

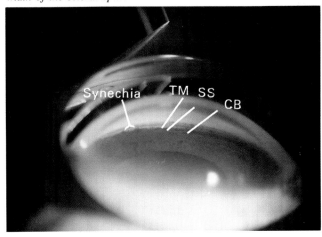

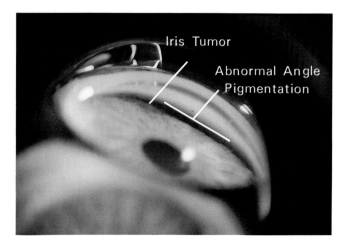

Plate 32   Iris nevus with abnormally heavy angle and trabecular meshwork pigmentation. Height of tumor and angle involvement makes lesion suspicious for a melanoma.

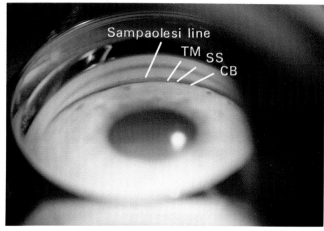

Plate 33   Sampaolesi's line. Example of this wavy line of pigmentation located just above Schwalbe's line. This is characteristic of the exfoliative syndrome and is also seen in pigment dispersion.

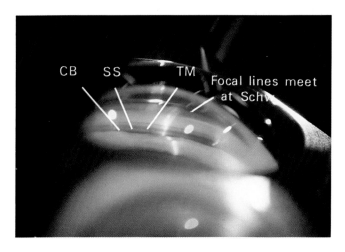

Plate 34   Focal line. Open angle with focal lines meeting at the ciliary body (CB). Notice the heavy pigmentation of Schwalbe's line (Schw). This can be confused for the pigmented trabecular meshwork, but the focal line split along the angle wall identifies this as Schwalbe's line. (Photo courtesy R. Gutner, O.D.)

Plate 35   Axenfeld's sign. Iris tissue is attached to Schwalbe's line (prominent posterior embryotoxin). Gonioscopy appearance would be similar to that shown on Plate 30. (Photo courtesy R. Gutner, O.D.)

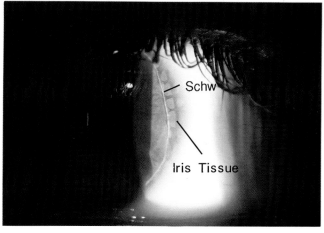

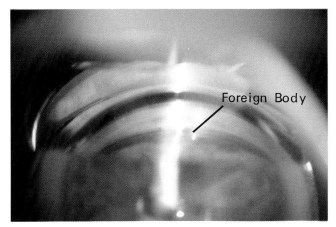

Plate 36   Angle foreign body.

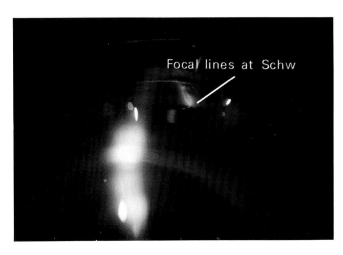

Plate 37   Focal lines in closed angle. In a closed angle, the focal line along the iris meets the focal line along the angle wall above the filtering trabecular meshwork. In this photograph, they meet right at Schwalbe's line. The iris is bowed forward.

Plate 38   Closed angle from pupil block. Notice the bombé appearance to the iris contour. No structures are visible.

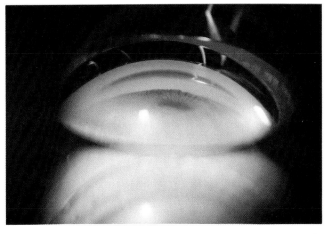

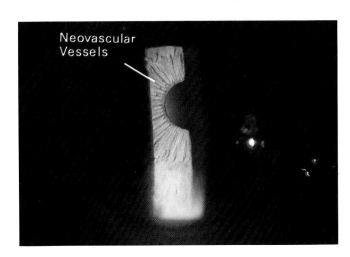

Plate 39   Fine iris neovascularization. Early stage of iris neovascularization located within the iris surface near the pupil border. Gonioscopy is necessary in this presentation.

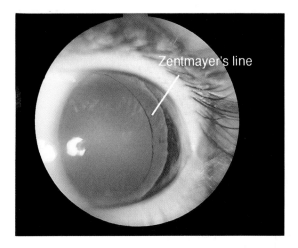

Plate 40   Zentmayer's line. Pigment line located on the posterior lens capsule. This is seen in pigment dispersion syndrome. (Photo courtesy R. Gutner, O.D.)

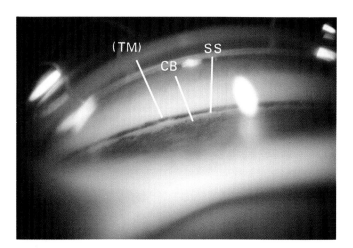

Plate 41   Pigmented trabecular meshwork. Grade 4 trabecular pigmentation in pigment dispersion syndrome.

Plate 42   Ghost cells. The anterior chamber has a hyphema and a khaki-colored layer of ghost cells above the red blood cells. (Photo courtesy C. Scott, O.D.)

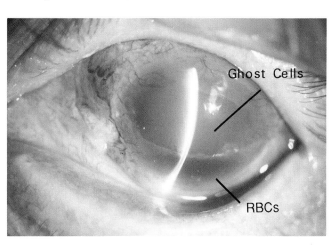

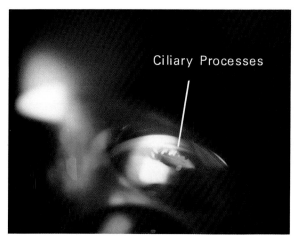

A

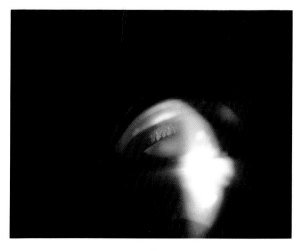

B

Plate 43   (A) Iridodialysis. The ciliary processes are discernible through the iridodialysis. (Photo courtesy C. Scott, O.D.) (B) Ciliary processes. (Photo courtesy G. Selvin, O.D.)

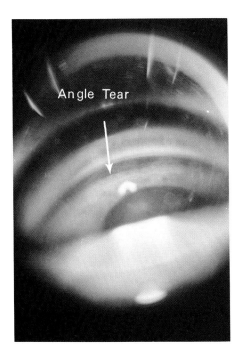

Plate 44 *Angle recession early phase. There is a tear along the angle wall with evidence of blood. (Photo courtesy C. Scott, O.D.)*

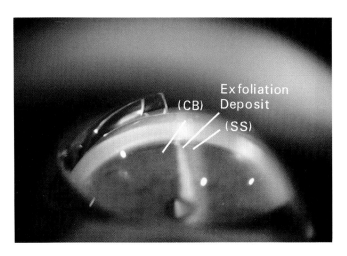

Plate 46 *Exfoliation in the angle. Rare observation of white exfoliative material in the angle.*

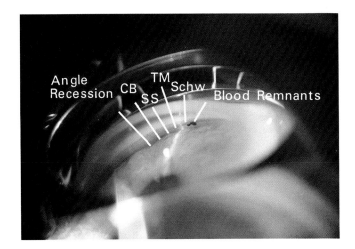

Plate 45 *Angle recession. The oval black ball is remnant of an old hyphema.*

Plate 47 *Iris tumor. Gonioscopic appearance of a raised vascularized tumor. (Photo courtesy R. Gutner, O.D.)*

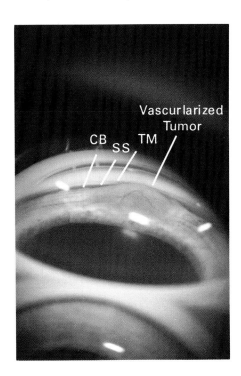

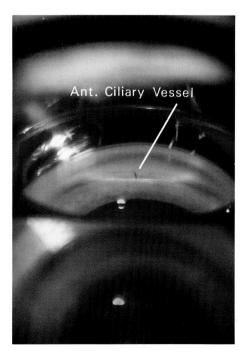

Plate 48   Ciliary artery vessel. An unusual presentation of this normal anterior chamber vascular supply.

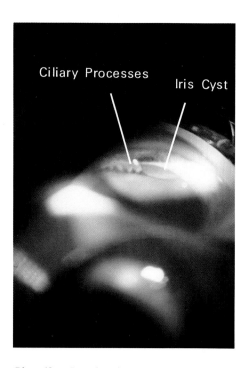

Plate 49   Peripheral iris cysts. Multiple cysts sitting in front of the iris processes. This was first observed during an active episode of recurrent acute anterior uveitis. Presented as a raised iris lesion.

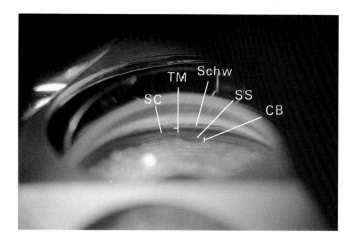

Plate 50   Pigment dispersion syndrome. Heavy pigmentation to the angle wall. Notice the gray appearance to a section of the deep ciliary body.

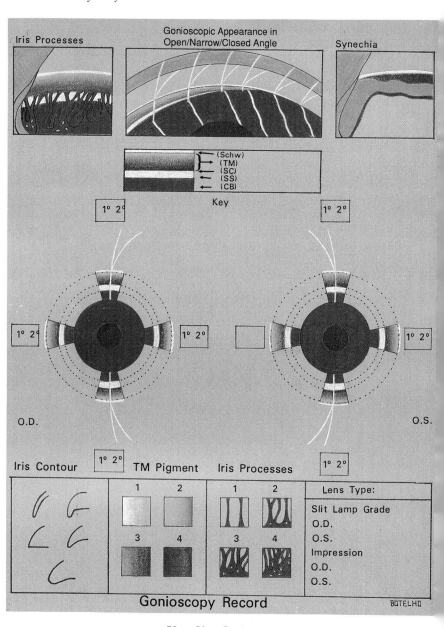

Plate 51   Goniogram.

It appears that angle closure glaucoma is inherited by polygenic inheritance. That is, the various factors involved, such as lens position and corneal diameter, are related to different genes. When the wrong combinations of these factors take place, angle closure occurs. The fact that one family member has developed angle closure is not very predictive that another member will develop it; however, the predisposing shallow anterior chamber depth is a familial tendency that may place members of the same family at risk (64,65).

Prevalence

The prevalence of angle closure glaucoma depends on the population studied being common in Japan, Southeast Asia and among Eskimos (2). It varies from 5% in the Greenland Eskimo population to 1% in the African black population to as low as 0.1% in the Rhondda Valley in Wales (25). The inheritence of certain characteristics may predispose some races to a greater prevalence and type of angle closure glaucoma. Screenings of the Greenland and Alaskan Eskimos reveal frequent observations of shallow anterior chambers and narrow angles (66,67). The Chinese have thick irides located close to the angle wall and shallow chambers, causing them to suffer a particularly destructive form of angle closure (12). The racial variations in the prevalence of angle closure glaucoma may be explained by the genetic influence of biometric variables.

Acute angle closure appears to be rare in blacks but chronic angle closure in blacks is as common as in Caucasians (58, 68). When blacks suffer angle closure, signs and symptoms may be less severe. This may produce unfortunate delays in seeking care. When blacks thought to have open-angle glaucoma were gonioscoped, a number were found to have chronic angle closure glaucoma (1). Angle closure glaucoma is more common in women than in men, by as much as three to one and is most often detected in 50- to 70-year-old patients (25,58). The frequency of angle closure appears to peak between the ages of 53 and 58 and 63 and 70 (55). Which patients predisposed to angle closure will actually suffer an attack is not possible to predict accurately since we know that not all individuals with narrow angles develop angle closure. In one study only 5% of patients age 78 to 88 years had angles capable of closing and only 10% of that group went on to develop angle closure (54). Synechia in an eye deemed at risk for angle closure is probably the most predictive of the potential of future closure (5).

Provocative Testing

There are a number of provacative tests that have been employed over the years to aid in the diagnosis of angle closure glaucoma. Some tests rely on the use of pharmacologic agents, and some attempt to provoke an attack by physiological means. The aim of the provocative test is to identify patients who would benefit from prophylactic treatment (Table 5.10).

TABLE 5.10
Candidate for Provocative Testing

Shallow chamber and narrow angle
Signs or symptoms of intermittent (subacute angle) closure
Fellow eyes
Chronic angle closure
Mixed mechanism glaucoma

This would include patients with suspected intermittent angle closure glaucoma who present for examination between attacks, asymptomatic patients with anterior chamber configurations suggesting a high risk for future angle closure, patients who have suffered an attack in one eye and for whom treatment is being considered for the fellow eye, patients suspected with chronic angle closure, and patients suspected with mixed mechanism glaucoma. Factors that may increase the chances of a positive provocative test in an at-risk eye are active pupil, thick hyperplastic iris root, redundant folds in the iris periphery, and/or a prominent last roll of the iris (69).

Provocative Tests

Unfortunately there is no ideal provocative test (Table 5.11). Any such test should be as physiological as possible to mimic natural living conditions. In many instances, provocative test results are too variable to be predictive. The current tests are generally not reproducible, and a positive test is no assurance that the patient will develop angle closure in the future, nor is a negative test an assurance that the patient will not develop angle closure.

There are many instances of both false positive and negative results with all the provocative tests, even the standard clinical provocative tests, the dark room test, and the mydriatic provocative test (70). Test results may be so variable that they show normal results one day and marked positive results on another day in the same eye (71). The anticholinergic drugs themselves may cause elevation of IOP and decreased outflow in an open angle, confusing the results (72,73). Thus a positive test should be accompanied by a gonioscopically closed angle to be considered reliable and to avoid false positive results.

TABLE 5.11
Provocative Testing

Criticism	Example
Some not physiological	Use of pharmacologic agents
Variability	Same eye can have varying results
Reliability	Not always predictive
Sensitivity	Negative results in eyes with angle closure
Unsafe	Adrenergic agents may precipitate difficult to break attack
False positive results	Anticholinergics can raise IOP in open angle
False negative results	Widely dilated eye becomes free of pupil block

The tests themselves are not without danger as there is the risk of inducing an attack that may be difficult to break, particularly when adrenalin-type drugs are used (69,74). These agents tend to create greater pupil block than is the case with the dark-room test or anticholinergic agents. There is added danger when cholinergic agents are used to break a mydriatic provocative-induced angle closure. The cholinergic agents may exacerbate the angle closure by increasing pupil block. They cause this by creating posterior pulling of the iris, increasing sphincter rigidity and pupil block, causing constriction of the circular muscle of the ciliary body, which relaxes the zonules and allows the forward movement of the lens, and increasing aqueous outflow from the anterior chamber (which lowers the pressure in the anterior chamber with respect to the posterior chamber, thus promoting further anterior movement of the iris (70). Thus the routine use of pilocarpine to constrict pupils after dilation, particularly in eyes at risk for relative pupillary block where Neo-Senephrine® or other mydriatic agents have been used, is not advisable. Rev-Eyes® (dapiprazole), which is an alpha adrenergic receptor blocker, produces miosis by blocking the action of the dilator muscle without the unwanted side effects of cholinergic agents.

There are practitioners who rarely perform provocative tests and rely instead on patients' signs and symptoms in determining the need for prophylactic treatment. Others will not treat a patient prophylactically unless the patient has had a positive provocative test. In addition, some patients need the reassurance of a positive provocative test before agreeing to have surgery or believing in the necessity for the surgery. Possibly the best provocative test, particularly in cases of intermittent angle closure, is to reproduce the situation that creates the patient's symptoms. This, however, may not be practical.

Dark-Room Test

The dark-room test is performed by having patients sit in a dark room with their eyes opened for about 60 minutes. The patient must remain awake to avoid sleep-induced miosis. A light, tight patch can be placed over the eyes to ensure darkness. An 8 mm Hg rise in ocular pressure is considered a positive test. In conclusive tests, the pressure may rise to 40 to 60 mm Hg, with evidence of gonioscopic narrowing and closure (69). Some older individuals with miotic pupils may need to remain in the room for as long as 2 hours in order for the pupils to dilate sufficiently. When a rise in pressure if found, gonioscopy is performed to confirm angle closure. Whenever possible, it is better to do the provocative tests on a day subsequent to the initial gonioscopic evaluation. This avoids the potential of the gonioscopy altering the anterior chamber characteristics prior to the test. Posttest pressure measurements and gonioscopy should be carried out in a darkened room to avoid inducing pupil constriction from bright lights. Some have tried to use infrared slit lamp observation, which can be used in total darkness (75). The dark-room test is positive in about 50% of cases of angle closure (76). A

negative test does notremove the potential for angle closure (1). Some consider this test to simulate normal physiological conditions best.

Prone-Provocative Test

In this test, the patient is placed in a prone position with the forehead, not the chin, resting on a pillow. The patient should remain awake to avoid sleep-induced miosis. Theoretically, placing the head in the prone position will cause pupillary block in a susceptible eye by shallowing the chamber from forward movement of the lens against the iris although this has never been proven (77). The test is done in a lighted room. A pressure rise of 8 mm/Hg is considered positive. In one study, 53 out of 57 eyes with positive responses had their IOPs return to baseline without treatment within one hour, indicating the safety of this test. The results are positive in 50% to 70% of cases of angle closure and closure of the angle is demonstrable by gonioscopy in positive cases (78). In one study comparing provocative tests, it was found that, for narrow-angle glaucoma patients, lying prone for one hour was more sensitive than a dark-room provocative test or dilation using 10% phenylephrine. This test, however, only produces 70% positive results in eyes with angle closure (25).

Dark-Room Prone-Provocative Test

Some examiners attempt to increase pupil blocking forces by combining the dark-room test and the prone-provocative test. Patients place their heads down as in the prone-provocative test in a darkened room for one hour. The test is considered positive when the IOP is elevated 8 mm Hg and the angle is closed or more narrow than it was before the test (69). In one report of 114 dark-room prone tests performed in eyes at risk for angle closure, all patients with negative results were followed for six months, with no cases of angle closure occurring during that period. One conclusion in this study was that it is safe to release the patient and repeat provocative testing at six month intervals. The dark-room prone-provocative test is considered physiological and safe (76) (Table 5.12).

Patients with shallow chambers on long-term miotic therapy may fail to dilate sufficiently in the dark-room test. In these cases, a mydriatic provocative test may be more informative; however, generally the dark-room test appears to be more sensitive than the mydriatic test.

Pharmacologic Provocative Tests

The choice of dilating agent is important because different pupil-iris responses occur with different agents. According to Mapstone's results, pharmacologic provocative tests are best done using a weak anticholinergic agent such as 1% tropicamide (Table 5.13). If closure occurs, it tends to be easier to break and less complete, and when it does occur, it is usually within the first hour after the drop was instilled. Mapstone suggests the avoiding cyclopentolate as an agent

TABLE 5.12
Dark Room Prone-Provocative Test

If possible gonioscopy on visit prior to actual test
Measure IOP
Head prone
Forehead rests on pillow
Darken room
Patient remains awake
Measure IOP after one hour*
Positive if IOP elevated = > 8 mm Hg
Gonioscopically, confirm angle narrowing or closure*
If negative, repeat in six months

*Always minimize room and slit lamp illumination.

for provocative testing because attacks occurring with this agent are difficult to break and can occur as much as 6 hours after the drops are instilled (79).

In cases of bilateral narrow angles, the test should be done in one eye at a time. (Gonioscopy should have been performed at a prior examination, if possible). After tensions are measured, the drop is instilled in one eye. The pressure should be measured while the pupil enlarges. If there is a significant rise in the pressure and gonioscopy confirms narrowing and closure of the angle, the effects of the drop can be reversed with an alpha-adrenergic such as Rev-Eyes® (dapiprazole). The appropriate time to measure the pressure in pharmacologic provocative tests in suspected cases of relative pupillary block is when the pupil is mid-dilated, on its way up and on its way down. In some instances, if the examiner measures the ocular tension when the eye is fully dilated, the test will result in a false-negative result. As the pupil widens and the iris moves toward the wall, the relative pupil blocking forces are relieved. The wide dilation may in fact cause a deepening of the angle because the iris is now beyond the position of apposition to the lens and the iris is able to move posterior. Slit lamp observation at this time will present a picture of a deep angle. The examiner assumes a normal provocative test.

TABLE 5.13
Pharmacologic Provocative Test

Use tropicamide (0.5%)
Measure IOP when: Mid-dilated on way up
Dilated: Look for plateau iris etiology
Mid-dilated on way down
If IOP increased, do gonioscopy to confirm angle closed and to reverse dilation
Reverse with dapiprazole; avoid pilocarpine
False-positive IOP increase from tropicamide in open-angle
Gonioscopy will confirm angle open and not narrowed or closed
False negative   Some wide dilations will relieve pupil blocking forces. Therefore: Measure IOP and use gonioscopy when mid-dilated (4.5–5.0 mm)
Discharge patient when pupil returns to normal size, angle open, IOP at baseline

Test each eye on a separate day.

Actually, the eye is at greatest risk for pharmacologic-induced relative pupillary block when the effects of the drug are resolving rather than when they are most effective. The iris is more lax on the way down in comparison to when it is on the way up. Additionally, when the iris is dilating (on the way up), it is moving more quickly; therefore, it is in the appositional position for a shorter time. When the pupil size decreases, the iris is placed in a position of pupillary block for a potentially longer period of time. Thus, the most important time to look for closure is when the pupil is on its way down from dilation, at approximately 4.5 to 5.0 mm in size (70,79). Evidence of gonioscopic closure should accompany elevated IOP of approximately 8 mm Hg for the test to be considered positive (80). If the test is negative at this time, it is prudent to keep the patient in the office until the effects of the dilating drops have resolved and the pupil has returned to its normal size and is reactive.

Plateau Iris Provocative Tests

Some cases of angle closure secondary to plateau iris can be identified by provocative testing. In these cases the elevated IOP and the angle closure occur secondary to the bunching of the iris root against the wall while the pupil is fully dilated. Some of these cases may suffer attacks that are difficult to break. The use of cholinergic agents is indicated to pull the iris away from the angle wall; however, these agents may not be strong enough to break the attack, particularly when the iris periphery is redundant (56). Because cases of plateau iris angle closure may have some amount of pupil block, the use of dapiprazole may be a better choice for breaking these attacks. Once the IOP is lowered, gonioscopy should be done to confirm that the iris is away from the wall.

Provocative Test Sensitivity

In order for a provocative test to be reliable, it should be very sensitive. Unfortunately, the dark-room tests and the mydriatic tests are not. In one group of patients who previously had an angle closure attack, only 75% had a positive dark-room test; 25% with a history of angle closure had a negative test. Thus, it is likely for a patient to have a negative test and still go on to have an attack (81). In addition, dark-room tests performed on normal eyes have been known to elicit increases of IOP as much as 9 mm Hg, and in patients with open-angle glaucoma as high as 14 mm Hg. Overall, the differences in mean IOP elevation in normal eyes, eyes with open-angle glaucoma, and eyes with angle closure do differ. The normal eye and the eye with open-angle glaucoma measure a mean IOP elevation of 2.1 mm Hg, and the eye with angle closure glaucoma measures a mean rise of 16.2 mm Hg (71).

Mapstone observed that 30% of eyes of patients who have suffered an angle closure attack in their fellow eye will not have a positive mydriatic provocative but will have significant gonioscopic closure, producing a false-negative test (82).

TABLE 5.14
Action of Iris with Mydriatic Pilocarpine Provocative Test

Mydriatic stimulates iris dilator:	Moves iris laterally and posterior
Cholinergic stimulates iris sphincter:	Moves lens forward in some
	Moves iris tightly against protruding lens, increasing pupil block.

He reported on a case in which he provoked the left eye of a patient who had a suffered an acute angle attack of the right eye. During the test, he noted that the angle became gonioscopically closed, but the pressure remained normal. He explains this by theorizing that only a small portion of opening to the trabecular meshwork is necessary to maintain normal IOP, and that could account for a number of patients who undergo provocative tests being gonioscopically closed but experiencing no IOP elevations. This effect may be related to the iris contacting the cornea away from the peripheral cornea, thus leaving a space between the cornea and iris peripherally, where aqueous can have access to the trabecular meshwork. Thus, gonioscopically, the angle recess will not be visible because of the iris cornea contact, but the IOP remains normal because of the open passageway. It seems that if the iris were to remain in this position long enough, the remaining angle would close off, producing a positive provocative test. Mapstone disagrees with this. This response would also require a normal-functioning trabecular that had not been previously compromised by intermittent atacks of closure.

Attempts to increase the sensitivity of provocative testing have led some investigators to search for a better test; however, one problem is that as the sensitivity increases, the number of false positives may increase (81). Mapstone found an 80% rate of angle closure in narrow-angle eyes when using phenylephrine and pilocarpine (31). This mydriatic miotic pharmacologic provocative test consisted of repeated instillation of pilocarpine after Neo-Synephrine had created a mid-dilated pupil (Table 5.14). This produces a very unnatural situation and may induce an angle closure attack that is difficult to break. (Provocative testing should mimic normal circumstances as much as possible.) The adrenergic agent stimulates the iris posterior vector forces, moving the iris and sphincter. The cholinergic agent causes the sphincter to tighten, stimulates the sphincter muscle's medial vector forces, and causes the anterior lens to move forward. This results in the iris being pulled tightly against the forward protruding lens. Thus, with the iris pulled posterior, the lens moved anterior, and the pupil mid-dilated, the optimal position for pupil block is created (39,82).

Kirsch described a triple test where the pupil is dilated with cycloplegics. The patient then drinks one liter of water, and one drop of 4% pilocarpine is added every five minutes. Tonometry and gonioscopy are then repeated every 0.5 mm decrease in pupil size. If the IOP increases 10 mm/Hg or the angle closes gonioscopically, the test is positive (70). Both (Mapstone's and Kirsch's) tests produce very unnatural situations and may induce an angle closure attack that is very difficult to break. Thus these tests are not recommended.

Based on the poor predictive value in terms of false positive and negative results and inherent problems associated with provocative testing, the importance of a careful history and examination must be stressed as an additional and important guide for deciding on the efficacy of prophylactic treatment (83).

Prophylactic Treatment

Today argon or Nd: YAG laser iridotomy is the prophylactic treatment most widely used. Laser iridotomy treatment, however, is not always curative, particularly in chronic angle closure where gonioplasty may be more suitable, and complications, including corneal burns, foveal burns, transient or permanent IOP elevation, lenticular myopia, cataract formation, malignant glaucoma, hyphema hypopyon, pigmented pupillary pseudomembranes, or closure of the iridotomy, may result (84,85,86). If provocative tests are negative and if there is no evidence of synechia, conservative management in chronic angle closure, fellow eyes, and asymptomatic narrow angles may be appropriate. This would include educating the patient about the potential signs and symptoms of acute and subacute angle closure and the judicious use of weak miotics if they widen the angle and do not decrease chamber depth. The patient should be examined every six months, and provocative tests should be repeated at that time (84). Some authors recommend prophylactic laser treatment in all fellow eyes (2) as some studies estimate that as many as 80% of the noninvolved eyes eventually develop an angle closure attack. The use of miotics may help in postponing surgery, but they are not curative because as many as 40% of fellow eyes treated with miotics eventually develop angle closure attacks (87).

Prophylactic treatment for at-risk eyes is often a clinical decision based on the examiner's own bias as there is no definitive way of determining whether a patient with an at-risk eye will actually develop an angle closure attack. Thus one strict recommendation is that prophylactic treatment for eyes that are deemed narrow is usually not recommended unless there is evidence of appositional closure or of previous closure or there are symptoms associated with past closure, or a positive provocative test with evidence of angle closure (1) and laser iridotomy in all fellow eyes (88) (Table 5.15).

Treatment of Acute Angle Closure

The initial short-term goal in treating a primary acute angle closure attack is to lower the IOP, clear the cornea, protect

TABLE 5.15
Recommendation for Prophylactic Iridotomy Treatment

Angle is narrow and chamber is shallow and there is
  Evidence of appositional closure
  Evidence of previous closure
  Symptoms associated with past closure
  Positive provocative test with evidence of angle closure
All fellow eyes receive treatment

TABLE 5.16
Medical Treatment for Primary Acute Angle-Closure Glaucoma

Goal	Normalize IOP Clear the cornea Protect the optic nerve Open angle Prevent PAS Prepare for laser iridotomy or iridoplasty
Aggressive treatment if	IOP >50 mm Hg Evidence exists of nerve damage Congested and painful eye
Lower IOP	Oral carbonic anhydrase inhibitors, for example, acetazolamide 500 mg PO 1 drop 0.5% timolol or equivalent beta blocker 1 drop of 1% hourly prednisolone acetate Oral osmotic agent, for example, 45% isosorbide 1.5 ml/lb 2% Pilocarpine one drop every 30 min for 90 min once the IOP is in 40s

If unsuccessful, use IV osmotics or carbonic anhydrase inhibitors

Most cases resolve in 4–6 hours

the optic nerve, and reduce congestion to prevent PAS. The long-range goal includes neutralizing the precipitating factor and restoring normal aqueous flow. The height of the IOP is unimportant in predicting the long-term outcome, however; the longer the delay in presentation and the longer it takes to break the attack, the worse the outcome. The time delays may allow for more peripheral anterior synechia formation, pigment deposition in the angle, and iris atrophy—all of which may contribute to later interference with the normal aqueous filtration (89).

Medical Treatment for Acute Angle Closure Glaucoma

The level of medical treatment will depend on the amount of pressure increase, the amount of trabecular closure, and amount of synechia (Table 5.16). Efforts should be made to determine the status of the optic nerve and the presence and extent of visual-field loss. The degree of the symptoms and the systemic status of the patient will also influence the choice of treatment. Poor cardiac function, pulmonary status, or impaired kidney function may contraindicate the use of carbonic anhydrase inhibitors, topical beta blockers, or osmotic agents.

Medical treatment is directed toward decreasing aqueous production and/or osmotically dehydrating the eye by shrinking the volume of the vitreous. Lowering the IOP, however, is no assurance that the attack is broken as PAS may remain and continue to form even if the IOP is normalized.

Aggressive treatment may include the use of 500 mg of a carbonic anhydrase inhibitor (Diamox®) and/or an oral hyperosmotic agent such as 45% isosorbide 1.5 ml per lb of body weight. A drop of a topical beta blocker and hourly instillation of 1% prednisilone acetate is also recommended. Once the IOP is lowered so that the iris sphincter will function, usually in the range of 40 mm Hg 2% pilocarpine may be

used. This will pull the iris away from the angle and also increase outflow. Because of the potential for miotics to increase pupil block in some eyes, excess use of miotics is discouraged, and one drop every 30 minutes for 90 minutes is recommended. In hospital environments or when the IOP remains elevated, 500 mg of intravenous acetazolamide and or intravenous mannitol 1 to 1.5 gm/kg over a 40-minute period can be administered. Depending on the level of IOP and associated signs and symptoms, less aggressive treatment may be sufficient to lower the IOP and break the attack (1). This will include the use of one dose of 500 mg of an oral carbonic anhydrase inhibitor (Diamox®) or 50 mg of methazolamide (Neptazine®), one drop of a topical beta blocker, hourly use of 1% prednisolone acetate, and judicious use of 2% pilocarpine. Apraclonidine has also been reported to aid in lowering the IOP in angle closure attacks, although it is not FDA-approved for this purpose (47). Once the IOP is lowered, gonioscopy should be repeated to insure that the angle has opened. Most cases are broken within four hours (2). If the angle is opened, medical treatment should be continued, including the use of topical steroids, which will help reduce patient symptoms and reduce inflammation (1). When the eye is quiet and the cornea is clear, laser iridotomy can be performed. Both argon and Nd: YAG lasers are used for this therapeutic modality (90).

If medical treatment is unsuccessful, the cornea will remain edematous and the iris will be inflamed, dilated, and flaccid. Laser iridotomy in such a case may increase inflammation and potentially promote PAS. There is also the likelihood that the iridotomy will close rapidly. Argon laser peripheral iridoplasty or pupilloplasty may be beneficial in these cases as it will cause the iris to contract, pulling it centrally, and thus may break the synechia (91).

Some cases of angle closure may be broken with the use of a selective alpha-adrenergic agonist such as thymoxamine, which is not available in the United States, or dapiprazole (Rev-Eyes®), which is available but has not been studied for this purpose, although it was shown to be ineffective in a case of angle closure induced by 10% phenylephrine (92). Instillation of this type of agent causes inhibition of the dilator muscle without increasing pupil block (52,93). Compression gonioscopy has also been reported to break an attack of angle closure.

Surgical Treatment

The surgical treatment of choice in patients who have suffered a primary angle closure attack is a laser peripheral iridotomy. Patency can be assured by observation of the anterior lens capsule. Relying on transillumination may result in the false impression of a patent iridotomy. There may be intact iris stroma or iris atrophy over the transilluminating opening, which will prevent aqueous flow (81). Direct observation of the iridotomy with a gonioscopy lens is helpful in determining the absence of tissue over the transilluminating area.

Relieving the pupil block forces with an iridotomy will not significantly change the axial depth of the chamber as the lens will keep this portion of the iris in its presurgical location. The angle width, however, will usually increase as the peripheral iris is able to move posterior without restriction from posterior pressure as the pupil blocking forces are relieved by the patent iridotomy. Gonioscopy will document the increase in angle width, confirming the success of the iridotomy.

Predicting the success or failure of an iridotomy may be aided by presurgical gonioscopic evaluation once the cornea is cleared to determine the presence of synechia, its extent, and the firmness of adhesion. In the 1950s operating-room gonioscopy was utilized to determine the extent of synechia. In these instances, a peripheral iridectomy was done with one knot in the suture; after refilling the anterior chamber, the angle was examined with a Koeppe lens. If little or no synechia was found, the suture was tied and the operation completed. If there was significant synechia present, a filtering type of procedure or synechialysis was performed.

Chandler performed an anterior chamber deepening-procedure by evacuating the anterior chamber and then reforming it by injecting saline and deepening the chamber slightly more than it would be in its natural state. With the deeper chamber, he was better able to determine the extent of actual synechia. He felt that, if after deepening the angle one third or less of it was closed, an iridectomy could be performed. If more than half of the angle was closed by synechia, a filtering procedure was a better option (94). Today compression gonioscopy can be utilized for obtaining this information. Forbes, using compression gonioscopy, concluded that succesful pressure control could be attained by iridectomy even if 70% of the angle was closed preoperatively (95). Patients with 50% to 70% preoperative PAS, however, would require medication to control their pressure. If only 50% or less of the angle was closed, there was a good chance of pressure control with a surgical iridectomy and no medical management afterward. Other factors that cannot be predicted by gonioscopy will also influence the success of the surgery such as the level of function of the visible trabecular meshwork once the angle is opened (81). In cases where repeated attacks have occurred and/or where there is evidence of peripheral anterior synechia of greater than 70% or trabecular damage has occurred, the patient may have greater success with a trabeculectomy or goniosynechialysis followed by argon-laser gonioplasty (81,96). In cases where a 100% closure has taken place with evidence of field loss, and raised pressure 38% will remain with uncontrolled IOP after iridectomy, trabeculectomy should be done initially (73). Iridotomy seems less likely to succeed the longer the attack, the more congested the eye, the greater the nerve damage and field loss and the more synechia present.

Some eyes will continue to have elevated IOP immediately after laser iridotomy. The patency of the iridotomy must be confirmed by direct observation of the opening because trans-illumination can be misleading. If the IOP remains elevated in an eye with a patent peripheral iridotomy, the examiner must perform gonioscopy to determine if the angle is open or if a majority of the angle has PAS. If a majority of the angle is still open and the pressure remains elevated, the trabecular meshwork may be damaged from the previous attack, or the patient may have a mixed-mechanism glaucoma and will require treatment for the open-angle glaucoma component. Other possibilities include the presence of plateau iris, development of malignant glaucoma, postlaser inflammation or pigment debris clogging the meshwork, or a positive steroid response although it is unusual to get a steroid response before two weeks have passed. In the presence of a patent PI, if the IOP becomes elevated upon dilation, consider the presence of plateau iris syndrome. Plateau iris syndrome is managed either with a weak cholinergic miotic agent to keep the iris away from the wall or by laser iridoplasty or pupilloplasty. In some cases, a miotic like pilocarpine may narrow the angle further so slit lamp examination and gonioscopy should be performed routinely to look for shallowing of the chamber and narrowing of the angle. In eyes where angle closure was unrelieved by a patent iridotomy, compression gonioscopy performed early after completion of laser iridotomy will identify persistent synechia. Argon laser gonioplasty has been shown to relieve the pressure effectively by reducing synechia. This is most beneficial when the procedure is performed shortly after recognizing failure of the iridotomy. Compression gonioscopy performed immediately after laser iridectomy is recommended for early detection of iridotomy failure secondary to PAS. Approximately three hours of angle opening by gonioplasty will provide clinical benefit (91).

Gradual loss of IOP control and recurrent acute and subacute angle closure may occur in eyes with patent iridotomies. This may be secondary to progressive PAS greater than 180 degrees and gross trabecular damage, subtle trabecular damage accompanied by less than 180 degrees of PAS, or plateau iris syndrome. Nd:YAG laser gonioplasty has been shown to be effective in these cases. Success should be expected in cases of plateau iris syndrome or subactue angle closure when visible widening of the angle can be observed during the gonioplasty (97). Argon laser trabeculoplasty was found effective in two-thirds of patients with chronic angle closure glaucoma and uncontrolled IOP following laser or surgical iridotomy (98). This should be considered in eyes with uncontrolled IOP after gonioplasty if 50% or less of the angle has PAS.

At present, both argon and Nd:YAG lasers are useful for angle closure laser treatment although the Nd:YAG is gaining in popularity, possibly because iridotomies created with it are less likely to close and because there is less need for retreatment. Nd:YAG laser is not complication-free as there is risk for hyphema, lens dislocation, and rupture of the anterior lens capsule. Even so some feel it may replace argon laser for iridotomy treatment (99).

References

1. Greenidge KC. Angle-closure glaucoma: Definitions, detection, distinctions, decisions, and dissolution. In: Starita RJ, ed. *Clinical signs in ophthalmology.* St. Louis: CV Mosby, 1988.
2. David R. The management of primary acute glaucoma. *Glaucoma.* 1985;8:64–68.
3. Fourman S. Differential diagnosis of acute angle-closure glaucoma in an emergency department. *Glaucoma.* 1989;1:135–138.

4. Chandler P, Grant WM. *Glaucoma*. Philadelphia: Lea & Febiger, 1979.
5. Spaeth G. Distinguishing between the normally narrow, the suspiciously shallow, and the particularly pathological, anterior chamber angle. *Perspect Ophthalmol*. 1977;1:3.
6. Gorin G. *Clinical glaucoma*. New York: Marcel Dekker, 1977.
7. Tornquist R. Angle-closure glaucoma in an eye with a plateau type iris. *Acta Ophthalmol*. 1958;36:419–423.
8. Epstein D. *Chandler & Grant's glaucoma*, 3d ed. Philadelphia: Lea & Febiger, 1986.
9. Pavlin CJ et al. Ultrasound biomicrosciopy in plateau iris syndrome. *Am J Ophthalmol*. 1992;113:390–395.
10. Lowe P, Ritch R. Angle closure glaucoma. In Ritch R et al, eds., *The glaucomas*. St. Louis: CV Mosby, 1989.
11. Barkan O. Narrow angle glaucoma. *Am J Ophthalmol*. 1954; 37:332–350.
12. Lowe R. *Angle closure glaucoma*. Singapore: PG Medical Books, 1989.
13. Wand M et al. Plateau iris syndrome. *Trans Am Acad Ophthalmol Otolarygol*. 1977 (January);83:122–130.
14. Harris LS. Cycloplegic-induced intraocular pressure elevations: A study of normal and open-angle glaucomatous eyes. *Arch Ophthalmol*. 1968;79:242–246.
15. Shaw BR, Lewis RA. Intraocular pressure elevation after pupillary dilation in open angle glaucoma. *Arch Ophthalmol*. 1986;104:1185.
16. Harris LS, Galin MA. Cycloplegic provocative testing effects of miotic therapy. *Arch Ophthalmol*. 1969;81:544.
17. Gorin G. Shortening of the angle of the anterior chamber in angle-closure glaucoma. *Am J Opthalmol*. 1960;49:141.
18. Lowe RF. Primary creeping angle-closure glaucoma. *Br J Ophthalmol*. 1964;48:544–550.
19. Hillman JS, Turner DC. Association between acute glaucoma and the weather and sunspot activity. *Br J Ophthalmol*. 1977; 61:512–516.
20. Mapstone R, Clark CV. Diurnal variation in the dimensions of the anterior chamber. *Arch Ophthalmol*. 1985;103:1485–1486.
21. Sugar S. The mechanical factors in the etiology of acute glaucoma. *Am J Ophthalmol*. 1941 (August);24:P851.
22. Shah P et al. Lesson of the week; acute angle closure glaucoma associated with nebulised ipratropium bromide and salbutamol. *Br Med J*. 1991;304:41–42.
23. Fazio DT et al. Acute angle-closure glaucoma associated with surgical anesthesia. *Arch Ophthalmol*. 1985;103:360–362.
24. Hyams SW et al. Mixed glaucoma. *Br J Ophthalmol*. 1977; 61:105.
25. Hyams S. *Angle-closure glaucoma*. Berkeley, Calif.: Kugler & Ghedini, 1990.
26. Watson NJ, Kirkby GR. Acute glaucoma presenting with abdominal symptoms. *Br Med J*. 1989;299:254.
27. Hung PT. Provocation and medical treatment in post-iridectomy glaucoma. *J Ocular Pharm*. 1990;6(4):279–283.
28. Wohl T et al. Atypical chest pain presumed secondary to acute-angle closure glaucoma. *Glaucoma*. 1989;11:77–81.
29. Ravits J, Seybold M. Transient monocular visual loss from narrow-angle glaucoma. *Arch Neurol*. 1984;41:991–993.
30. Posner A. Angle-closure glaucoma: Its high incidence in relation to chronic simple glaucoma. *Eye Near Nose Throat Mon*. 1964;43:84–114.
31. Mapstone R. Mechanics of pupil block. *Br J Ophthalmol*. 1968; 52:19–25.
32. Douglas G et al. The visual field and nerve head following acute angle closure glaucoma. *Can J Ophthalmol*. 1974;9:404.
33. Zimmerman LE et al. Pathology of the optic nerve in experimental acute glaucoma. *Invest Ophthalmol*. 1967;6:109.
34. Sonty S, Schwartz B. Vascular accidents in acute angle closure glaucoma. *Ophthalmology*. 1981;88:225–228.
35. Leibowtitz, H. *Cornea disorders: Clinical diagnosis and management*. Philadelphia: WB Saunders, 1984.
36. Duke-Elder S. *System of ophthalmology*, vol XI. London: Kimpton, 1969.
37. Cogan D. Clearing of edematous corneas by glycerine. *Am J Ophthalmol*. 1943;26:551.
38. Gorin G, Posner A. *Slit lamp Gonioscopy*, 3d ed. Baltimore: William & Wilkins, 1967.
39. Markowitz S, Morin JD. The endothelium in primary angle-closure glaucoma. *Am J Ophthalmol*. 1984;98:103–104.
40. Bigar F, Witmar R. Cornea endothelial changes in primary acute angle closure glaucoma. *Ophthalmology*. 1982;89:596–599.
41. Krontz D, Wood T. Corneal decompensation following angle closure glaucoma. *Ophthalm Surg*. 1988 (May);19:334–338.
42. Patel BCK, Tullo AB. Corneal sensation in acute angle closure glaucoma. *Acta Ophthalmol*. 1988;66:44–46.
43. Ritch R. Argon laser treatment for medically unresponsive attacks of angle-closure glaucoma. *Am J Ophthalmol*. 1982;94: 197–204.
44. Winstanley J. Iris atrophy in primary glaucoma.
45. Jones BR. Cataracta glaucomatosa and its role in the diagnosis of the acute glaucomas. *Trans Ophthalmol Soc UK*. 1959; 79:753–756.
46. Yanoff M, Fine B. *Ocular pathology*. Philadelphia: JB Lippincott, 1989.
47. Krawitz PL. Podos SM. Use of apraclonidine in the treatment of acute angle closure glaucoma. *Arch Ophthalmol*. 1990;108: 1208–1209.
48. Fourman S. Differential diagnosis of acute angle-closure glaucoma in an emergency department. *Glaucoma*. 1989;11:135–138.
49. Phillips R. Closed-angle glaucaoma. *Br J Ophthalmol*. 1956; 40:136.
50. Tornquist R. Peripheral chamber depth in shallow anterior chamber. *Br J Ophthalmol*. 1959;43:169.
51. Campbell DF. A comparison of diagnostic techniques in angle-closure glaucoma. *Am J Ophthalmol*. 1979;88:197–204.
52. Wand M, Grant WM. Thymoxamine test. Differentiating angle-closure glaucoma from open angle glaucoma with narrow angles. *Arch Ophthalmol*. 1978;96:1009–1011.
53. Tornquist R. Shallow anterior chamber in acute glaucoma. *Acta Ophthalmol*. Suppl XXXIX, 1953.
54. Alsbirk PH. Primary angle-closure glaucoma. *Acta Ophthalmol*. 1976;Suppl 127.
55. Markowitz S, Morin D. Angle closure glaucoma; relation between lens thickness, anterior chamber depth and age. *Can J Ophthalmol*. 1984;19:7.
56. Romano J. Anterior chamber depth in medically-treated open angle glaucoma. *Brit J Ophthalmol*. 1968;52:361.
57. Panek W et al. Biometric variables in patients with occludeable anterior chamber angles. *Am J Ophthalmol*. 1990;110:185–188.
58. Lowe RF. Anatomical basis for primary angle-closure glaucoma. *Br J Ophthalmol*. 1970;54:1961.
59. Markowitz S. Morin JD. The clinical course in primary angle closure glaucoma. *Can J Ophthalmol*. 1986;21(4):130–133.
60. Fontanna ST, Brubaker RF. Volume and depth of the anterior chamber in the normal aging human eye. *Arch Ophthalmol*. 1980;98:1803.
61. Markowitz SN, Morin JD. Ratio of lens thickness to axial length for biometric standardization in angle-closure glaucoma. *Am J Ophthalmol*. 1985;99:400.
62. Lee DA et al. Anterior chamber dimensions in patients with narrow angle and angle-closure glaucoma. *Arch Ophthalmol*. 1984;102:46.
63. Spaeth G. Gonioscopyy: Uses old and new the inheritence of occludable angles. *Ophthalmology*. 1978;85(22):222.
64. Lowe RF. Primary angle-closure inheritence and environment. *Br J Ophthalmol*. 1972;56:13.

65. Tomlinson A, Leighton DA. Ocular dimensions in the heredity of angle-closure glaucoma. *Br J Ophthalmol*. 1973;57:475–486.

66. Van Rens GHMB et al. Primary angle-closure glaucoma among Alaskan eskimos. *DC Ophthalmol*. 1988;70:265–276.

67. Clemmesen V. Gonioscopic screening in Greenland. *Can J Ophthalmol*. 1973;8:270–273.

68. Alper MG, Laubach JL. Primary angle closure in the American Negro. *Arch of Ophthalmol*. 1968;79:663–668.

69. Gorin G. Provocative tests in angle-closure glaucoma. *Am J Ophthalmol*. 1965;60:235.

70. Kirsch R. A study of provocative tests for angle closure glaucoma. *Arch Ophthalmol*. 1965 (December);74:P770.

71. Higgitt AC. The dark-room tests. *Br J Ophthalmol*. 1954;38:242.

72. Galin M. The mydriasis provocative tests. *Arch Ophthalmol*. 1961;6:353.

73. Playfair T, Justin, Watson PG. Management of chronic or intermittent primary angle-closure glaucoma. *Br J Ophthalmol*. 1979;63:23–28.

74. Lowe RF. Primary angle-closure glaucoma. *Am J Ophthalmol*. 1965;60:415–419.

75. Becker S. *Clinical gonioscopy*. St. Louis: CV Mosby, 1972.

76. Wand M. Provocative test in angle-closure glaucoma: A brief review with commentary. *Ophthalmic Surgery* 1974;5(2):32–37.

77. Hyams SW et al. Elevated intraocular pressure in the prone position. *Am J Ophthalmol*. 1968 (October);6(64):661.

78. Neumann E, Hyams SW. Gonioscopy and anterior chamber depth in the prone-position provocative test for angle-closure glaucoma. *Ophthalmologica*. 1973;167:9–14.

79. Mapstone R. Dilating dangerous pupils. *Br J Ophthalmol*. 1977;61:517–524.

80. Lowe RF. Primary angle-closure glaucoma: Investigation after surgery for pupil block. *Br J Ophthalmol*. 1967;51:727–732 and Lowe RF. Primary angle-closure glaucoma: Investigation after surgery for pupillary block. *Am J Ophthalmol*. 1964;57:931–938.

81. Lichter P, Anderson D. *Discussions on glaucoma*. New York: Grune & Stratton, 1977.

82. Mapstone R. One gonioscopic fallacy. *Br J Ophthalmol*. 1979;63:221–224.

83. Lowe RF. Angle-closure glaucoma; Acute and subacute attacks. *Trans Ophthalmol Soc Aust*. 1961;21:65–75.

84. Hyam S. Laser iridotomy—think first. *Glaucoma*. 1991;13:122–125.

85. River AH et al. Laser iridotomy vs surgical iridectomy. Have the indications changed? *Arch Ophthalmol*. 1985;103:1350.

86. Geyer O et al. Pigmentary pupillary pseudomembranes as a complication of argon laser iridotomy. *Ophthalmic Surgery*. 1991;22:162–164.

87. Bain WES. *Br J Ophthalmol*. 1957;41:193.

88. Shields MB. *Textbook of glaucoma*, 3d ed. Baltimore: William & Wilkins, 1992.

89. David R et al. Long-term outcome etc. *Br J Ophthalmol*. 1985;69:261–262.

90. Moster M et al. Laser iridectomy: A controlled study comparing argon and neodymium; YAG. *Ophthalmology*. 1986;93:20–24.

91. Weiss H et al. Argon laser gonioplasty in the treatment of angle-closure glaucoma. *Am J Ophthalmol*. 1992;114:14–18.

92. Doro D et al. How safe is safe—Mydriasis in high-risk eyes. *Glaucoma*. 1988;10:178–181.

93. Hoskins HD Jr, Kass MA. *Becker-Shaeffer's diagnosis and therapy of the glaucomas*. St Louis: CV Mosby, 1989.

94. Chandler PA, Simmons RJ. Anterior chamber deepening for gonioscopy at time of surgery. *Arch Ophthalmol*. 1965;74:177.

95. Forbes M. Indentation gonioscopy and efficacy of iridectomy in angle closure glaucoma. *Trans Am Ophthal Soc*. 1974;72:488.

96. Tanihara H, Makoto N. Argon-laser gonioplasty following goniosynechialysis Graefe's. *Arch Clin Exp Ophthalmol*. 1991;229:505–507.

97. Kumar H, Sood NN. Gonioplasty in angle-closure glaucoma uncontrolled with a patent neodynium: yttrium aluminum garnet laser iridotomy. *Glaucoma*. 1991;13:149–151.

98. Shirakashi M et al. Argon laser trabeculoplasty for chronic-angle closure glaucoma uncontrolled by iridotomy. *Acta Ophthalmol*. 1989;67:265–270.

99. Greenidge KC. Angle-closure glaucoma. *Int Ophthalm Clin*. 1990;30(3):177–186.

CHAPTER 5. PRIMARY ANGLE CLOSURE GLAUCOMA

Chapter 6

Seconday Angle Closure Glaucoma

The most common mechanism of angle closure glaucoma is pupillary block. In one recent report of acute angle closure glaucoma presenting in an emergency room, as many as 40% of cases had a secondary form of angle closure glaucoma (1). In most of these cases, the mechanism for closure was not pupil block, and the use of miotics was contraindicated. Recognizing that the mechanism for closure is unrelated to pupil block will help in establishing appropriate treatment. In most of these situations, observation of the fellow eye will reveal that it has a normal central chamber depth and normal iris contour without iris bombe. This chapter will discuss secondary forms of angle closure without pupil block.

Secondary Angle Closure without Pupil Block

The glaucomas associated with tumors of the anterior and posterior chambers will be included in this section. It should be understood, however, that these lesions may induce open-angle glaucoma as well as angle closure glaucoma.

Anterior Chamber Angle, Iris, and Ciliary Body Tumors

Observation of suspicious lesions on the iris, especially if they encroach upon the angle, requires gonioscopic evaluation. This will enable the examiner to determine the characteristics, extent, and exact borders of the lesion. On routine slit lamp examination, evidence of a localized iris elevation requires further gonioscopic examination, undilated and dilated, searching for the etiology of the raised iris (Figure 6.1). Sometimes on routine gonioscopy, an examiner may detect a mounded appearance to the iris (Figure 6.2). The mounded appearance may be a sign of an isolated lesion

within or posterior to the iris, and the area adjacent to the mound should not be confused with a focal area of angle recession. In these instances, full wide dilation will allow gonioscopic evaluation of the posterior chamber through the space between the lens periphery and the iris. The anterior ciliary processes and lens periphery become visible (Plate 43). Any space-occupying lesion causing iris elevation from this area, such as cystic lesions, melanomas, leiomyomas, and inflammatory lesions, will become visible on gonioscopy (2)(Plates 2,12, and 49). Goniophotography is essential for following lesions of the anterior chamber, particularly pigmented lesions, since documented growth of a pigmented lesion may be the strongest evidence of melanoma (3,4) (Plates 32 and 47).

Tumors

A *tumor* is a localized or focal swelling or mass that may consist of some or all of the following: fluid, inflammatory cells, vascular dilations, and/or an accumulation of neoplastic cells (a neoplastic tumor—cells that no longer respond to the normal growth-suppressing mechanisms of the body). Neoplastic tumors may be benign, and as such they are slow growing lesions consisting of mature cells resembling the cells and tissue of derivation. They are often circumscribed, well-demarcated, and encapsulated. Benign tumors grow by expansion rather than by infiltration and do not metastasize. Unlike benign tumors, malignant tumors are made of pleomorphic, rapid growing cells that are poorly differentiated and have many mitotic figures. In addition to expansion, malignant tumors can infiltrate, intravasate, disseminate, and metastasize and as such are a threat to survival (5). Cancers may be broadly classified as carcinomas or sarcomas. Mesothelial cells are the cells of origin of sarcomas and epithelial cells are the cells of origin for carcinomas. Leukemia, lymphoma, and rhabdomyosarcoma are examples

77

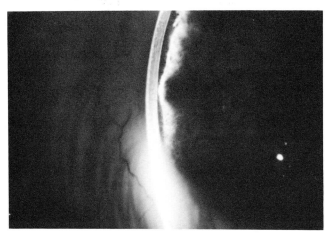

Figure 6.1 Raised iris surface. Gonioscopy is indicated to view into angle and posterior chamber to determine etiology. (Photo courtesy R. Gutner, O.D.)

of sarcoma; basal cell, squamous cell, and melanoma are examples of carcinomas (6).

Iris Nevus

The preponderance of iris tumors are melanocytic tumors, either nevi or melanomas (7), and are made up of uveal melanocytes located within the stroma of the iris, ciliary body, or choroid and are embryologically derived from the neural crest. Nevi and melanomas differ from extremely rare tumors of the iris pigment epithelium known as adenomas and adenosarcomas (4,8). Melanocytic tumors are rare in blacks and Asians but have a strong predisposition in whites with blue irides (8).

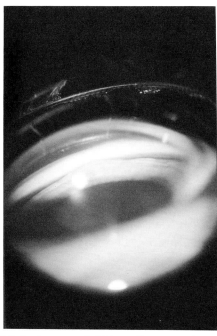

Figure 6.2 Raised or mounded iris surface on gonioscopy. A mass or cyst is located in the posterior iris or ciliary body. (Photo courtesy R. Gutner, O.D.)

Nevi differ from iris freckles in that freckles do not alter the iris architecture and are made up of normal iris melanocytes. Freckles are not elevated, tend to have the texture of the surrounding tissue, and have no malignant potential, whereas nevi do (4,7).

An iris nevus is a solid benign mass of abnormal melanocytes that replaces the anterior iris stroma and alters its architecture. The cells are present at birth and become pigmented around the time of puberty. Clinically, Shields classifies iris nevi according to size (4). His means of classification provides the clinician with a useful initial guideline. He bases this upon his review of the literature and histopathologic examination, where lesions smaller than 3 mm by 3 mm in diameter by 1 mm in height are typically benign. If the lesion is flat, it is considered a nevus regardless of extent. If it is less than 1 mm in height and smaller than 3 mm in diameter, it is also classified as a nevus. Once the diameter is greater than 3 mm and raised, even if less than 1 mm, it is considered suspicious for melanoma.

Size, however, is not an absolute means of defining a nevus, as shown by conditions such as iris nevus syndrome, ocular melanocytosis, or oculodermal melanocytosis. In these cases, the entire iris can be diffusely involved (8). Iris nevus syndrome is one of the clinical manifestations of the ICE syndrome. Ocular melanocytosis is characterized by episcleral and uveal tract hyperpigmentation. Oculodermal melanocytosis (nevus of Ota) is characterized by hyperpigmentation of the episclera, the facial skin, and the mucous membrane in the distribution of the ophthalmic, maxillary, and mandibular branches of the trigeminal nerve. These latter two conditions are examples of congenital melanocytic uveal lesions. They may predispose the eye to uveal melanoma (8,9). As with melanomas, most iris nevi are located inferior.

Iris nevi can be localized, rough, and irregular or diffuse, involving a sector or the entire iris creating heterochromia (8). Sector iris nevi, extending from the pupil border to the iris root, are usually congenital and can be associated with choroidal nevi in the same quadrant (8). Most nevi are pigmented, but they can be nonpigmented and appear gelatinous and transparent. When located near the pupil, they can cause an ectropion irides and also can be associated with sectoral cortical lens changes; neither necessarily implies malignant changes, but they do make the lesion more suspect (Figure 6.3). Invasion of the angle by a melanocytic iris tumor is not necessarily a sign of malignancy, but malignancy should strongly be considered (4,10). Nevi can in fact extend into the angle, into the trabecular meshwork, or as high as the Schwalbe's line or cornea and still be benign (4) (Figure 6.4). Most nevi remain unchanged in size, with little tendency for malignancy.

Iris nevi can cause glaucoma by extension across the trabecular meshwork; however, unilateral elevated intraocular pressure (IOP) in an eye with a pigmented iris tumor should be concern for malignancy (11). In addition to direct observation of the mass, gonioscopic examination will reveal heavy pigmentation (Plate 32) to the trabecular meshwork in these instances (11). The iris nevus does not have to be contiguous with the heavy pigmentation in the angle (12) (Figure 6.5).

CHAPTER 6. SECONDARY ANGLE CLOSURE GLAUCOMA

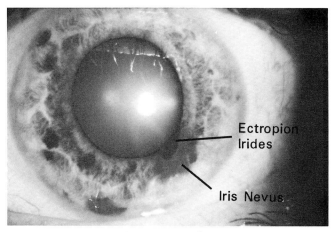

Figure 6.3 Iris nevus with ectropion irides.

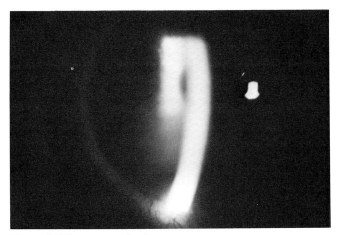

Figure 6.5 Spontaneous hyphema.

Most nevi do not produce a secondary glaucoma. Rarely, they may produce a secondary glaucoma when a necrotic iris nevus liberates pigment into the anterior chamber (4). Macrophages laden with melanin will then block the trabecular meshwork (13). This will happen most often with an iris melanocytoma (14). Examination of the trabecular meshwork will reveal marked pigmentation (11).

Melanocytoma is a term traditionally used to describe benign, deeply pigmented tumors of the optic nerve head, but have been reported in the uveal tract, including the iris. In one retrospective clinicopathological study, they accounted for 5% of excised lesions suspected for melanoma (10). They are made up of heavily pigmented cells. Histopathologically, they are made up of plump polyhedral cells that reflect a spectrum of uveal nevi with minimal capacity for malignant

transition (10,11). Rarely, malignant transformation of an iris melanocytoma may occur, and glaucoma has been reported when this occurs (13). According to Cialdini and colleagues, three clinical features suggest malignancy of an iris melanocytoma: (1) an increase in the size of the lesion, (2) the presence of satellite lesions, and (3) the onset of glaucoma (11).

Nevi can be managed by photodocumentation and close observation. If they are observed located into the angle, yearly gonioscopic examination and photodocumentation is advisable, looking for evidence of growth. If growth is documented, melanoma should be suspected as most uveal melanomas arise from preexisting benign uveal nevi (8). Clinically, nevi are the most difficult lesion to differentiate from a melanoma (4).

Iris Melanomas

Shields classifies melanocytic iris lesions greater than 3 mm in diameter and 1 mm in height as melanomas (4) (Plate 12). They tend to grow anteriorly since posterior growth is inhibited by the dilator muscle (7). Other factors than size, such as prominent vascularity, alteration of adjacent structures such as the lens, iris splinting on dilation, pigment cells in the anterior chamber, spontaneous hyphema, trabecular pigmentation (Plate 32), unilateral glaucoma, large size, corneal compression with edema, and documented growth should all be considered as making the lesion more suspect for melanoma and that most cases defined by size alone will not be confirmed as melanomas by histological examination (Table 6.1) (4,8). The clinical diagnosis of malignant melanoma is difficult, and positive identification requires histologic examination (12). Most melanomas are located inferior temporal, and if a superior melanoma is suspected, an anterior extension of a ciliary body melanoma is a more likely diagnosis (4).

Clinically, iris melanomas may be diffuse or circumscribed (Figure 6.6). Glaucoma is rare with either type. The circumscribed types are well defined, irregular, and elevated and typically dark brown to tan in color (5). They have a predilition for the inferior portions of light-colored irides, implicating an association with sun exposure (6). The diffuse type,

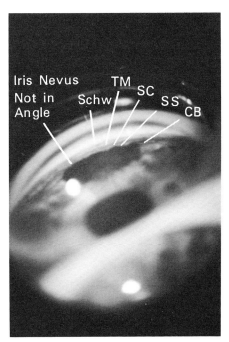

Figure 6.4 Nevus in the angle at the level of the cilairy body. (Photo courtesy M. Garston, O.D.)

TABLE 6.1
*Characteristics Making an Iris Lesion
Suspicious for Melanoma*

Color
Size (greater than 3 mm in diameter and 1 mm in height)
Documented growth
Prominent vascularity
Alteration of adjacent structures (lens, pupil, angle)
Trabecular pigmentation (nodular pattern)
Unilateral glaucoma
Spontaneous hyphema
Unilateral acquired heterochromia
Corneal edema from lesion compression
Inferior location

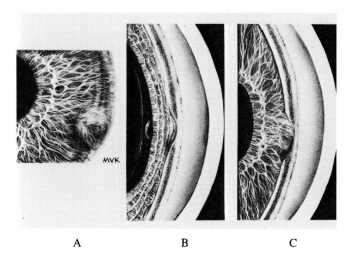

A   B   C

Figure 6.7 Peripheral uveal tract cyst. (A) External view of raised iris surface created by cyst. (B) Gonioscopic view. (C) Dilated gonioscopic view. The cyst is visible under the iris. (Reprinted with permission from Kozart DM, Scheie HG. Spontaneous cysts of the ciliary body. Trans Am Acad Ophthalmol Otolaryngol. 1970;74: 534.)

is rarer than the circumscribed type, may produce more diagnostic problems. Classically, it causes a unilateral acquired heterochromia (darkening) with unilateral painless glaucoma, resulting from direct tumor tissue invasion of the trabecular meshwork, which is visible on gonioscopy. Gonioscopically, the iris will have an irregular nodularity, the trabecular meshwork may also become deeply pigmented in an irregular nodular pattern (8). These tumors may bleed spontaneously, resulting in a spontaneous hyphema, which may be the presenting finding in an eye with iris melanoma (Figure 6.7).

The differential of diffuse iris melanomas includes conditions that produce acquired heterochromia, including pigment dispersion syndrome (Plate 50), heomosiderosis, siderosis, congenital melanocytoma, congenital heterochromia, melanosis oculi, nevus of Ota, and iris nevus syndrome (15). Circumscribed iris melanomas must be differentiated from iris atrophy, benign iris tumors, and iris cysts (14). Amelanotic melanomas with apparent nodular vascularity are referred to as "tapioca" melanomas. They have multiple translucent nodules sitting above the iris plane projecting into the anterior chamber (10,16). At one time, these were thought to be variants of iris melanoma and signs of malignancy, but they are now also recognized as capable of being benign nevi (8). They may mimic leiomyoma (sphincter or dilator muscle tumors), metastatic tumors, or granulomatous iridocyclitis (4). History will aid in differentiating tapioca melanomas from metastatic

lesions. Granulomatous lesions should clear after resolution of the inflammation, and this differentiates them from tapioca melanomas. Leiomyomas may need electron microscopy for differentiation and are extremely rare (9,14,15).

Iris melanomas, which constitute 3% to 10% of all uveal malignant melanomas, (4) usually appear in a younger patient population than choroidal melanomas (10,12). Prognosis for life is favorable for patients with iris melanoma, especially when compared to the relatively poor prognosis associated with choroid or ciliary body melanomas (10). Mortality rates are reported at between 1% and 4% with only 37 cases of death reported in the literature, attributed to metastases from primary iris melanomas (4,17).

The Callender classification is the traditional histological classification system used for uveal melanomas. There are five variations: spindle A, spindle B, fascicular, epitheliod mixed, and necrotic where there is signficant necrosis and the tumor cell type cannot be identified. Histologically the epitheliod cell type is the most malignant, and the mixed cell type is second in malignancy with no cases of metastatic malignant melanoma being reported from spindle A cells (17,18). Most iris tumors are benign, being either nevi or spindle A melanomas (19).

Elevations of IOP may be present in as many as 7% of eyes with iris melanomas (20). Slit lamp observation of diffuse pigmentation of the inferior peripheral iris in a case of unilateral elevated IOP warrants careful gonioscopy. If a melanoma is present, gonioscopy will often reveal the lesion and characteristic pigmentary changes to the trabecular meshwork (Plate 32). The trabecular meshwork is very susceptible to an invading iris melanoma. This is more likely to occur with a diffuse melanoma (4). The trabecular cells may also become replaced by melanoma cells obstructing outflow, causing a secondary open-angle glaucoma (14). Open-angle glaucoma may also occur secondary to pigment dispersion,

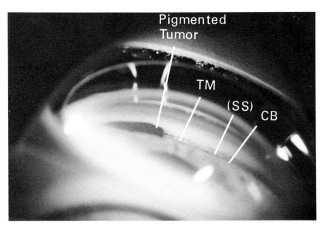

Figure 6.6 Iris melanoma. (Photo courtesy R. Gutner, O.D.)

TABLE 6.2
Mechanisms by Which Unilateral Iris Melanoma Precipitates Glaucoma

Open-angle glaucoma
  Pigment dispersion
  Trabecular cells replaced by melanoma cells
  Macrophages clog meshwork

Angle closure glaucoma
  Invasion of tumor into the angle
  PAS
  Neovascularization

by clogging of the meshwork by melanin-laden macrophages (melanomalytic glaucoma) or from a secondary hyphema (13,20,21). Secondary angle closure glaucomas may occur associated with melanomas. Gonioscopy will reveal the direct invasion of the tumor or any associated peripheral anterior synechia, PAS, or neovascularization as the secondary causes (10,20) (Table 6.2).

Ciliary Body Melanomas

Ciliary body melanomas may produce a localized anterior displacement of the iris detected on slit lamp examination or on gonioscopy. They may cause refractive changes because of lens tilting, subluxation, or cataract formation. Ocular inflammation including episcleritis, (dilated episcleral vessels) iridocyclitis, uveitis, endophthalmitis, panophthalmitis, and vitreous or anterior chamber hemorrhage may be initial presenting manifestations of ciliary body melanomas (23). Direct slit lamp observation of a ciliary body lesion is not possible unless it extends anteriorly to the iris surface. Gonioscopically, it will not be detectable in an undilated eye, unless the lesion has invaded into the anterior chamber or is so large that it is gonioscopically visible under the pupil. When it does penetrate into the anterior chamber, the tumor will be evident as a mass, possibly vascularized, with pigmentation of the trabecular meshwork adjacent to the mass (12). It may cause an appearance of a local dialysis of the iris root and be accompanied by pigmented tissue obscuring the angle root (24). Once the pupil is dilated, the lesion will become visible behind the iris (Plate 20).

Usually ciliary body melanomas are circumscribed, but they may be circumferential (ring melanomas) and extend extrasclerally as localized episcleral pigmentation, producing an external sign of a ciliary body melanoma. Prominent episcleral vessels (Episcleritis) is another external sign of ciliary body melanoma or of ciliary body involvement of an iris melanoma (5,7,10,23).

Ciliary body melanomas can cause dense cataracts that will obscure the tumor from clinical observation. Conventional B-scan ultrasound will aid in the diagnosis in these instances and should be performed in all cases of unexplained dense unilateral cataracts obscuring the posterior segment from view. Recent reports of ultrasound biomicroscopy suggest this new imaging technique may be beneficial for following small

ciliary body tumors and for differentiating ciliary body tumors from iridociliary cysts (25).

Ciliary body tumors are most likely to affect outflow when the mass involves the angle or iris (12) resulting in unilateral increased IOP. Elevated IOP will occur in 17% of eyes with ciliary body melanomas (20). They can cause glaucoma by closing the angle by pushing the iris or the iris and lens against the angle wall, by invasion into the meshwork by a necrotic-induced inflammatory PAS or posterior synechia, or by pigment dispersion (20). Generally tumors of the ciliary body and iris tend to induce glaucoma by direct infiltration of the trabecular meshwork with malignant pigmented tissue or by seeding of the trabecular meshwork with tumor cells (12,14). When a melanoma is isolated to the ciliary body, it is possible for the IOP to be lowered when the ciliary processes become involved because the ability of the nonpigmented epithelium to produce aqueous may be compromised or the outflow and inflow affects by the melanoma may balance each other out, (the mass induces inhibition of outflow but also reduces production) resulting in a normal IOP (12,26,27).

Treatment

The tendency today is to manage iris melanoma by observation, but this will vary depending on whether the lesion is diffuse or circumscribed (8). Diffuse lesions often require enucleation. Documented growth, along with the presence of trabecular seeding associated with uncontrolled glaucoma or other associated complications such as vitreous hemorrhage or lens subluxation, indicates a need for surgical intervention, particularly in iris lesions (4) (Plate 13). Most anterior segment tumors do not contribute to vision loss unless secondary glaucoma occurs (4). Once growth of a melanoma is documented, the surgical procedure will depend on the location and size of the tumor, with enucleation considered when there is no restorable vision and it cannot be treated by any other means (17,28). Enucleation should also be considered in iris melanomas when the melanoma involves more than half of the iris and angle and there is evidence of growth, the melanoma involves more than half of the iris and secondary glaucoma is uncontrollable, or the melanoma involves at least one-quarter of the iris in any eye that is blind or glaucomatous (4,17). In addition to surgery, radiation, chemotherapy, and photoradiation therapy using dihematopophyn ether (DHE) have been used (28).

The detection, evaluation, and observation of lesions located within the anterior chamber is enhanced by the use of gonioscopy. Gonioscopy will allow the examiner to delineate the extent of the lesion and determine whether it is localized, whether it extends into the angle structures, whether it originates from the posterior chamber, whether vascularization is present and its extent, if the lesion is a solid mass or cystic, and the texture of the lesion. In some cases, gonioscopy may be the only means available to observe the mass directly and to document its growth. Any eye presenting with dilated episcleral vessels, unexplained and nonresponsive inflammation, spontaneous hyphema, spontaneous subluxated lens, unexplained dense unilateral cataract, acquired heterochromia, unilateral pigment dispersion, unilateral elevated IOP, unilateral hypotension, and unilateral unexplained angle closure glaucoma should undergo gonioscopy, undilated and dilated in some instances, looking for an iris or ciliary body tumor as the cause.

Cystic Uveal Tract Lesions

Cystic lesions of the uveal tract, which are confined to the iris and ciliary body, should be suspected when there is local shallowing of the chamber and/or a raised or undulated appearance to the iris surface on slit lamp examination or gonioscopy (Figure 6.7). When they are located in the posterior iris or ciliary body, they can produce shallowing to the chamber, similar to ciliary body melanomas.

Classification and Pathogenesis

Shields has classified anterior uveal cysts into primary and secondary cysts. *Primary cysts* of the iris and ciliary body emerge spontaneously from the epithelial layers and are an epithelial-lined space. They may be of congenital origin, representing a persistence of the space of the primary optic vesicle or arise from proliferation of cells of the inner neuroepithelial layers (29). Other theories suggest that they develop from a fluid accumulation between the two layers of neuroepithelium and/or from an inability of the tissue in the area to dehydrate (30). Another theory proposes that ciliary body cysts arise from traction on the zonular fibers during accommodation, producing separation between the pigmented and nonpigmented ciliary body epithelium (31). Secondary iris cysts are also epithelial lined spaces but result from surgical or nonsurgical trauma, miotics, parasites, or secondary inflammation. They are more likely to enlarge than are congenital cysts and lead to complications such as glaucoma or inflammation, but primary cysts can also be associated with glaucoma and inflammation (29,30,32,33,34). The identification of cysts in an eye with an active inflammation, history of inflammation, or glaucoma brings into question whether the cyst is primary or secondary.

The primary uveal tract cysts may manifest anywhere between the pupil and ciliary body. They may be observed and classified by their location on the pupillary margin on the posterior iris epithelial layers, in the corona ciliaris between the ciliary processes, in the aqueous or vitreous as free-floating cysts (Plate 2) or, more rarely, in the iris stroma (29). The fluid within the cyst is clear and appears to be similar in content to the aqueous (32). Iris stroma cysts are observable on slit lamp examination as raised, clear, nonpigmented cysts. They are extremely rare and usually occur unilaterally in infants and young children. When they are large and rapidly progressive, they can be surgically excised (29, 35,36,37). Ciliary body pars plana cysts have been described associated with multiple myeloma (15).

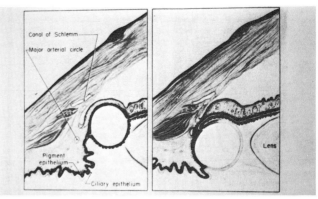

Figure 6.8 Pigmented posterior iris epithelium. The posterior epithelium of the ciliary body has two layers. The inner layer (closest to the vitreous) is nonpigmented; the outer layer is pigmented. The location (which layers) of the iris/ciliary body involved will determine whether the inner walls of the cyst are pigmented. (Reprinted with permission from Scheie HG. Gonioscopy in the diagnosis of tumors of the iris and ciliary body with emphasis on intraepithelial cysts. Trans Am Ophthalmol Soc.1953;51:313.

Clinical Characteristics

Most iris pigment epithelial cysts are stationary and rarely progress or cause compromise of vision, and patients can be followed routinely without treatment (29). The clinical observation of these cysts is rare, and even more rarely is glaucoma associated with them (30). Clinically they are a problem, however, when they are mistaken for a melanoma or when they do in fact induce a secondary glaucoma. Dislodged cysts (Plate 2) may be gonioscopically observed in the anterior chamber, and their glistening, smooth surface should differentiate them from an iris tumor. These dislodged cysts can be made to move with movement of the patient's head (4). Once they are dislodged, the original location of the cyst cannot be determined by slit lamp or gonioscopic examination.

Iris cysts are often misdiagnosed as melanomas. This is because the potential space between the posterior layers of the iris is lined by pigmented epithelium (Figure 6.8). The pigmented layer produces a dark appearance to the cyst, giving it the appearance of a solid mass. This is particularly true for midzonal epithelial cysts, located between the pupil and the iris root. The midzonal cysts are lined with pigment and do not transmit light as well as the peripheral (iridociliary sulcus) cysts. The most peripheral cysts located on the ciliary body are lined with nonpigmented ciliary tissue, and thus light is more easily transmitted (2,29) although the nonpigmented layer has the potential to produce melanin. They can be visualized between the ciliary processes and can at times gonioscopically have a brownish-red coloration from the reflected light from the underlying uveal vessels (31).

In differentiating pigmented cysts from melanomas, Shields notes that in some cases the absence of pigmentation, absence of prominent episcleral vessels, the smooth anterior placement of the iris, and the transillumination of the cysts help differentiate them from a melanoma (4). Also aiding in the differential is the fact that cysts may be tremulous, and when

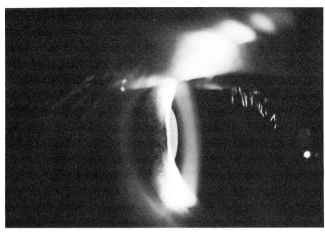

Figure 6.9 Iris cyst visible behind the iris. The pupil dilates normally, and the cyst transilluminates.

the pupil is dilated, iris cysts also evert and become visible in the pupil (2) (Figure 6.9). Additionally cysts are often multiple and bilateral and do not cause local interference with dilation or splitting of the pupil (7,37).

Diagnostic difficulty between iris cysts and melanomas can also occur when the iris cyst is in contact with the cornea and secondary pigment proliferation has occurred on the iris surface (4). On slit lamp examination, this gives the appearance of mass supplanting iris stroma rather than the usual appearance of iris stroma thinning over an iris cyst (2,4). When a cyst is detected, transscleral transillumination should also be done to confirm that the visible iris cyst is not an extension of a solid tumor from the ciliary area (4). The presence of an anterior uveal melanoma should be considered whenever a cyst of the iris if found (12).

Uveal Tract Cysts and Glaucoma

Peripheral cysts may be unilateral or bilateral, single or multiple, and located in the valleys between the ciliary processes or in front of the tips of the ciliary processes (2) (Plate 49). They can be pigmented or nonpigmented when they are located in this region. Implantation cysts secondary to penetrating trauma or surgery may form in this area, but they usually have translucent walls and are filled with observable debris (33). When peripheral uveal tract cysts push forward beyond the tips of the ciliary processes, the iris bulges. The cysts may be large enough to produce a shallowing of the chamber and/or a narrowing of the angle. They produce variability to the angle width, occasionally heavy pigmentation to the angle structures, and a lumpy appearance to the angle (34). Occasionally the cyst may push the peripheral portion of the iris against the chamber wall and block aqueous outflow, causing an acute angle closure glaucoma. There are reports of familial cases of iris ciliary body cysts theorizing a genetic association and suggesting the need for careful gonioscopic evaluation of family members of patients presenting with this condition (30,33,38). In some cases of angle closure caused by these cysts, the diagnosis was made retro-

spectively only after the observation of the cysts after an iridectomy was done to relieve suspected pupil block angle closure (33). The iridectomy was not curative because pupil block was not the cause of angle closure in these cases (30).

Temporary treatment of uveal tract cyst–induced angle closure glaucoma with pilocarpine is sometimes effective, although in one case it caused an increase in pressure in an eye being treated for presumed plateau iris angle closure. It also presumably caused a change in the position of the cyst, resulting in its visibility in the pupil and enabling a proper diagnosis (34). Long-term use of pilocarpine may not inhibit synechial closure (34). Argon laser therapy for nonpigmented ciliary body cysts has a poor prognosis, but with pigmented cysts, it is quite effective, although an inflammatory response may occur postoperatively and the cysts may re-form (30,34). Neodymium (Nd)-YAG laser therapy may be effective for nonpigmented ciliary body cysts. Observation of an oily fluid rather than a clear aqueous-like fluid emanating from the cysts during laser treatment may be a sign of an associated malignant melanoma (12).

When the eye is dilated and the cyst is large enough, it will be visible on slit lamp examination, protruding from behind the iris. Slit lamp observation of the more peripheral cysts can be enhanced by having the patient look into the extreme field of gaze to the side of the iris elevation; the slit lamp illumination and oculars are then moved in the opposite direction and directed, obliquely, into the area of suspicion. In some instances, the peripheral cysts can be detected only on gonioscopic examination, and in other cases, the cysts may not be observable even after dilation (29,36,38). Gonioscopically, iris and ciliary body cysts cause the angle width to be variable, although when the cyst is circumferential, this variability will be absent (34). The trabecular meshwork may be heavily pigmented, with evidence of PAS (30). In some cases, pigment may be sufficient to induce obstruction to outflow, causing a secondary open-angle glaucoma (33).

In general, no treatment is necessary for iris and ciliary body cysts when the patient is symptom-free and vision and ocular function are not compromised. Routine examinations, including photographic documentation, should suffice. Eyes that develop angle closure or secondary open-angle glaucoma should receive laser therapy in an attempt to rupture the cysts (30,38).

Iridocorneal Endothelial Syndrome

The iridocorneal endothelial syndrome (ICE syndrome) is a progressive disease consisting of three clinical entities (Table 6.3): the Cogan-Reese syndrome (iris nevus syndrome), Chandler's syndrome, and essential iris atrophy (progressive iris atrophy) (39). All are associated with an angle closure glaucoma without pupillary block. This is the result of iris contracture PAS caused by an abnormal membrane formed from corneal endothelial degeneration, possibly virally acquired or from an embryological abnormality of neural crest cell proliferation (39,40,41). The affected corneal endothelial cells migrate into the angle and iris, resulting in changes to

TABLE 6.3
Iridocorneal Endothelial Syndrome

Major Clinical Variations	Characteristic Features
Progressive iris atrophy	Iris features predominate, with marked corectopia, atrophy, and hole formation, high PAS
Chandler's syndrome	Changes in the iris are mild to absent, corneal edema, often at normal IOP, is typical; fine, hammered-silver appearance of corneal endothelium
Cogan-Reese syndrome	Nodular, pigmented lesions of the iris are the hallmark and may be seen with the entire spectrum of corneal and other iris defects

Adapted from Shields, MB. *Textbook of glaucoma*, 3d ed. Baltimore: Williams & Wilkins, 1992.

their structure and function (42). Clinically this will manifest as a fine hammered-silver appearance and/or microguttata to the corneal endothelium, often with an associated corneal edema (Figure 6.10). The abnormal endothelium may also form a membrane that will induce a characteristic PAS and iris pupil abnormalities. The clinical proportion of these structural changes and the degree exhibited define which of the categories of ICE is present. Yanoff and Eagle in the late 1970s proposed *iridocorneal endothelial (ICE) syndrome* as an umbrella term to classify this disorder because of the common features of corneal endothelial and iris abnormalities (43,44).

PAS and Glaucoma

Glaucoma is a usual sequela in the ICE syndrome, the result of blockage of the trabecular meshwork by an abnormal endothelial membrane and/or contracture of the membrane, causing PAS, which blocks access to the trabecular meshwork. The contracture of the PAS causes corectopia in the direction of the PAS. Thus an early sign may be the appearance of a pearlike or slitlike pupil pointing to an area of synechia (33). Observation of the iris collarette's becoming displaced locally toward the PAS is also an early sign of this membrane-

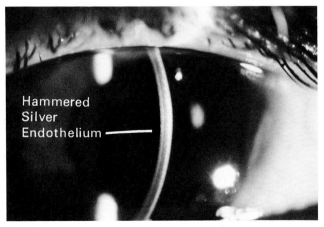

Figure 6.10 Fine hammered-silver appearance to endothelium in Chandler's syndrome. (Photo courtesy C. Scott, O.D.)

induced change. Eventually the collarette disappears as it is drawn into the progressive synechia (40).

The degree of glaucoma manifested usually corresponds to the degree of angle closure from PAS, but this is not always true. Some cases can have marked glaucoma without significant clinical evidence of PAS. This may be the result of the clinically undetectable membrane covering over significant portions of the angle and blocking outflow, without evidence of PAS (40). In some presentations even with marked synechia, glaucoma may not exist. This occurs because of a bridging of the PAS, resulting in tunnels of open trabecular meshwork below the PAS (33).

Patient Signs and Symptoms

Each form of ICE syndrome has a somewhat different characteristic initial clinical presentation (Table 6.4). Depending upon which form is present, changes of the pupil, iris, or visual disturbance from corneal edema may be the first signs or symptoms. The corneal edema is mostly related to the endothelial changes present in all forms and not from glaucoma, although the associated glaucoma can cause or exacerbate the edema. Some patients may experience pain from the corneal edema or, later in the disease, from increased pressure. In some instances, patients may first notice iris changes such as dark spots, the result of tractional or full thickness hole formation, or they may become primarily concerned about changes in the size and shape of their pupils, and this may prompt them to seek care. Patients with Chandler's syndrome are more likely to complain of blurred vision. Patients with iris atrophy and iris nevus syndrome are more likely to complain of iris/pupil abnormalities.

Clinically ICE is unilateral; however, the contralateral eye may show evidence of subclinical endothelial abnormalities appreciated with specular microscopy (15). It is more common in women than men, whites more than blacks, and is probably as noted, an acquired disease, possibly of viral origin, with abnormalities occurring possibly two to three decades before clinical detection (39).

A recent study evaluating the serologic profiles of patients with and without ICE syndrome suggested an association between ICE and the Epstein-Barr virus. The patients with ICE

TABLE 6.4
ICE: Correlating Patient Signs, Symptoms and Form of ICE

Patient Complaints	Form of ICE	Clinical Signs
Visual disturbance: Reduced vision, colored halos, especially in A.M. Pain secondary to corneal edema	Chandler's	Beaten metal fine silver appearance to the corneal endothelium (unilateral)
Change in pupil size and shape	Progressive or essential iris atrophy	PAS, iris melting holes, possibly full thickness
Dark spots on iris	Iris nevus or Cogan-Reese syndrome	Iris pigmented nodules

*Any form may have characteristics of another. All share an abnormality of the corneal endothelial cell layer.

CHAPTER 6. SECONDARY ANGLE CLOSURE GLAUCOMA

syndrome had serologic profiles that suggested a cellular immune abnormality sufficient to allow reactivation of latent Epstein-Barr virus, suggesting an association of ICE with the virus (45). Investigators have previously conjectured on the role of a virus in this syndrome because of its unilateral presentation and evidence of ultrastructure lymphocytic inflammation of the endothelium, representing a low-grade endothelitiis (39,44).

Chandler's Syndrome

Of the three entities making up the ICE syndrome, Chandler's syndrome is clinically the most common (46). It is unilateral and occurs mostly in young females. Early clinical signs are difficult to detect in this disorder because, typically in a quiet eye, very subtle corneal changes occur first, consisting of a fine hammered-silver appearance of the corneal endothelium. These changes are easy to miss, especially if the patient lacks other signs and is symptomless. There is often only slight pupil distortion with limited iris atrophy and no iris hole formation. Histologically, the abnormal corneal endothelium is observed to grow over the anterior chamber angle and onto the iris stroma. This causes the later additional clinical presentation of a distorted pupil resulting from PAS. The pupillary displacement is in the direction of the PAS. Depending on the amount of PAS and the degree of angle involvement glaucoma may develop, but this is usually a late finding in Chandler's syndrome, and is more mild than in the other forms of ICE (15,46).

The predominant clinical sign in Chandler's syndrome is corneal edema. The edema is related to the "dystrophy" of the endothelial layer rather than to the level of IOP. Thus, the edema may be present at normal or even low tensions (44). The edema is often sufficient to result in symptoms of blurred vision and colored halos around lights and may be sufficient to prompt a person to seek care (33). Classically a patient with Chandler's syndrome may present with early morning blurred vision and/or signs of corneal edema in one eye, not related to any IOP abnormality in an otherwise normal-appearing eye should prompt a detailed comparative exam-

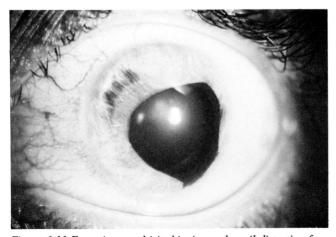

Figure 6.11 Ectropion uveal iris thinning and pupil distortion from iris displacement in essential iris atrophy.

ination of the corneal endothelium in each eye looking for characteristic, subtle hammered-silver endothelial changes in the symptomatic eye. Treatment is aimed at keeping the IOP low enough to eradicate corneal edema. The level of treatment may vary with the extent of endothelial dystrophy and may change as the problem worsens or as glaucoma develops.

Progressive or Essential Iris Atrophy

In essential or progressive iris atrophy, the corneal changes and glaucoma occur around the same time (Figure 6.11) (45). The initial signs are the displacement or distortion of the pupil, usually first noticed in midlife. The iris is displaced in the direction of a synechia usually found in an otherwise open angle (44).

The finding of synechia is a main feature in this disorder and they are characteristically attached at the cornea and may be visible by slit lamp. This type of high synechia may occur in other conditions such as iris bombe from pupil occlusion, penetrating injury, postoperative flat chambers, and the result of postsurgical or traumatic epithelial downgrowth (Plate 23). Based on history, these are usually easy to differentiate. This type of synechia may also be present in congenital iridocorneal dysgenesis; however, this is usually bilateral, present at birth, nonprogressive, and associated with a prominent Schwalbe's line.

Synechia associated with angle closure glaucoma, inflammation, and neovascular glaucoma is more often confined to structures more posterior along the angle wall, possibly only as high as the trabecular meshwork but usually not extending to the cornea (Plates 13 and 31). In essential iris atrophy, the synechia initially are narrow and become broader as the disease progresses. At the point where the iris attaches to the cornea, a small, translucent, yellowish material may be present, possibly representing spread of the synechia since it does not seem to appear when synechia is static (33).

As additional synechia develop, they cause the iris to become stretched, and holes develop in the iris between synechia opposite the distorted pupil. Sometimes the holes are full thickness, including the pigment epithelium (15). Two types of holes have been described. One is the result of local obstruction of the vasculature within the contracting iris, causing small, melting holes. This type is probably secondary to ischemia. The second type, which is much larger, is caused by stretching of the iris, resulting in iris tearing (40).

As the synechia increases, an intractable glaucoma may develop; however, elevated IOP may exist without observation of synechia (15). This may be the result of the endothelial membrane's covering the angle but not as yet contracted to cause permanent synechia (21). The iris abnormalities are related to the endothelial proliferation. Electron microscopy studies of an eye with essential iris atrophy revealed an extracellular matrix secreted by the endothelial layer between the iris and cornea in the areas of synechia and an endothelial membrane on the anterior iris surface (44). The corneal endothelium shows a hammered-silver appearance similar to guttata but not as coarse in appearance (15). The iris atrophy in essential iris atrophy is not the same graylike mothy appearance as the atrophy in other conditions such as acute angle closure glaucoma but is more a melting away of the iris. The primary defect is assumed to be in the iris stroma.

Iris Nevus Syndrome

This form of the ICE syndrome is characterized by iris pigmented nodules. These are present in only about 10% of essential iris atrophy cases and are very rare in Chandler's syndrome, if present at all (47). The nodular lesions may resemble Lisch nodules found in neurofibromatosis; however, in iris nevus syndrome, the iris lesions are unilateral, tend to be pedunculated and mushroomlike, and are more localized than Lisch nodules (48,49). The nodules in iris nevus syndrome are a clinical marker of the presence of an abnormal endothelial membrane common to all forms of ICE (40). The nodules may be produced by a proliferation of the melanocytes in the anterior border layer of the iris or may be a result of the abnormal endothelial membrane binding off portions of the iris stroma and encircling them (47). The nodules tend to be multiple and located on the iris surface. Two cases of isolated iris nevi extending into the stroma, however, have been reported (50).

In contrast to essential iris atrophy, the iris atrophy in this form rarely results in hole formation. There are a number of secondary iris abnormalities that may manifest in this form, which may include stromal effacement, distortion of the pupil, ectropion uvea, diffuse iris lesions, heterochromia, matted velvety appearance of the iris stroma, and a loss of iris crypts (15,44).

In the iris nevus syndrome (Cogan-Reese syndrome), glaucoma occurs early and corneal changes later (45). The corneal endothelial abnormality in this disorder manifests clinically as a slit lamp appearance of fine hammered-silver and an iridescent quality to Descemet's membrane (26,40). The age of disease presentation is usually middle age. Conditions that may resemble iris nevus syndrome include diffuse malignant melanoma, nevus of Ota, and neurofibromatosis. In iris nevus syndrome, the distortion of the pupil margin, PAS, fine pedunculated nodules, and velvety iris help differentiate it from malignant melanoma. The lack of ipsilateral hyperpigmentation of the lid, conjunctiva, sclera, and fundus differentiates it from nevus of Ota. The presence of pupil distortion and PAS differentiates it from neurofibromatosis (48).

Treatment

In general, glaucoma treatment is aimed at reducing IOP and the accompanying corneal edema by medical means using aqueous suppressants whenever possible. In more advanced cases, surgical procedures such as cyclotherapy, cyclodialysis, or trabeculectomy may be needed to control the IOP (51). In some cases, failure of the trabeculectomy may be the result of progressive endothelial proliferation, which hinders bleb functioning. Eyes that fail conventional filtering surgery even with the use of 5-fluorouracil may need to undergo drainage implant surgery (52). Penetrating keratoplasty may be indicated to relieve pain and improve vision in cases with severe corneal edema (53). The corneal edema may be the result of endothelial cell loss rather than the elevated IOP, and thus lowering of the IOP may not reduce corneal edema, especially in the presence of significant loss of endothelial function (53).

Conditions Confused for ICE Syndrome

Because the clinical presentation of the ICE syndrome is so inconsistent, a number of clinical entities can be confused with it. These include Fuch's endothelial dystrophy, posterior polymorphous endothelial dystrophy, and iridoschisis. Fuch's corneal dystrophy and posterior polymorphous endothelial dystrophy share clinical features with this syndrome but differ in that they are usually bilateral and do not have iris involvement and do not have as strong an association with glaucoma. Fuch's is found predominantly in elderly women and is bilateral; clinically it can be differentiated by the presence of Hassal-Henle warts (guttata) present centrally at the level of Descemet's membrane.

The ICE syndrome and posterior polymorphous endothelial dystrophy have some similarities. The literature indicates that there may be clinical observation of iridocorneal adhesions, pupillary ectropion, and glassy membranes bridging the angle and adhering to the iris observed in posterior polymorphous endothelial dystrophy (PPD). These are features of ICE syndrome as well and thus blur somewhat the differential diagnosis between the two. However, ICE, unlike PPD, is usually progressive, frequently is associated with glaucoma, and is not familial. One study showed that specular microscopy, a clinical tool, could differentiate morphological changes specific to PPD and ICE at the layer of the corneal endothelium and Descemet's membrane (54).

Iridoschisis is a separation of the anterior iris stroma from its deeper layers. It occurs later in life than the ICE syndrome—around the seventh decade of life—but has been reported in children. It affects males and females equally. It is usually bilateral and tends to involve the inferior iris quadrants. Unlike ICE, the pupil is not displaced. It is thought to be an age-related phenomenon or related to trauma. Glaucoma may occur in 50% of cases and may develop if PAS forms from the loosened stromal fibers or from release of pigment and debris (15,21).

Summary

In general, the three clinical entities of the ICE syndrome are considered three distinct processes; however, it may be more a continuum of one disease, and a patient's particular condition may change from one form to another in the course of time (Figure 6.12) (51). Therefore, it may be difficult to distinguish a particular form in any one patient at any particular time, especially early in the disease. The three syndromes share an abnormality of the cornea involving the corneal endothelial cell layer. A hammered-silver appearance of the posterior cornea and corneal edema is a primary clinical characteristic of this disorder. The endothelial membrane layer migrates across the anterior chamber angle and across the iris surface, resulting in characteristic membrane-induced iris changes and IOP elevation. Contracture of the abnormal membrane results in a unique form of synechia and induces

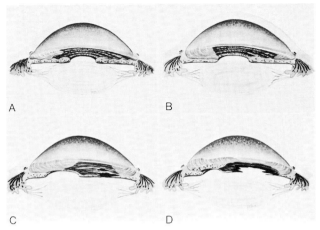

Figure 6.12 Membrane theory of Campbell for pathogenesis of the ICE syndrome. (A) Extension of the membrane from corneal endothelium over anterior chamber angle and onto iris. (B) Contraction of membrane, creating PAS and corectopia. (C) Thinning and atrophy of the iris in quadrants away from corectopia. (D) Hole formation in area of atrophy (in progressive iris atrophy), ectropion uvea in direction of corectopia, and nodules in area of membrane (in Cogan-Reese syndrome). (Reprinted with permission from Shields MB. Progressive essential iris atrophy, Chandler's syndrome, and the iris nevus (Cogan-Reese) syndrome: A spectrum of disease. Surv Ophthalmol. 1979;24:3.)

a unilateral angle closure glaucoma. The different manifestations may be the result of differences in the type of endothelial proliferation. In essential iris atrophy, the endothelialization is more focal; in iris nevus syndrome, it is more diffuse; and in Chandler's syndrome, the changes are primarily confined to the cornea (47). It is generally believed that this is a unilateral clinical condition; bilateral cases have been reported, however, although no details of these cases were provided (55).

Neovascularization of the Iris and Angle

Neovascularization of the iris was described in 1868 by Bader, and in 1928 Salus named it *rubeosis iridis diabeticus*. Later,

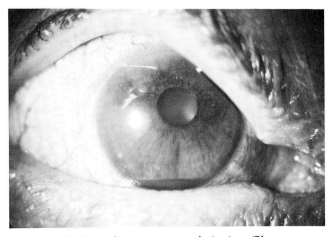

Figure 6.13 Hyphema from iris neovascularization. (Photo courtesy R. Gutner, O.D.)

it became apparent that there were other causes of neovascularization, and the name was changed to *rubeosis irides*. Today *rubeosis irides* refers to the presence of new iris blood vessels without consideration for the presence of neovascularization of the angle or the presence or absence of glaucoma (Figure 6.13) (21). The glaucoma associated with neovascularization has been called thrombotic glaucoma, hemorrhagic glaucoma, congestive glaucoma, and rubeotic glaucoma. Most observers today use the term *neovascularization of the iris* to describe new iris vessels and *neovascular glaucoma* to describe the glaucoma associated with it (21,56,57). Some have suggested doing away with the term *rubeosis* completely (56).

Pathogenesis

The most accepted hypothesis for the pathogenesis for iris and angle neovascularization is the presence of retinal ischemia (hypoxia), which liberates some angiogenic factor forward into the anterior chamber via the aqueous (58,59,60). This results in stimulation of blood vessel growth at its primary site of contact with a receptive vascular bed, most often at the capillary bed of the minor arterial circle at the pupil. The new blood vessel buds turn into tufts of vessels on the iris, at the pupil margin. These tufts actually leak flourescein, proving that they are new vessels with fenestrated endothelium. The vessels eventually extend along the iris into the angle, although they may be visible only at the pupil border and/or in the angle (59). Wand speculated that the normal balance between stimulation and inhibition of vessel formation is altered when hypoxia occurs to the eye and stimulatory factors predominate, resulting in new blood vessel formation (58). Most observers believe that retinal capillary occlusion or ischemia initiates the process. Others have postulated vascular leakage or chronic vascular dilation, either in response to hypoxia or from the dilation itself, as the initiating process (21,22,61). Other factors may also exist, such as oxygen-consuming tumors or scleral buckles that may induce mechanical interference of the vortex vessels causing anterior segment ischemia (22,60).

Discovery of neovascularization of the iris and/or angle is achieved by meticulous slit lamp evaluation and gonioscopy of those eyes at risk (Plate 20). Therefore, a familiarity with the conditions most likely to manifest neovascularization is important. Most often, neovascularization is associated with eyes that have suffered ischemic central retinal vein occlusions, diabetic retinopathy (with a greater prevalence in eyes with proliferative retinopathy), postcataract extraction in eyes with diabetic retinopathy, ocular ischemia secondary to some form of reduced blood flow to the eye, such as carotid occlusive disease, or, more rarely, aortic arch syndrome (56,62). Less common associations include chronic ocular inflammation, ocular neoplastic disease, and chronic retinal detachment (62,63). In neovascularization associated with retinal detachments, the RPE cells may act as modulators carrying the serum factors for neovascularization (60). It also has been reported in cases of exfoliation, pigment dispersion, and Fuch's heterchromic cyclitis, probably the result of localized anterior segment reduction of blood flow (Plate 18) (56,64,65). (These conditions rarely, if ever, cause neovascularization of

TABLE 6.5

Diseases and Conditions Associated with Neovascularization of the Iris and Neovascular Glaucoma

Ocular vascular disease
  Central retinal vein occlusion
  Central retinal artery occlusion
  Branch retinal vein occlusion
  Branch retinal artery occlusion
  Sturge-Weber syndrome with choroidal hemangioma
  Leber's miliary aneurysms
  Sickle cell retinopathy
  Diabetes mellitus

Extraocular disease
  Carotid artery disease/ligation
  Aortic arch syndrome
  Carotid-cavernous fistula
  Giant cell arteritis
  Pulseless disease

Assorted ocular diseases
  Retinal detachment
  Eales' disease
  Coat's disease
  Retinopathy of prematurity
  Persistence and hyperplasia of the primary vitreous
  Retinoschisis
  Glaucoma
    Open angle
    Angle closure
    Secondary
  Norrie's disease
  Stickler's syndrome
  Trauma
  Essential iris atrophy
  Neurofibromatosis
  Lupus erythematosus
  Marfan's syndrome
  Recurrent hemorrhages
  Vitreous wick syndrome

Ocular neoplasms
  Malignant melanoma
  Retinoblastoma
  Optic nerve glioma associated with venous stasis
  Metastatic carcinoma
  Reticulum cell sarcoma
  Medulloepithelioma
  Squamous cell carcinoma conjunctiva
  Angiomatosis retinae

Ocular inflammatory disease
  Chronic uveitis
  Endophthalmitis
  Sympathetic ophthalmia
  Syphilitic retinitis
  Vogt-Koyanagi-Harada (V-K-H) syndrome

Ocular therapy
  Cataract excision (especially in diabetics)
  Vitrectomy (especially in diabetics)
  Retinal detachment surgery
  Radiation
  Laser coreoplasty

Adapted from Gartner S, Henking P. Neovascularization of the iris (rubeosis iridis). *Surv Ophthalmol.* 1978;22:291 and Wand M. Neovascular glaucoma. In Ritch R, Shields MB, eds. *The secondary glaucomas.* St. Louis: CV Mosby, 1982. Reprinted with permission from Hoskins HD Jr, Kass MA. *Becker-Shaffer's diagnosis and therapy of the glaucomas,* 6th ed. St Louis: CV Msoby, 1989.

the angle and neovascular glaucoma.) In a recent prospective study, neovascularization of the iris was found to be present in 18% of patients suffering acute central retinal artery occlusions (66). It has also recently been reported to occur relatively quickly following Nd:YAG laser posterior capsulotomy in diabetic patients, possibly related to the capsulotomy's disrupting the protective barrier for the anterior movement of vasoproliferative factor (67). For this reason, it is recommended that patients with a history of central retinal vein occlusion (CRVO) or diabetics who undergo cataract extraction be followed carefully for postsurgical development of rubeosis irides. This includes diabetics even if they are noninsulin-dependent, have posterior chamber lenses, have an intact posterior capsule, and have no signs of proliferative retinopathy preoperatively (68).

Over 40 entities have been associated with neovascularization of the iris and severe glaucoma, and unfortunately, its complications are a common cause for enucleation (Table 6.5) (56). It is important to understand the current theories regarding the pathophysiology of the disease so eyes at risk can be followed closely for the signs of neovascularization. Any process that causes significant capillary nonperfusion, decreased ocular perfusion, decreased anterior segment perfusion, increased oxygen consumption, or chronic retinal detachment has the potential to incite iris neovascularization and eventual neovascular angle closure glaucoma (58). Duane has classified these processes under four broad headings: vascular, inflammatory, neoplastic, and retinal diseases (69).

Clinical Detection

The full blown case of neovascular glaucoma—with a steamy, cloudy cornea, pain, conjunctival congestion, markedly elevated IOP, frank evidence of new blood vessels everywhere on the iris surface and along the angle wall, and PAS—is usually not a diagnostic dilemma; in some cases, however, corneal clouding may prevent observation of the iris and angle. In these cases, glycerin can be applied to the corneal surface to clear the cornea temporarily, providing a view of the neovascularization. Examination of the fellow eye will also provide useful information because the predisposition to primary angle closure from relative pupillary block is usually a bilateral condition. The slit lamp observation of normal depth to the central and peripheral chamber and the absence of iris bombé in the fellow eye is strong evidence that the involved eye is suffering a secondary form of angle closure, and most cases of nonpupil block secondary angle closure are related to neovascular glaucoma (1).

It is important to detect the signs of iris neovascularization before the eye develops secondary angle closure. Unfortunately, there is no regular pattern to the temporal sequence and severity in the development of neovascularization, although it has been suggested that cases secondary to CRVO appear to be more severe and rapid in their development and that the angrier the new vessels look, the more quickly the neovascularization will result (58,59). When it occurs in eyes with CRVO, it also tends to present quickly, sometimes within six weeks (56). Comparatively, early neovascularization in a nonsurgically disrupted phakic diabetic eye tends to progress slowly (70). Thus, total synechia in some eyes may develop in days, while in other cases, neovascularization may remain stationary for years or even regress (56,59). Thus, it is imperative that the clinician be diligent in inspecting the iris and angle wall in patients at risk for neovascularization. Aphakic diabetics are particularly vulnerable as they may develop rapidly progressive neovascularization in the angle before evidence at the pupil margin or prior neovascularization of the disc or retina (70).

Use of red-free filters with slit lamp high illumination often aids in the early identification of new vessels along the pupil margin and iris root. Pressure with a gonioscopy lens should be avoided because light gonioscopic pressure may collapse the small vascular tufts at the pupil margin (58). Dark irides require more careful inspection as the new vessels may not be as apparent (71). Fluorescein angiography will reveal early neovascularization before it is even visible by slit lamp and could be helpful in unclear cases (72). Neovascularization of the iris is not confined to the anterior surface although clinically this is how it is perceived. Rarely it can extend through the pigment epithelium and grow behind the iris or extend across the pupil to form a pupillary membrane (56). Sometimes the neovascular vessels may disappear from view because of shrinkage of the connective tissue, which may compress the embedded vessels and obscure them from direct observation, erroneously suggesting that the vessels have resolved (56). Probably the most important factor in identifying early neovascularization is the clinician's index of suspicion. Simply put, if you don't look for it, you won't see it.

Normal Angle and Iris Vasculature

The examiner should be familiar with the normal iris and angle vasculature in order to prevent mistaking the normal angle and iris vessels as neovascular vessels (Plates 18 and 27). The major and minor vascular circles are located at the root of the iris and at the pupillary margin, respectively, with the arterial circle of the ciliary body being the arterial source for the angle. The major arterial circle is usually located posterior to the peripheral iris within the ciliary muscle. It is formed by the long posterior ciliary artery and the anterior ciliary artery. The anterior ciliary artery penetrates from the outer sclera to join the long posterior ciliary arteries running along the inner scleral surface (33). Fine vessels arising from the circle supply the ciliary muscle and the larger branches; the radial iris arteries course toward the pupil, forming the minor arterial circle.

Gonioscopically, four types of normal angle vessels may be observed corresponding to the major arterial circle, its branches, and branches of the anterior ciliary vessels (see Figures 2.7 and 2.8). Henkind described three distinct types of normal vessels. He named them the *circular ciliary band vessels*, *radial iris vessels*, and the *radial ciliary band vessels* or *trabecular vessels* (73). The first two are more commonly seen than the latter.

The circular ciliary band vessel is the most common and is often seen beyond the last roll of the iris or upon the surface of the ciliary body (Plates 18, 25, and 27). It runs circumferentially and represents the major arterial circle of the iris. It is often observed in a light-colored eye and appears to undulate along with the iris root undulations, appearing and disappearing along the circumference of the angle. It is usually thick and sometimes can rise as high as the scleral spur or trabecular meshwork.

The radial iris vessels originate from the arterial circle. They usually run a short distance from their origin and then disappear into the iris stroma. They can be observed to "hook over the last roll of the iris" (73). In light-colored irides, they may be observed as far as the mid-iris before they dip into the stroma. They usually run in a straight line without anastomosing or coursing diagonally (33). These vessels may be confused for neovascular vessels when they become dilated in an inflamed eye. Unlike neovascular vessels, the radial iris vessels and the circular ciliary body vessels are thick and usually surrounded by a white sheath.

The radial ciliary band or trabecular vessels are probably branches of the arterial circle in the area of Schlemm's canal or extensions of the anterior ciliary arteries. They may be observable in lightly pigmented eyes or in eyes that have suffered an angle recession. They appear to lie within the ciliary body or trabecular region and run as a thin linear streak perpendicular to the iris. Because of this appearance, they can be easily confused with neovascular vessels; however, they cannot be observed to be connected to any other vessels, nor are there branching vessels running off them. Additionally, the lack of rubeosis irides at the pupil border and the lack of associated neovascular-inducing conditions aid in differentiating these vessels from neovascular vessels.

I have seen gonioscopically a fourth type of vessel coursing along the angle wall, almost appearing imbedded into the wall (Plate 48). It is similar in thickness to the circular ciliary band vessels, without a white sheath. It runs perpendicular to the iris, runs along the wall without branching, and then abruptly dives into the sclera. It probably is one of the ciliary arteries (33).

Neovascular vessels are fine, thin vessels, without sheathing, that course along the surface of the iris in an irregular fashion, and when they reach the wall, they run perpendicular to the ciliary body and climb up to the trabecular meshwork, branching out along the meshwork surface. They often appear to dive into the filtering segment of the angle. In the early stages, they have a strawberry-like coloration rather than a deep, dark-red hue.

Nonprogressive Neovascular Iris Tufts at the Pupil Ruff

Pupillary vascular abnormalities that have been referred to as vascular tufts, microhemangiomas, hemangiomas, and neovascular iris tufts have been described (74,75,76,77). Microscopically they have been reported to be neovascular vessels although clinically they do not tend to change or cause neovascularization of the iris surface or angle (78). They can be a cause of blurred vision from associated spontaneous anterior chamber hemorrhage, have rarely been associated with acute glaucoma, and can be confused with progressive

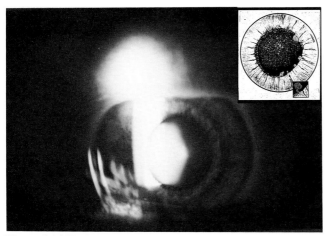

Figure 6.14 Nonprogressive neovascular tufts at pupil border.

neovascularization (74,76,77,78,79,80) (Figure 6.14). Unlike neovascular vessels, which lie on the iris surface and grow into the angle, these tufts are adjacent to, or overlap, the pupil ruff. They typically protrude from the iris in single or multiple loops and are separate from each other without forming a vascular network (74,75,77,80). On slit lamp examination, they will appear as distinct raised red dots, consisting of coils of blood vessels with thin, transparent walls, spiralled into glomular or mulberry tufts (80,81,82). The individual vessels are small, 15 to 25 microns in size, with a single tuft being approximately 150 microns in size (83). Pressure against the globe may result in the blood emptying from the vessel, making them harder to detect. In a majority of cases, they are bilateral and appear in patients over 45 years of age (80).

There appears to be no consistent systemic abnormality associated with these tufts. In addition to occurring in healthy individuals, they have been reported in patients with elevated blood glucose levels, diabetes, congenital heart disease, hypertension, central retinal vein occlusion, and myotonic dystrophy (75,81,82,84). If the tufts are detected on routine examination, gonioscopy should be performed looking for evidence of iris surface and angle neovascularization, and the patient should be followed closely for progression of the vascularization as some observers feel these vascular tufts serve as an indication of ocular and systemic disease (81,85). It should be noted that some diabetics may have neovascularization at the pupil region that remains stable for many years; therefore when the pupil ruff tufts (microhemangiomas) are found in eyes of diabetics, fluoresceine angiography should be considered, looking for evidence of capillary nonperfusion (ischemia) (69). This will aid in differentiating these vessels from the progressive neovascular vessels. The pupil ruff tufts have been observed in a number of eyes, some in diabetic patients, which have remained stable for many years.

Neovascularization in Uveitis

Almost all instances of iris neovascularization are associated with retinal vascular occlusive disease and retinal anoxia however anterior uveitis may precipitate neovascularization. In most instances, the presumed neovascular vessels are actually dilated normal vessels. Clinically the dilated vessels are difficult to differentiate from neovascularization (86) (Plate 1). Usually the dilation and prominence of the vessels will resolve after the inflammation has subsided. If the vessels remain dilated, however, they may well be neovascular. One recent study found that 26% of patients with Fuch's heterochromic uveitis had glaucoma and that 20% of the glaucomatous cases in the late stage were associated with neovascularization (87).

Gonioscopically the vessels often appear as fine, sparse, solitary angle vessels, running circumferentially and radially, they rarely branch along the trabecular meshwork and even more rarely proceeed to PAS (33,88,89). The prevalence of true angle and iris neovasculaarization in Fuch's heterochromic uveitis is unclear probably because, as the iris atrophies, the normal vasculature, particularly the radial ciliary vessels, becomes more prominent and confused for neovascular vessels (90). Clinically the observation of iris and angle neovascularization in Fuch's heterochromic uveitis is rare but chronic anterior ischemia is common even in early cases (64). Gonioscopy has been reported commonly to produce anterior chamber hemorrhage in heterochromic cyclitis from two locations, the canal of Schlemm and the radial ciliary vessels (90).

Stages of Iris Neovascularization

Classifying the stages of neovascularization will aid in predicting clinical prognosis, will simplify communication and records, and can be used for evaluating the efficacy of treatment (59). The following stages are adapted from Gartner and Henkind's, Wand's, and Weiss and Gold's classifications (56,59,71,91,92).

Stage 1. Early neovascularization (Plate 39) is detected by the observation of tiny tufts of new vessels at the pupil margin in less than two quadrants. These are the first signs of neovascularization. Histologically, they appear as an aneurysm of preexisting capillaries. They enlarge over time. In this stage it may be difficult initially to differentiate the nonprogressive pupil ruff iris tufts (microhemangiomas) from the more progressive ones (59,93). Although the angle is usually not involved at this stage, angle neovascular vessels may precede pupil margin, iris surface, and/or retinal neovascularization. Henkind has noted that the iris vessels are more likely to be stimulated to form new vessels than are the retina or optic nerve vessels (94). This emphasizes the need for gonioscopic evaluation in suspect eyes even when there is no obvious iris or retinal neovascularization (56,59,73).

Stage II. As the process continues, the new vessels extend on the iris surface in an irregular pattern. When the vessels reach the collarette, the normally present collarette vessels may become engorged and become part of the neovascular vasculature. The angle is usually not involved; if it is, however, more than two quadrants will be neovascularized. This stage will also differentiate true progressive neovascularization from the nonprogressive pupil ruff tufts as the progressive vessels are observed to run along on the iris surface.

CHAPTER 6. SECONDARY ANGLE CLOSURE GLAUCOMA

Stage III. If the process continues, the ciliary iris portion becomes involved and the vessels reach the angle, join the normal circumferential ciliary artery where new vessels emanate from, and proceed to cross the ciliary body and course along the angle wall perpendicular to the ciliary body band, and spread out in a branching fashion along the trabecular meshwork. The vessels along the angle wall may be somewhat difficult to detect at this time unless careful gonioscopy is done, preferably with a large Goldmann-type lens, which provides a parallel, stable, detailed view of the angle wall. Open-angle glaucoma may exist at this stage secondary to a clinically invisible fibrovascular membrane covering the trabecular meshwork that is invisible on gonioscopy. Three quadrants of the iris and angle are involved in this stage. Ectropion uvea is present, involving one to three quadrants. The ectropion uvea results from contraction of the fibrovascular tissue that pulls the pigmented layer of the iris forward (56). Isolated areas of synechial closure (PAS) from fibrous contraction may be observed. The neovascularization may continue to progress, sometimes quite rapidly, eventually leading to complete synechial closure and the next stage.

Stage IV. PAS involves at least three quadrants of the angle. In some eyes with burned out neovascularization, the vessels may be less evident, with only an occasional vessel visible as connective tissue surrounding the vessels covers the iris. The iris loses it sponginess. It becomes thin and flat, losing its normal delicate and wavy anterior surface and the crypts disappear. Ectropion uveae involve more than three quadrants of the pupil border. Three hundred and sixty degrees of ectropion uvea is characteristic for neovascularization of the iris (56).

Glaucoma Treatment with Angle Neovascularization

Glaucoma associated with angle neovascularization may be an early open-angle form or a later angle closure form (71). In some eyes, small buds of vessels on the iris at the pupil margin will be present with normal IOP. It is important to differentiate clinically very early the neovascular vessels from the normal vessels of the iris circulation because the new blood vessels may become associated with a clinically invisible fibrovascular membrane that forms on the surface of the iris and in the angle. When this membrane is present, the eye will look gonioscopically normal, particularly if no new vessels have yet formed in the angle. The IOP, however, may be elevated because of the membrane, and thus, an open-angle glaucoma will be present. This membrane has the potential to grow and contract and cause an intractable glaucoma by means of circumferential peripheral anterior synechia. In some cases, until the trabecular meshwork is significantly covered by the new vessels, the IOP may remain normal because it is not the vessels themselves that cause the glaucoma (4,59). With neovascularization secondary to carotid occlusive disease, the IOP may remain normal or low, possibly related to secondary ciliary body atrophy and decreased aqueous production (58,95). In rare instances, blood vessels may be present in the angle before being detected at the pupil margin, and they may also be present in eyes devoid of retinal neovascularization, indicating the need for gonioscopic evaluation in suspect eyes even when there is no observable iris neovascularization or retinal neovascularization (56,59,73).

It has been suggested that the best treatment for neovascular angle closure glaucoma is prevention (Table 6.6) (71). Diabetic patients may help by controlling their blood glucose level and blood pressure. Some suggest prophylactic PRP in high-risk eyes such as those suffering CRVO with evidence of capillary nonperfusion, eyes with diabetic retinopathy undergoing cataract or vitrectomy surgery, and eyes with rubeosis of the iris even without angle involvement and without evidence of increased pressure (61,71).

Panretinal photocoagulation (PRP) and panretinal cryotherapy (PRC) result in stabilization or regression of iris neovascularization and improvement of the neovascular glaucoma (59,96). The destruction of the hypoxic retinal tissue is assumed to eliminate or decrease the stimulus for new vessel growth (94). The success of PRP is strongly related to the amount of pretreatment PAS. It has been shown to be effective for eyes with neovascularization in stages I, II, and III. The prognosis is poor when PAS involves more than 270 degrees of the angle, stage IV, leading some to recommend other treatments; PRP will still decrease the stimulus for the neovascularization, however, and allow for safer surgical treatment (59,96). Evidence of iris/angle neovascularization and PAS stabilization and regression can be observed within one to four weeks following completed PRP (59,96). In eyes with dark irides, the neovascular vessels are replaced by atrophic white fibrous strands. In eyes with light irides, the abnormal vessels will become clinically undetectable (96).

PRC can be used as an alternative treatment when PRP fails or when the retina cannot be visualized properly for PRP, because of either an opaque media or poor patient cooperation (71). Goniophotocoagulation, direct argon laser application to angle blood vessels, has limited use. This technique

TABLE 6.6
Treatment for Neovascular Glaucoma

Goal	Method
Prevention by early recognition in an at-risk eye	Careful slit lamp and gonioscopic examination, prophylactic PRP
Decrease stimulus for neovascularization	PRP, cryopexy
Stop progression of neovascular angle vessels	Goniophotocoagulation
Medical treatment to lower IOP	Atropine, topical steroids, aqueous suppressants (avoid miotics)
Surgery to lower IOP	Filtering surgery with 5 FU, drainage implants
Reduce aqueous production and reduce pain in blind eye	Medical treatment, nd:YAG cyclotherapy, bandage soft lens for bullous keratopathy, retrobulbar alcohol injection, enucleation

has been recommended as a first level of treatment prior to retinal cryopexy. It has also been used when PRP is not possible as a temporary treatment before PRP and in eyes with neovascularization before undergoing cataract or glaucoma surgery. The goal of goniophotocoagulation is to stop the progression of angle closure. This treatment, however, will not stop the stimulus for new vessel growth (97).

Conventional filtering procedures in eyes with neovascular glaucoma are often unsuccessful because of intraoperative complications and postoperative progression of the fibrovascular membrane but the use of antimetabolites such as 5-fluorouracil (5-FU) with anterior chamber drainage implants may be considered as an alternative in eyes with uncontrolled neovascular glaucoma and useful vision (71,98) (Figure 6.15). As a last resort when pain persists in a blind eye, cyclotherapy, using trans-scleral YAG cyclophotocoagulation, causes destruction of the ciliary epithelium and will reduce aqueous production and relieve pain (71).

Medical therapy for neovascular glaucoma is aimed at lowering the IOP and reducing pain. It should include the use of antiglaucoma medications with the exception of cholinergic and epinephrine agents, which may increase pain and are often not effective in lowering the IOP (21). Miotics also stretch the iris, which may lead to hemorrhage and hyphema. They also contribute to iris vessel congestion (99). Atropine helps decrease ocular congestion and increases uveal scleral outflow, and topical steroids help reduce inflammation. Both are recommended. Close observation must be used when prescribing carbonic anhydrase inhibitors or osmotic agents for diabetic patients, watching for systemic side effects (99).

In cases of end stage glaucoma where synechia is total and the eye is blind, keeping the patient pain free is the primary goal. In some patients this can be accomplished by medical means, using 1% atropine twice a day, and topical steroid solutions four times daily. In addition topical beta blockers and/or carbonic anhydrase inhibitors may be helpful. When pain exists secondary to bullous keratopathy, bandage soft lenses are often helpful. When pain cannot be relieved medically or surgically, a retrobulbar injection of alcohol will often provide relief (100). If pain persists, enucleation may be necessary.

Malignant Glaucoma

Classic malignant glaucoma was described as a rare postoperative complication following surgery for angle closure glaucoma by von Graefe in 1869 (101). Over the years, a number of cases have been reported to result in a similar clinical form of secondary angle closure glaucoma with the following characteristics: a flat-to-shallow anterior chamber both centrally and peripherally, lack of iris bombé, poor or no response to miotics, elevated IOP, positive response to mydriatic agents, and ineffectiveness of iridectomy as treatment (102–111) (Table 6.7). The slit lamp appearance of uniform marked shallowing of the central (flat to 2.5 corneal thickness) and peripheral chambers, which corresponds to the relative position of the crystalline lens and produces an iris contour appearing parallel to the cornea, is crucial for differentiating this type of angle closure in phakic, pseudophakic, and aphakic forms (111). (In aphakic forms the iris contour assumes this configuration secondary to forward movement of the anterior hyaloid).

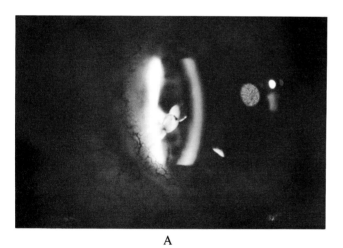

A

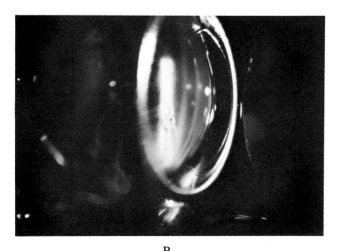

B

Figure 6.15 (A) Slit lamp view of anterior chamber filtering tube with Molteno implant. (B) Gonioscopic view of the same eye.

TABLE 6.7
Malignant Glaucoma Clincial Characteristics

Unilateral flat central and peripheral anterior chamber
  (flat to 2.5 corneal thicknesses centrally)
Absence of iris bombé
Absence of pupil block
Unilateral myopic refractive shift
IOP usually elevated
Poor response to miotics
Poor response to iridotomy, iridectomy
Requires mydriatic-cycloplegic therapy
Gonioscopically closed angle
No change to iris contour on compression gonioscopy

CHAPTER 6. SECONDARY ANGLE CLOSURE GLAUCOMA

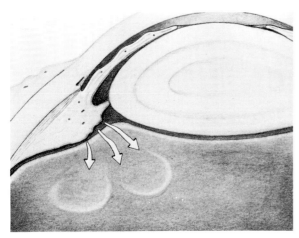

Figure 6.16 Aqueous flow in malignant glaucoma misdirected posterior. Notice the contour of the iris parallel to the cornea and the forward rotation of the ciliary body. (Reprinted with permission from Obstbaum SA. Glaucoma surgery. Norwalk, Conn.. Appleton and Lange, 1991.)

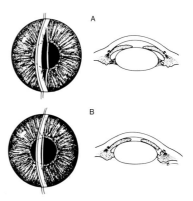

Figure 6.17 Distinction between pupillary block glaucoma and malignant glaucoma. (A) In pupillary block glaucoma, there is moderate depth to the central anterior chamber, with forward bowing of the peripheral iris. (B) In malignant glaucoma, the entire lens-iris diaphragm is shifted forward with marked shallowing or loss of the central anterior chamber. This configuration persists even with a patent peripheral iridectomy. (Reprinted with permission from Shields MB. Textbook of glaucoma, 3d ed. Baltimore: Williams & Wilkins, 1992.

In addition to the term *malignant glaucoma*, these cases have been named *aqueous misdirection syndrome, ciliary block glaucoma, cilio-vitreo-lenticular block*, and *direct lens block*, an indication of the varied mechanisms, considered to be involved in producing this form of glaucoma as well as its varied site of pathology (26,34,104,112). In all cases there appears to be an impediment to the forward flow of aqueous, resulting in the collection and entrapment of aqueous within the vitreous (Figure 6.16). The most likely locations for this interference is the lens-ciliary body sinus or the anterior vitreous. Evidence that the ciliary tips are rotated anterior to the anteriorly placed lens equator suggests that the blockage of aqueous occurs in the area. The site for this blockage, however, may be different in different forms of this condition (112,113,114). The ensuing expansion of the vitreous leads to the forward movement of the iris-lens diaphragm, which results in angle closure. Swelling or forward rotation of the ciliary body or ciliary tips may initiate this process by causing lens-ciliary body apposition or lens-ciliary body-vitreous adhesions. In addition to being a complication of glaucoma surgery, this clinical form of angle closure has been described to occur secondary to the use of miotics, ciliary body edema or uveal effusion, or from an increase to the posterior segment volume (109,113). An increase in the posterior segment volume itself may induce an anterior movement of the iris lens diaphragm, resulting in a similar clinical picture (115,116). This has been described in eyes suffering spontaneous subretinal or choroidal hemorrhages (116).

Direct lens block from a forward shifting of the crystalline lens, causing the lens periphery to force the peripheral iris into the angle, has also been proposed as a primary factor in the pathogenesis of malignant glaucoma (26,117). Luntz and Rosenblatt feel that any emphasis placed on the lens as a primary mechanism is flawed because it underestimates the role of the vitreous, which has been shown to have altered permeability in some forms of this disorder (113,118). Cases where the glaucoma persists after lens extraction when the cataract surgery is not accompanied by vitreous loss, incision, or aspiration exemplifies this point. It is likely that there are a number of different factors involved in producing this clinical presentation, and in some cases, it may be just one mechanism while in others it may be a combination of mechanisms; common to all, however, are the clinical characteristics already noted and the absence of pupillary block as the primary mechanism for restricted forward aqueous flow and the lack of iris bombé as a clinical sign (105,113,118, 119) (Figure 6.17).

Another important diagnostic characteristic is the initial unilateral presentation of this disorder (although a rare case of a bilateral presentation has recently been reported) (120). This corresponds to the clinical appearance of asymmetrical chamber depths and configurations between the eyes. The fellow eye has a normal or slightly shallow chamber depth when compared to the marked anterior chamber shallowing of the involved eye. In contrast, cases of primary angle closure with pupil block typically have eyes with symmetrically shallow anterior chambers axially (not as shallow as eyes with malignant glaucoma) and narrow angles. Thus comparison of the anterior chamber configuration between the eyes aids in identifying this form of angle closure and illustrates its secondary nature. In addition, forward movement and thickening of the crystalline lens induces a significant unilateral myopic shift in refraction (104,105,107).

Gonioscopy

Gonioscopically the angle structures may not be visible because the iris surface is usually too convex to see over and the iris lens diaphragm has shifted anteriorly (107). Compression gonioscopy assists in differentiating this form

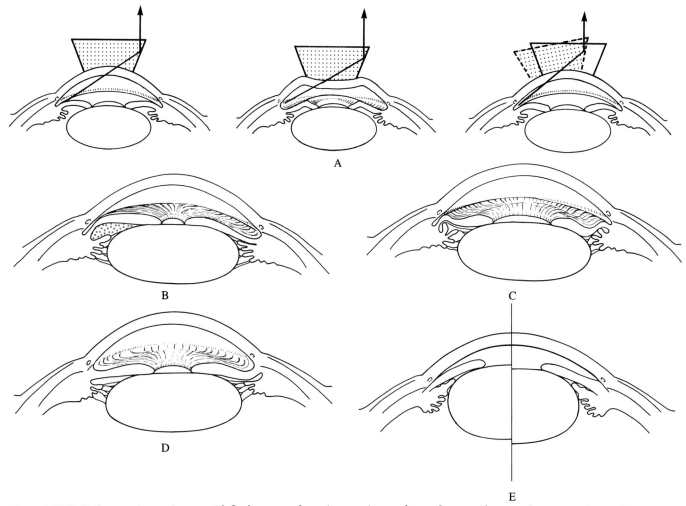

Figure 6.18 (B–E) Compression gonioscopy with flat-base curve four-mirror gonioscopy lenses. In eyes with narrow but open angles, avoid compression to see into the angle recess when evaluating the angle's natural status. (A) Left: Unable to view into angle recess of narrow but open angle. Middle: Avoid full corneal contact and unwanted compression to view into the angle. Right: Gently tilt and raise the lens slightly toward the angle of observation. This will place the gonioscopy mirror closer to the angle and will position the mirror slightly higher, providing a higher vantage point. This will enable the observer to see over the bowed iris without inducing unwanted compression.

Compression gonioscopy in closed angles. Left side of drawing represents a closed angle. Right side represents appearance with compression gonioscopy. (B) Left: Primary angle closure with pupil block and without PAS. The iris is being pushed into the angle. Right: Compression gonioscopy pushes the peripheral iris posterior and opens the angle. (C) Left: Plateau iris angle closure. Notice the anterior placement of the ciliary processes. Right: Compression gonioscopy will move posteriorly the peripheral iris free of the ciliary processes. The portion of the iris held forward by the ciliary processes will not move posterior. (D) Left: Secondary angle with PAS, for example, neovascular glaucoma, ICE syndrome. The peripheral iris is pulled into the angle and attached to the angle wall. Right: With compression the iris root will remain attached to the angle wall; however, the midperipheral iris free from attachment will bow posterior. (E) Left: Angle closure in phakic malignant glaucoma. The iris-lens diaphragm is anteriorly placed. Compression gonioscopy may open the angle slightly by pushing the entire iris-lens diaphragm posteriorly; however, the iris will not change contour.

of angle closure from pupil block angle closure and plateau iris (Figure 6.18). In pupil block unless the IOP is very high, compression gonioscopy will widen the angle by forcing the peripheral iris posterior where it is free of the lens and PAS. This creates a volcanolike iris contour. In plateau iris, the midperipheral iris will have the greatest posterior movement because the peripheral iris is held forward by the anteriorly placed ciliary processes. In malignant glaucoma, compression gonioscopy may in fact allow the wall structures to become visible (where PAS is absent), but the iris surface contour retains its convex shape, conforming to the crystalline lens,

and will not bow backward in the periphery, suggesting an absence of a formed posterior chamber (107,111). The lens-iris diaphragm and or iris-vitreous-lens diaphragm and ciliary body prevents the iris root from dropping posterior.

Classic Postoperative Malignant Glaucoma

Classically malignant glaucoma is defined as an elevation of IOP occurring in patients who have had angle closure glaucoma surgery or after glaucoma filtering surgery in the presence of a flat anterior chamber, patent iridectomy, and nonresponsiveness or worsening with miotic therapy or topical hypotensive agents (118). (It is malignant in the difficulty in treatment, not in the sense of neoplastic disease. [121,122]). The malignant glaucoma may develop early after the surgery or some time later, typically when cycloplegic agents are stopped and/or miotic agents are instituted. It is believed to be the result of misdirection of the aqueous into the vitreous cavity and the presence of an increased resistance to forward flow of the trapped aqueous from a thickened, less diffusible vitreous (112,118). The vitreous cavity expands and pushes the lens, iris, and ciliary body forward, shallowing the chamber and narrowing and closing the angle. It occurs in less than 1% to 4% of eyes subsequent to filtering or iridectomy surgery (114,118).

This condition can occur in both phakic and aphakic eyes, and it ultimately occurs postoperatively in both eyes (74,80). Thus, the diagnosis in one eye makes the second eye suspect, and if surgery is required in the fellow eye, the patient should have a course of medical therapy prior to surgery (113). This consists of the same regimen used for treatment in active cases (discussed below). Whenever possible, surgery should be avoided in the fellow eye.

If the patient is undergoing cataract extraction in the fellow eye, the risk for malignant glaucoma can be reduced if a prophylactic disruption of the posterior capsule and anterior vitreous can be performed at the time of the surgery (105). The etiology of malignant glaucoma is considered similar for phakic and pseudophakic eyes with anterior chamber or iris fixed lenses. In an eye with a PC-IOL after ECCE, the barrier to aqueous flow may be a cellular and fibrin reaction secondary to residual lens cortex and fibrocellular material causing an inflammatory membrane, adhesions of capsular material to the iris, the peripheral hyaloid, or some deeper vitreous abnormality (123,124,125).

According to Simmons and colleagues, the greatest chance for developing malignant glaucoma occurs in eyes with some portion of the angle still closed after surgery for angle closure (122). This risk seems to have little relationship to the type of conventional surgery or to the presurgical IOP. Recently it has been reported in cases after laser iridotomy, suggesting that the risk is not limited to conventional surgery (102,103, 110). Identification of eyes that experience increased angle narrowing and chamber shallowing on miotics is important because they may be more prone to postoperative malignant glaucoma (121).

Asssuming other causes of a flat anterior chamber have been ruled out, such as a wound leak or overfiltration in postoperative cases, this form of flat chamber angle closure glaucoma needs to be differentiated from angle closure from choroidal separation, suprachoroidal hemorrhage, plateau iris, or pupillary block (Table 6.8). In pupillary block, a patent iridotomy will relieve the pressure, and the central chamber is usually not flat or, for that matter, altered from its preoperative depth, because the central chamber depth does not change after successful iridotomy (111). Also, primary pupil block angle closure tends to be bilateral, and although the chamber may be shallow in the nonoperated eye, the operated eye will tend to have a much shallower central chamber (2.5 corneal thicknesses or less), with an iris contour conforming to the lens, without iris bombé. The absence of a shallow-to-flat axial chamber and the effectiveness of mydriatic agents in deepening the chamber and lowering the IOP rules out the presence of plateau iris (105,110).

Choroidal detachments can cause a shallow or flat anterior chamber, but the IOP is usually "soft" (121). In rare cases, angle closure glaucoma may result from choroidal detachments because of anterior rotation of the ciliary body or pressure on the vitreous forcing the lens-iris diaphragm forward (107,118) (Table 6.9). The light-brown ophthalmoscopic appearance of the separated choroid and B-scan ultrasound evidence of choroidal separation will aid in the differentiation. If the choroidal separation occurs with hemorrhage, the

TABLE 6.8
Differential Diagnosis

	Malignant Glaucoma	Choroidal Separation	Pupillary Block	Suprachoroidal Hemorrhage
Anterior chamber	Flat or shallow	Flat or shallow	Iris bombé—not as shallow as others	Flat or shallow
Intraocular pressure	Normal or elevated	Subnormal	Normal or elevated	Normal or elevated
Fundus appearance	No choroidal elevation	Large, smooth, light brown choroidal elevations	Normal	Dark brown or dark red choroidal elevations
Suprachoroidal fluid	Absent	Straw-colored fluid present	Absent	Light red or dark brown blood present
Relief by drainage of suprachoroidal fluid	No	Yes	No	Yes
Relief by iridectomy	No	No	Yes	No
Patent iridectomy	Yes	Yes	No	Yes

Adapted from Simmons RJ, Thomas JU, Yaqub MK. Malignant glaucoma. In Ritch R, Shields MB, Krupin T, eds. *The glaucomas*, vol 2. St Louis: CV Mosby, 1989.

TABLE 6.9
Angle Closure Glaucoma Complicating Ciliochoroidal Disorders

Inflammatory
  Scleritis
  Pars planitis
  Harada's disease (V-K-H syndrome)
  Hemorrhagic fever with renal syndrome
  Autoimmune deficiency syndrome

Vascular
  Post-central retinal vein occlusion
  Nanophthalmos
  Arteriovenous malformation

Postoperative
  Cataract extraction, aphakia
  Trauma
  Scleral buckling
  Post-panretinal photocoagulation

Neoplastic
  Malignant melanoma
  Pseudomotor
  Pseudotumor
  Ocular metastases

Physiologic
  Ciliary body spasm

Idiopathic
  Uveal effusion syndrome

Reprinted with permission from Fourman S. Angle-closure glaucoma complicating ciliochoroidal detachment. *Ophthalmology.* 1989;96:646–653.

patient usually experiences a deep, sudden, acute pain, flattening of the anterior chamber, and hyperemia to the eye; ophthalmoscopically, the detachment will appear dark reddish-brown (121). The characteristic ophthalmoscopic appearance and ultrasound evidence of choroidal detachments also differentiate this form of acute angle closure glaucoma complicating nonsurgical choroidal detachments.

Malignant Glaucoma Not Associated with Glaucoma Surgery

Malignant glaucoma has been reported in cases other than those occurring after surgery for angle closure (103,104,108).

This includes cases developing after cataract surgery with the use of miotics or carbonic anhydrase inhibitors, in cases of cyclitis, scleritis, and even spontaneous presentations in unoperated eyes (104–107,109,126). Some prefer to call these *related cases*, reserving the classification of malignant glaucoma for cases associated with invasive surgery, usually for angle closure or cataracts. The related cases have similar clinical characteristics to those found in classically described malignant glaucoma, respond to the same treatments, and are therefore usually classified as malignant glaucoma (118).

Two mechanisms have been proposed to explain the blockage of forward aqueous movement and posterior misdirection in these related cases. In some instances, a forward rotation of the ciliary body around the scleral spur may cause aqueous forward flow obstruction. This can occur from ciliary body edema, ciliary body cellular infiltration, or spasm of the ciliary muscle (Figure 6.19). The ciliary muscle thickens and rotates forward, blocking flow, obliterating the posterior chamber, and inducing a ciliary block angle closure (114). Interference of uveal tract venous drainage has also been implicated as one of the causes of this scenario. This can occur after a CRVO, panretinal photocoagulation, or scleral buckling procedures (107).

In other instances, the inciting mechanism may be an increase in pressure in the posterior segment from increased posterior volume (118). This causes forward movement of the lens-iris diaphragm, blocking aqueous flow forward and closing off the posterior chamber and resulting in a non-pupillary block form of angle closure. (In some of these cases, pupil block may develop secondarily.)

Either of these mechanisms may cause a form of malignant glaucoma reported after panretinal photocoagulation, central retinal vein occlusions, retinal surgery with encircling buckles, from tumors, in pars planitis, with arteriovenous fistulas, in acquired immunodeficiency syndrome, in (choroidal, retinal, or vitreous) hemorrhages, in dural shunt syndromes, or in posterior scleritis, some of which are associated with or without choroidal effusions (107,114,115,116,120,126,127). Hyams notes that the risk for this type of glaucoma developing

TABLE 6.10
Anatomical Blocks to Fluid Flow Causing Aqueous Diversion and Loculation in Malignant Glaucoma

Location of Block	Area of Aqueous Accumulation	Treatment Aimed at Aqueous Pool and Abnormal Flow
Irido-lens capsule block (irido-vitreal block in aphakes)	Vitreous	Lysis of adhesions, re-creation of posterior chamber, iridectomy, posterior sclerotomy, and vitreous tap (or anterior vitrectomy)
Ciliolens block*	Vitreous	Cycloplegia, hypersomotics, posterior sclerotomy, and vitreous aspiration (formerly lensectomy)
Iridovitreal, ciliovitreal in aphakes	Vitreous	As for ciliolens block
Suprachoroidal effusion with possible rotation of ciliary body and processes	Initially suprachoroidal space, possibly vitreous	Posterior sclerotomy, drainage of suprachoroidal fluid with or without vitreous aspiration

Miscellaneous related entities, of unclear pathogenesis, which may behave clinically as part of the truly malignant glaucoma entity

  Central vein occlusion
  Retrolental fibroplasia
  Buckling in retinal detachment surgery
  Fungal infections

*"Classic" malignant glaucoma is most commonly felt to be a subtype of ciliary lens block with aqueous diversion into the vitreous.
(Adapted from Luntz MH, Rosenblatt M. Malignant glaucoma. *Surv Ophthalmol.* 1987;32(2):73–93.

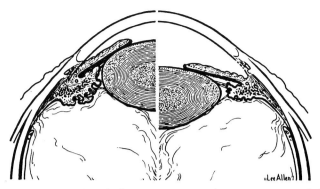

Figure 6.19 Right side demonstrates normal anterior segment. Left side demonstrates changes from ciliary body swelling. The ciliary body is rotated about the scleral spur, producing an angle closure, lens displacement forward, and lens thickening. (Reprinted with permission from Phelps CD. Angle closure glaucoma secondary to ciliary body swelling. Arch Ophthalmol. *1974;92:287–290 c/r 1974, American Medical Association.*

after central retinal vein occlusions and panretinal photocoagulation suggests that caution should be exercised when performing panretinal photocoagulation in an eye with a shallowed chamber subsequent to a CRVO. It is probably preferable for these eyes to have laser treatment done in stages (114). In nonoperated eyes, malignant glaucoma must be differented from pupil block, plateau iris, synechial closure, and posterior space occupying lesions, pushing the lens-iris diaphragm forward (105).

Treatment

As has been already noted, malignant glaucoma and related cases have similar clinical presentations, and although the site of aqueous blockage may be at different locations and from different mechanisms, the treatment strategy is similar for all cases. According to Luntz and Rosenblatt, the principles of treatment are (1) to relieve the aqueous obstruction by medical means, and (2) if necessary to correct the obstruction surgically, to reestablish a normal pathway for the aqueous, and to drain the aqueous from its trapped location (118) (Table 6.10).

Medical treatment for malignant glaucoma and related cases consists of using mydriatic and cycloplegic agents and avoiding miotic agents. The cycloplegic-mydriatic agents tighten the zonules and gradually pull the lens posterior against the vitreous. This relieves the vitreous pressure against the iris, lens, and ciliary processes and allows the posterior chamber to form and aqueous to filter forward. In some cases, these agents are not adequate, and reduction of aqueous production using carbonic anhydrase inhibitors and topical beta-blockers is added as well as hyperosmotic agents to reduce vitreous volume. Topical steroids are also used to reduce inflammation particularly to the ciliary body. They also reduce the risk for inflammatory synechial closure (121). Simmons and colleagues recommend that early medical therapy includes mydriatics, cycloplegics, carbonic anhydrase inhibitors, hyperosmotics, and topical beta-blockers until the anterior chamber forms and the IOP is lowered (122). This may take as long as five days and is successful in 50% of cases. Once the attack

is broken, the hyperosmotic agents and carbonic anhydrase inhibitors can be tapered and the mydriatic stopped with the cycloplegic agent being continued indefinitely (121).

If medical therapy fails, surgical intervention in an attempt to expel the captured aqueous and restore normal aqueous movement is necessary by removal of posterior vitreous fluid with disruption of the anterior hyaloid face. This can be accomplished by anterior pars plana virectomy, establishing an opening in the vitreous face for the aqueous to escape forward or by means of posterior sclerotomy with aspiration of fluid and air injection into the anterior chamber to deepen the anterior chamber. Conservative treatment involves Nd:YAG treatment to the hyaloid face, breaking the cycle of poor permeability of the vitreous. Laser application to the ciliary processes, if visible, has also been tried, and the success of this according to Hyams may be related to a small disruption of the anterior hyaloid, providing an avenue for fluid to move into the posterior chamber, rather than any shrinking of the ciliary processes (114,128). Lens extraction with incision into the anterior hyaloid face is the more traditional treatment and is still used.

In cases of angle closure with choroidal effusion, suprachoroidal drainage may be necessary to relieve the glaucoma although cases may respond to medical therapy (121). The higher the IOP (greater than 15 mm Hg) in an eye with a flat chamber, the greater the risk is for complications of corneal edema, endothelial cell decompensation, and PAS, so prompt treatment is necessary.

Malignant glaucoma also occurs in cases of aphakia and pseudophakia and should be differentiated from vitreopupillary block, which is the result of the posterior hyaloid face's contacting the posterior iris surface, blocking aqueous flow. In this case, the posterior chamber is still formed, iris bombé is evident, and an iridotomy will allow communication between the two chambers, relieving pupil block. In malignant glaucoma, the posterior chamber is abolished, the central and peripheral chamber is shallow and/or flat, and an iridotomy will not eliminate the problem. If malignant glaucoma is present, the use of Nd:YAG laser treatment for disrupting the anterior hyaloid face is considered effective (125,129).

Mixed Secondary Angle Closure Glaucoma

Miotic-Induced Angle Closure

Miotics can cause a nonpupil block angle closure by pulling the ciliary body forward and rotating it around the scleral spur or possibly by sufficiently increasing forward lens movement in predisposed eyes (130). This may reduce the space between the lens and the ciliary body, obliterating the posterior chamber and causing aqueous to flow posterior and increasing forward movement of the lens-iris diaphragm (109).

Miotics may also induce pupil block in narrow angles by causing forward movement of the lens in combination with sphincter tightening against the lens. This impedes the flow of aqueous from the posterior chamber to the anterior chamber, with resultant bombé and pupil block closure. Although rare, the potential does exist for even weaker miotics such as pilocarpine to induce a pupil block angle closure attack or worsen an ongoing attack (109,131). When miotics increase pupil block, the angle narrows, the iris has a bombé appearance, and gonioscopically the width of the recess narrows.

Inflammation

Inflammation may cause acute angle closure with or without pupil block. Pupil block occurs when there is an anterior chamber inflammation and the iris at the pupil border becomes attached to the lens by synechia 360 degrees, resulting in a secluded pupil. The aqueous becomes trapped in the posterior chamber, and the iris bows forward because of the pupil block and closes the angle. The depth of the central chamber remains unchanged; if it was normal before the inflammation, it remains that way. Depending on the status of the ciliary body, the IOP may be elevated or decreased.

This type of attack can be aborted by dilating the pupil and breaking the synechia. A laser iridotomy can be performed, but in the presence of inflammation, the opening can close quickly with fibrin, and a surgical iridectomy may need to be performed. The laser treatment may exacerbate inflammation, and prolonged frequent steroid application may be necessary after laser treatment (132).

Nonpupillary block closure can occur when the ciliary body becomes inflamed, swells, rotates forward, and blocks the posterior chamber, resulting in a flat chamber. A comparison of the depth of the central chambers in each eye will reveal the unilateral nature of this presentation. I have observed this in association with an anterior scleritis. Depending on the severity of the inflammation and the secondary glaucoma, treatment includes topical, subtenons, or systemic steroids; carbonic anhydrase inhibitors; and cycloplegic agents. Miotics should be avoided because they can promote posterior synechia and inflammation. Choroidal detachments may be present in this situation and have been noted in cases of posterior scleritis (105,133).

Nonpupillary block closure associated with anterior uveitis may occur when PAS develops and occludes a significant portion of the angle. The anterior chamber usually retains its normal depth. This type of synechia, however, tends to develop in eyes with shallow chambers and those with chronic granulomatous inflammation (21). The PAS may be broad based and insert high along the wall. Usually, however, the PAS associated with anterior chamber inflammation is not uniform in terms of height and shape and appears to occur abruptly along the angle wall (33). It alternates with normal-appearing segments and sometimes produces a tenting appearance of the iris when attached to the angle wall. In contrast, PAS that forms in primary angle closure tends to be more even (134). This aids in differentiating inflammatory-related PAS from chronic angle closure PAS. Inflammatory-induced PAS generally starts in the inferior angle, but I have observed it to occur initially in the lateral quadrants. This indicates the necessity to examine the entire angle circumference. There is

a risk for neovascularization with chronic inflammation, which can cause fibrovascular synechial angle closure.

Inflammation of the trabecular meshwork, a trabeculitis, may cause elevated IOP, particularly if the ciliary body is not inflamed and aqueous production remains normal. Gonioscopically, the angle will be open, but inflammatory precipitates will be evident on the meshwork.

In some cases, swelling of the trabecular meshwork may cause elevated IOP. This becomes a diagnosis of exclusion as gonioscopy is usually normal without signs of PAS or inflammatory debris blocking the meshwork; there is no iris bombé or posterior synechia, the chamber is not flat, yet the IOP is elevated. The possibility of steroid response should be considered, but it is rare for a steroid response to occur before 10 days of use. Possibly inflammatory debris, including fibrin, pigment cells, or macrophages, may be clogging the meshwork farther downstream (91). Sometimes the congestion of the meshwork is visible by gonioscopy, and this will aid in the diagnosis (26).

Fuch's heterochromic cyclitis and Posner-Schlossman glaucomato-cyclitic crisis are specific forms of anterior uveitis associated with elevated IOP, open angles, and characteristic gonioscopic abnormalities although Fuch's has been reported associated with PAS and angle closure (65,87). In Fuch's heterochromic cyclitis, there may be multiple fine vessels concentrically and radially arranged in the trabecular meshwork area (134). In glaucomato-cyclitic crises, Hart noted an anterior insertion of the iris, fine iris processes, cellophane tissue obscuring the trabecular meshwork, and fine, irregular vessels coursing across the angle (135). The IOP may be elevated by mononuclear cells in the trabecular interspaces, impeding outflow (136). Small trabecular precipitates have been reported in this syndrome. The angle, however, remains open. Trabecular precipitates have also been reported after laser trabeculoplasty and in granulomatous inflammations (137).

Chandler and Grant's textbook on glaucoma describes an uncommon form of glaucoma associated with angle precipitates (33). The inflammatory precipitates, which are located on the trabecular meshwork, may be visible before organization of PAS. There is an associated elevation of the IOP, which is not necessarily proportional to the number of precipitates present. Interestingly, the precipitates have been observed in eyes with elevated IOP without evidence of inflammation elsewhere. They are described as colorless or slightly yellow and somewhat broad and flat. The observation of an irregularity of the iris root with abrupt changes in the location of its attachment is suggestive of their presence. If the condition is not recognized, PAS may form while the patient is being treated for open-angle glaucoma. When there is no PAS and it is early in the course, the treatment consists of topical steroid. The precipitates will then often resolve in 1 to 2 weeks. If the IOP returns to normal levels, only observation is needed. If the IOP remains elevated, a course of topical aqueous suppressants and carbonic anhydrase inhibitors may be needed. Miotics are contraindicated when precipitates are present in the angle. The only associated disease noted with this uncommon form of glaucoma is sarcoidosis (33). These rare cases point out the importance of doing careful gonioscopy in all cases of glaucoma.

In treating glaucoma associated with inflammation, miotics customarily should be avoided; they may increase inflammation, increase ciliary spasm, and potentiate posterior synechia. In general, therapy is aimed at reducing aqueous production by beta-adrenergic antagonists and carbonic anhydrase inhibitors and quieting the inflammation with steriods.

Lens-Induced Angle Closure

Angle closure secondary to the crystalline lens can evolve from swelling of the lens (phacomorphic glaucoma) or from lens subluxation. This is different than phacolytic glaucoma, where leakage of lens protein from a relatively intact cataract causes secondary open-angle glaucoma, and it is also different than lens-particle glaucoma, where after trauma or cataract surgery lens material blocks outflow. In phakomorphic glaucoma, the intumescent lens may cause a secondary pupil block angle closure, or it may cause an angle closure by mechanically pushing the iris forward into the angle. Confirmation of pupil block will be evident if after iridotomy the peripheral iris drops posterior and the angle widens. If the peripheral iris remains in the same position (assuming a patent iridotomy and no significant PAS) and gonioscopically the angle remains closed, pupil block is not the cause and the swollen lens should be removed. Cataract extraction is the definitive treatment in either case. An iridotomy, however, may provide temporary relief when pupil block is present (138,139,140). Some systemic medications such as sulfa drugs, thiazide diuretics, carbonic anhydrase inhibitors, or spironolactone have been implicated in causing lens swelling and may induce this form of angle closure glaucoma (112).

Lenticular angle closure may also occur secondary to ectopia lentis, subluxation, or lens displacement (Figure 6.20). This can be secondary to trauma, occur spontaneously, or be related to a systemic abnormality, such as Marfan's syndrome, Weill-Marchesani syndrome, or homocystinuria. In Marfan's syndrome, the lens is usually displaced superiorly,

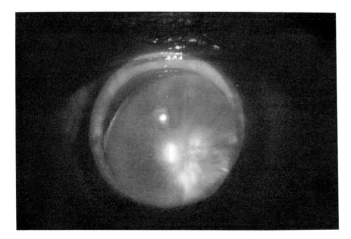

Figure 6.20 Subluxated lens. (Photo courtesy R. Gutner, O.D.)

and the angle may have a number of anomalies consisting of bridging iris processes, fraying of the iris root, abnormal vessels, and moundlike formations near the iris root (141). In homocysturnia, the lens is usually displaced inferior. In the Weill-Marchesani syndrome, a small, spherical lens (microspherophakia) is usually displaced more anteriorly than normal, blocking the pupil.

Liebman and Ritch define the terms *ectopia lentis, subluxation,* and *dislocation* in the following manner (142). Ectopia lentis is a displacement of the lens from its normal central position. Subluxation is the loosening or breaking of some zonules, resulting in a decentered lens located behind the iris and remaining at least partially within the pupil space. Lens dislocation occurs when there are no zonular attachments. In this situation, there is risk for the lens to relocate in the anterior chamber or into the vitreous.

When a lens is subluxated, there may be variable anterior chamber depths, changes in refraction, and/or a shallowed anterior chamber from forward lens movement. If the lens is dislocated into the posterior vitreous, the central chamber will deepen and the angle widen. A tilted lens may cause irregular chamber depth and variable angle width. When the lens is subluxated anterior or dislocated anterior and the lens is small, a volcano appearance of the iris has been described (142). This occurs when the lens causes the center of the iris to move forward and the peripheral iris drops posterior because there is no lens or zonules behind that iris portion (142). In some cases, vitreous may be located in the pupil space and contribute to pupil block. When the lens is displaced or subluxated, iridodenesis and movement of the lens, phakodenesis, may be observed.

Leibmann and Ritch recommend "individualized" treatment for cases of pupil block angle closure secondary to anterior placed subluxated lenses. They propose having the patient placed in a supine position and using concomitant hyperosmotic agents and topical beta-blockers. Pressing against the central cornea may encourage lens repositioning. Once the vitreous volume decreases and the lens moves posterior, one drop of 2% pilocarpine can be instilled. If the miotic does not shallow the chamber, the lens is totally dislocated with the absence of any zonular attachments, and further use of mydriatics or cycloplegics is contraindicated to avoid the lens dislocating into the anterior chamber.

If the miotics shallow the chamber, the lens is still partially attached to the zonules, and cycloplegics should be used. The cycloplegic agent will relax the ciliary muscle and tighten the remaining zonules, which will pull the lens posterior. Once the lens is posterior, laser iridectomy should be performed to break any pupil block and then miotics instilled to keep the lens from dislocating into the anterior chamber. In some cases, an initial laser iridotomy can be performed to relieve any pupil block. This will result in a lower IOP, making it easier to put the lens into place. Miotics should not be used unless a patent laser iridectomy is present as the chronic use of the miotic in this instance will promote pupil block.

Nanophthalmos is a rare condition in which the eye has a normal shape but is small. As such the eye is anatomically predisposed to angle closure glaucoma. It is a pure form of micro-ophthalmos not concurrent with other congenital variations (113). It may be recessively or dominantly inherited or occur sporadically (143). It is bilateral, and affects both sexes equally. The nanophthalmic eye is characterized by a short axial length, small corneal diameter, high hyperopia, a normal or large lens, a shallow chamber centrally and peripherally, and a thick sclera. In some cases, the thick sclera has been postulated to cause obstruction to aqueous outflow through the vortex veins, resulting in choroidal effusion and angle closure (21,143,144).

There is a question of whether pupil block plays a role in angle closure in nanophthalmic eyes as some think the mixed response to laser iridectomy does not favor this concept (111,145). Jin and Anderson, however, recently reported that laser iridotomies alone or in combination with laser iridoplasty is often sufficient to control the glaucoma in these eyes (146). In some cases, additional medical treatment is required. Caution should be exercised using miotics as they may narrow the angle. Angle closure usually occurs in the fourth to six decade of life in these patients. Nonrhegmatogenous retinal detachments also cause vision loss in these eyes, and associated uveal effusion can be treated by means of a sclerotomy or sclerectomy (143).

References

1. Fourman S. Differential diagnosis of acute angle-closure glaucoma in an emergency department. *Glaucoma.* 1989;11:135–138.
2. Schie HG. Gonioscopy in the diagnosis of the iris and ciliary body with emphasis on intraepithelial cysts. *Trans Am Ophthalmol Soc.* 1953;51:313.
3. Olsen O. Goniophotography. *Am J Optom Physiol Optics.* 1979;56(9):563–568.
4. Shields JA. *Diagnosis and management of intraocular tumors.* St Louis: CV Mosby, 1983.
5. Rao NA, Forster DJ, Augsberger JJ. The uvea uveitis and intraocular neoplasms. In Podos SM, Yanoff M, eds. *Textbook of ophthalmology,* vol 2. New York: Gower Medical Publishing, 1992.
6. Swanson MW. Metastatic tumor formation: Processes within the visual system. *J Am Opt Assoc* 1990;61:296–308.
7. Becker S. *Clinical gonioscopy: A text and stereoscopic atlas.* St Louis: CV Mosby, 1972.
8. Shields JA, Shields CL. *Intraocular tumors: A text and atlas.* Philadelphia: WB Saunders, 1992.
9. Teekhasanee C et al. Ocular findings in oculodermal melanocytosis. *Arch Ophthalmol.* 1990;108:1114.
10. Jakobiec FA, Silbert G. Are most iris "melanomas" really nevi? *Arch Ophthalmol.* 1981;99:2117.
11. Cialdini AP et al. Malignant transformation of an iris melanocytoma. *Graefe's Arch Clin Exp Ophthalmol.* 1989;227:348–354.
12. Shields MB, Klintworth GK. Anterior uveal melanomas and intraocular pressure. *Ophthalmology.* 1980;87:503–517.
13. Yanoff M, Schie HG. Melanomalytic glaucoma. *Arch Ophthalmol.* 1970;84:471.
14. Shields JA et al. Glaucomas associated with intraocular tumors. In Ritch R et al, eds. *The glaucomas.* St Louis: CV Mosby, 1989.
15. Yanoff M, Fine BS. *Ocular pathology,* 3d ed. Philadelphia: Lippincott; 1989.
16. Zaaka FA et al. Metastatic tapioca iris melanoma. *Br J Ophthalmol.* 1979;63:744–749.
17. Brown D et al. Diffuse malignant melanoma of iris with metastases. *Surv Ophthalmol.* 1990;34(5):357–364.
18. Powers T et al. Remote metastases from uveal melanoma. *J Tenn Med Assoc.* 1990;1:11–14.
19. Geisse LJ, Robertson DM. Iris melanomas. *Am J Ophthalmol.* 1985;99:638–645.
20. Shields CL et al. Prevalence and mechanisms of secondary intraocular pressure elevations in eyes with intraocular tumors. *Ophthalmology.* 1987;94:839–846.
21. Hoskins HD Jr, Kass MA. *Becker-Schaeffer's diagnosis and therapy of the glaucomas,* 6th ed. St Louis: CV Mosby, 1989.
22. Shields MB, Proia AD. Neovascular glaucoma associated with an iris melanoma. A clinicopathologic report. *Arch Ophthalmol.* 1987;105:672.
23. Fraser DJ, Font RL. Ocular inflammation and hemorrhage as initial manifestations of uveal melanoma. *Arch Ophthalmol.* 1979;97:1311–1314.
24. Kremer I, Ben-Sira I. Borderline spindle cell nevus of the ciliary body as a second primary melanoma—A clinicopathologic case. *Ann Ophthalmol.* 1989;21:217–221.
25. Pavlin CJ et al. Ultrasound biomicroscopy of anterior segment tumors. *Ophthalmology.* 1992;99:1220–1228.
26. Ritch R, Shields BM. *The secondary glaucomas.* St Louis: CV Mosby, 1982.
27. Gorin G. *Clinical glaucoma.* New York: Marcel Dekker, 1977.
28. Chambers RB et al. Treatment of iris melanoma with dihematoporphyn ether and an ophthalmic laser delivery system. *Contemp Ophthalmic Forum.* 1986;4:3.
29. Shields JA. Primary cysts of the iris. *Tr Am Ophthalmol Soc.* 1981;89:771–809.
30. Vela NA et al. The heredity and treatment of angle-closure glaucoma secondary to iris and ciliary body cysts. *Ophthalmology.* 1983;91:332–337.
31. Davidson SI. Spontaneous cysts of the ciliary body. *Br J Ophthalmol.* 1960;44:461.
32. Shields J et al. Primary iris cysts: A review of the literature report of 62 cases. *Br J Ophthalmol.* 1984;68:152–166.
33. Epstein D. *Chandler & Grant's glaucoma,* 3d ed. Philadelphia: Lea & Febiger, 1986.
34. Thomas R et al. Angle closure glaucoma due to iris and ciliary body cysts. *Aust and NZ J of Ophthalmol.* 1989;3:317.
35. Naumann GOH, Rummelt V. Congenital nonpigmented epithelial iris cyst removed by block-excision. *Graefe's Arch Clin Exp Ophthalmol.* 1990;228:392–397.
36. Semes LP, Amos JF. Idiopathic cysts of the anterior chamber. *Am J Opt Physiol Optics.* 1984;61:327–333.
37. Duke-Elder S. Perkins ES. Diseases of the uveal tract. In Duke-Elder S, ed. *System of Ophthalmology,* vol 9. St Louis: CV Mosby, 1966;754–937.
38. Primo SA. Iris cysts. *Clin Eye Vision Care.* 1990;2:124–128.
39. Alvarado A et al. Pathogenesis of Chandler's syndrome, essential iris atrophy and the Cogan-Reese syndrome, II. Estimated age at disease onset. *Invest Ophthalmol Vis Sci.* 1986;27:873–882.
40. Campbell DG et al. The corneal endothelium and the spectrum of essential iris atrophy. *Am J Ophthalmol.* 1978;86:317–324.
41. Bahn CF et al. Classification corneal endothelial disorders based on neural crest origin. *Ophthalmology.* 1984;91:558–563.
42. Pathogenisis of Chandler's syndrome, essential iris atrophy and the Cogan-Reese Syndrome, I. Alterations of the corneal endothelium. *Invest Ophthalmol Vis Sci.* 1986;27:853–872.
43. Yanoff M. Corneal edema in essential iris atrophy. *Ophthalmology.* 1979;86:1549–1550.
44. Eagle RC, Shields JA. Iridocorneal endothelial syndrome with contralateral guttate endothelial dystrophy ophthalmology. A light and electron microscopic study. *Ophthalmology.* 1987;94(7):862–870.

45. Tsai CS et al. Antibodies to Epstein-Barr virus in iridocorneal endothelial syndrome. *Arch Ophthalmol.* 1990;108:5172.

46. Wilson MC, Shields MB. Comparison of the clinical variations of the iridocorneal endothelial syndrome. *Arch Ophthalmol.* 1989;107(10):1465–1468.

47. Mackley TA, Kspetansky FM, Iris nevus syndrome. *Ann Opthalmol.* 1988;20:311–315.

48. Schie HG, Yanoff M. Iris nevus (Cogan-Reese) syndrome. *Arch Ophthalmol.* 1975;93:963–970.

49. Lewis RA, Riccardi VM. von Recklinghausen's neurofibromatosis: Incidence of iris harmatomas. *Ophthalmology.* 1981; 88:348–354.

50. Jakobiec FA et al. Solitary iris nevus associated with periphela anterior synechiae and iris endothelialization. *Am J Ophthalmol.* 1977;83:884.

51. Kidd M et al. Surgical results in iridocorneal endothelial syndrome. *Arch Ophthalmol.* 1988;106:199.

52. Wright MM et al. 5-fluorouracil after trabeculectomy and the iridocorneal endothelial syndrome. *Ophthalmology.* 1991;98: 314–316.

53. Crawford G et al. Penetrating keratoplasty in the management of iridocorneal endothelial syndrome. *Cornea.* 1989;8(1): 34–40.

54. Laganowski HC et al. Distinguishing features of the iridocorneal endothelial syndrome and posterior polymorphous dystrophy: Value of endothelial specular microscopy. *Br J Ophthalmol.* 1991;75(4):212–216.

55. Frangoulis ES et al. Clinical features of the irido-corneal endothelial syndrome. *Trans Ophthalmol Soc UK.* 1985;104:775.

56. Gartner S, Henkind P. Neovascularization of the iris. *Surv Ophthalmol.* 1978;22(5):291–311.

57. Weiss DJ et al. Neovascular glaucoma complicating carotid-cavernous fistula. *Arch Ophthal.* 1963;69:304–307.

58. Wand M. Neovascular glaucoma. In Ritch et al, eds. *The glaucomas,* vol 2. St Louis: CV Mosby, 1989.

59. Teich SA, Walsh JB. A grading system for iris neovascularization. Prognostic implications for treatment. *Ophthalmology.* 1981;88:1102–1106.

60. Comarrata MR et al. Iris neovascularization in proliferative vitreoretinopathy. *Ophthalmology.* 1992;99:898–905.

61. Shields BM. *Textbook of glaucoma,* 3d ed. Baltimore: William & Wilkins, 1992.

62. Brown GC et al. Neovascular glaucoma. Etiologic consideration. *Ophthalmology.* 1984;91:315–320.

63. Anderson DM et al. Rubeosis irides. *Can J Ophthalmol.* 1971; 6:183–188.

64. Berger BB et al. Anterior segment ischemia in Fuch's heterochromic cyclitis. *Arch Ophthalmol.* 1980;98:499.

65. Lerman S, Levy C. Heterochromic iritis and secondary neovascular glaucoma. *Am J Opthalmol.* 1964;57:479.

66. Duker JS et al. A prospective study of acute central retinal artery obstruction. The incidence of secondary ocular neovascularization. *Arch Ophthalmol.* 1991;109:39.

67. Weinreb RN et al. Neovascular glaucoma following neodynium–YAG laser posterior capsulotomy. *Arch Ophthalmol.* 1986;104:730.

68. Pavese T, Insler MS. Effects of extracapsular cataract extraction with posterior chamber lens implantation on the development of neovascular glaucoma in diabetics. *J Cataract Refract Surg.* 1987;13:197.

69. Duane TD. *Clinical Ophthalmology.* New York: Harper and Row, 1978.

70. Pavan PR et al. Diabetic vitrectomy in ocular manifestations of diabetes. *Internat Ophthalmol Clin.* 1984 (Winter);24:4.

71. Roth SM, Brown GC. The diagnosis and management of rubeosis irides glaucoma series. *Clin Signs Opthalmol.* 1989;10(4).

72. Sanborn GE et al. Fundus-iris fluorescein angiography: Evaluation of its use in the diagnosis of rubeosis irides. *Ann Opthalmol.* 1986;18:52.

73. Henkind P. Angle vessels in normal eyes. *Br J Ophthalmol.* 1964;48:551.

74. Welch RB. Spontaneous anterior chamber hemorrhage from the iris: A unique cinematographic documentation. *Trans Am Ophth Soc.* 1980;LXXCVIII:132–142.

75. Cobb B. Vascular tufts at the pupillary margin: A preliminary report on 4 patients. *Trans Ophthalmol Soc UK.* 1968;88:211.

76. Hagen AP-V, Williams GA. Argon laser treatment of a bleeding iris vascular tuft. *Am J Ophthalmol.* 1986;101:379.

77. Rosen E, Lyons D. Microhemangiomas at the pupillary border. *Am J Ophthalmol.* 1969;67:846.

78. Coleman S et al. Vascular tufts of the pupillary margin of iris. *Am J Ophthalmol.* 1977;83:881.

79. Savir H, Manor RS. Spontaneous hyphema and vessel anomaly. *Arch Ophthalmol.* 1975;93:1056.

80. Perry HD et al. Microhemangiomas of the iris with spontaneous hyphema and acute glaucoma. *Br J Ophthalmol.* 1977; 61:114–116.

81. Mason GI. Iris neovascular tufts. *Arch Ophthalmol.* 1979; 97:2346.

82. Sellman A. Hyphaema from microhemangiomas. *Acta Ophthalmol.* 1972;59:58.

83. Mason GI, Ferry AP. Bilateral spontaneous hyphema arising from iridic microhemangiomas. *Ann Ophthalmol.* 1979;11: 87–91.

84. Krarup JC. Atypical rubeosis irides in congenital cyanotic heart disease. *Acta Ophthalmol.* 1977;55:581.

85. Cobb B et al. Vascular tufts at the pupillary margin in myotonic dystrophy. *Am J Ophthalmol.* 1970;69:573.

86. Schachat A. Discussion in Duker JS, Brown GC. Iris neovascularization associated with obstruction of the central retinal artery. *Ophthalmology.* 1988;95:1244.

87. Jones NP. Glaucoma in Fuch's heterochromic uveitis: Aetiology, management and outcome. *Eye.* 1991;5:662–667.

88. Jones P. Fuch's heterochromic uveitis: A reappraisal of the clinical spectrum. *Eye.* 1991;5:649–661.

89. Perry HD et al. Rubeosis in Fuch's heterochromic iridocyclitis. *Arch Ophthalmol.* 1975;93:337.

90. Beggi IS. Significance of goniohaemorrhage in heterochromic cyclitis. *Br J Ophthalmol.* 1969;53:1–8.

91. Weiss DI, Gold D. Neofibrovascularization of iris and anterior chamber angle: A clinical classification. *Ann Ophthalmol.* 1978;10:488.

92. Wand M et al. Effects of panretinal photocoagulation on rubeosis irides, angle neovascularization and neovascular glaucoma. *Am J Ophthalmol.* 1978;86:332.

93. Laatikainen L. Development and classification of rubeosis irides in diabetic eye disease. *Br J Ophthalmol.* 1979;63:150.

94. Henkind P. Ocular neovascularization. *Am J Ophthalmol.* 1978;85:287–301.

95. Abedin S, Simmons RJ. Neovascular glaucoma in systemic occlusive vascular disease. *Ann Ophthalmol.* 1982;14:284.

96. Jacobson DR, Murphy RP, Rosenthal AR. The treatment of angle neovascularization with panretinal photocoagulation. *Ophthalmology.* 1979;86:1270.

97. Simmons RJ et al. The role of gonio-photocoagulation in neovascularization of the anterior chamber angle. *Ophthalmology.* 1980;87:79.

98. Molteno ACB, Hadda PJ. The visual outcome in cases of neovascular glaucoma. *Aust and NZ J Ophthalmol.* 1985; 13:329.

99. Carenini BB, Anfossi DG. Nonsurgical management of neovascular glaucoma. 1988;10:17–24.

100. Weiss RA, Ashburn FS Jr. Neovascular glaucoma: A review of current therapeutic modalities. *Glaucoma.* 1984;6:68.

101. von Graefe A. Beitrage zur pathologic and therapie des

glaucoms. *Archiv Ophthalmol.* 1869;15:108–252.

102. Brooks AMV et al. Occurrence of malignant glaucoma after laser iridotomy. *Br J Ophthalmol.* 1989;73:617–620.

103. Jacoby B et al. Malignant glaucoma in a patient with Down's syndrome and corneal hydrops. *Am J Ophthalmol.* 1990; 110(4):434.

104. Schwartz AL, Anderson DR. "Malignant glaucoma" in an eye with no antecedent operation or miotics. *Arch Ophthalmol.* 1975;93:379.

105. Phelps C. Angle-closure glaucoma secondary to ciliary body swelling. *Arch Ophthalmol.* 1974;92:287.

106. Weber PA et al . Central retinal vein occlusion and malignant glaucoma. *Arch Ophthalmol.* 1987;105:635–636.

107. Fourman S. Angle-closure glaucoma complicating ciliochoroidal detachment. *Ophthalmology.* 1989;96:646–653.

108. Fanous S, Brouillette G. Ciliary block glaucoma: Malignant glaucoma in the absence of a history of surgery and of miotic therapy. *Can J Opthalmol.* 1983;18(6):302–303.

109. Reiser JC. Miotic induced malignant glaucoma. *Arch Ophthalmol.* 1972;87:706–712.

110. Cashwell LF, Martin TJ. Malignant glaucoma after laser iridotomy. *Ophthalmology.* 1992;99:651–659.

111. Fourman S. Diagnosing acute angle-closure glaucoma; A flowchart. *Surv Ophthalmol.* 1989;33(6):491.

112. Shaffer RN, Hoskins HD Jr. Ciliary block (malignant glaucoma) *Ophthalmology.* 1978;85:215–221.

113. Hyams S. Nonpupillary-block angle-closure glaucoma. *Glaucoma.* 1991;13:153–156.

114. Hyams S. Angle-closure glaucoma. Berkeley, Calif.: Kugler & Ghendini, 1990.

115. Newton N Jr et al. Acute angle-closure glaucoma after panretinal photocoagulation. *Glaucoma.* 1989;11:105–107.

116. Pesin S et al. Acute angle-closure glaucoma from spontaneous massive hemorrhagic retinal or choroidal detachment. *Ophthalmology.* 1990;97:76–84.

117. Levene R. A new concept of malignant glaucoma. *Arch Ophthalmol.* 1972;87:497–506.

118. Luntz MH, Rosenblatt M. Malignant glaucoma. *Surv Ophthalmol.* 1987;32(2):73–93.

119. Weber P et al. Central retinal vein occlusion and malignant glaucoma. *Arch Ophthalmol.* 1987;105:635.

120. Batko KA. Bilateral malignant glaucoma. *Glaucoma.* 1990; 12:28.

121. Simmons RJ. Malignant glaucoma. In Epstein DL, ed. *Chandler & Grant's Glaucoma,* 3d ed. Philadelphia: Lea & Febiger,1986.

122. Simmons RJ, Thomas JV, Yaqub MK. Malignant glaucoma. In Ritch R et al, eds. *The glaucomas,* vol 2. St Louis: CV Mosby, 1989.

123. Vajpayee RB, Talear D. Pseudophakic malignant glaucoma in a child. *Ophthalm Surg.* 1991;22:266.

124. Lynch MG et al. Surgical vitrectomy for pseudophakic malignant glaucoma. *Am J Ophthalmol.* 1986;102:149–153.

125. Epstein D. Pseudophakic malignant glaucoma—Is it really pseudomalignant? Editorial. *Am J Ophthalmol.* 1987;103(2): 231–233.

126. Fiore PM et al. The dural shunt syndrome I. Management of glaucoma. *Ophthalmology.* 1990;97:56–62.

127. Nash RW, Lindquist TD. Bilateral angle-closure glaucoma associated with uveal effusion; presenting sign of HIV infection. *Surv Ophthalmol.* 1992;36(4):255.

128. Herschler L. Laser shrinkage of the ciliary processes. A treatment for malignant (ciliary block) glaucoma. *Ophthalmology.* 1980;87:155–159.

129. Brown RH et al. Neodynium-YAG vitreous surgery for phakic and pseudophakic malignant glaucoma. *Arch Ophthalmol.* 1986;104:1464–1466.

130. Abramson DR et al. Pilocarpine-induced retinal tear: An ultrasonic evaluation of lens movements. *Glaucoma.* 1981; 39:9–12.

131. Gorin G. Angle-closure glaucoma induced by miotics. *Am J Ophthalmol.* 1966;62(6):1063–1067.

132. Krupin T et al. Secondary glaucoma associated with uveitis. *Glaucoma.* 1988;10:85–90.

133. Quinlan MP, Hitchings RA. Angle-closure glaucoma secondary to posterior scleritis. *Br J Ophthalmol.* 1978;62: 330–335.

134. Krupin T. Glaucoma associated with uveitis. In Ritch R, Shields MB. *The secondary glaucomas.* St Louis: CV Mosby, 1982.

135. Hart CT, Weatherill JR. Gonioscopy and tonography in glaucomatocyclitic crises. *Br J Ophthalmol.* 1968;52:682.

136. Harstad HK, Ringvold A. Glaucomatocyclitic crises (Posner-Schlossman syndrome). A case report. *Acta Ophthlamol.* 1986;64:146–151.

137. Fiore PM. Trabecular precipitates and elevated intraocular pressure following argon laser trabeculoplasty. *Ophthalm Surg.* 1989;20(10):697.

138. Epstein D. Diagnosis and management of lens-induced glaucoma. *Ophthalmology.* 1982;89:227–230.

139. Tomey KF, Al-Rajhi AA. Neodynium: YAG laser iridotomy in the intial management of phacomorphic glaucoma. *Ophthalmology.* 1992;99:660–665.

140. van Buskirk EM. Hazards of medical glaucoma therapy in the cataract patient. *Ophthalmology.* 1982;89:238–241.

141. Burian HM et al. Chamber angle anomalies in systemic connective tissue disorders. *Arch Ophthalmol.* 1960;64: 671.

142. Liebmann JM, Ritch R. Glaucoma secondary to lens intumescence and dislocation. In Ritch R et al, eds. *The glaucomas.* St Louis: CV Mosby, 1989.

143. Martorina M. Familial nanophthalmos. *J Fr Ophthalmol.* 1988;11(4):357.

144. Shaffer RN. Discussion in Calhoun FP Jr. The management of glaucoma in nanophthalmos. *Trans Am Acad Ophthalmol.* 1973;63:97–119.

145. Kimbrough RL et al. Angle-closure glaucoma in nanophthalmos. *Am J Ophthalmol.* 1979;8:572–579.

146. Jin JC, Anderson DR. Laser and unsutured sclerotomy in nanophthalmos. *Am J Ophthalmol.* 1990;109(5):575–580.

Chapter 7

Open-Angle Glaucoma

Secondary Open-Angle Glaucomas

The normal gonioscopic appearance in primary chronic open-angle glaucoma and some forms of secondary open-angle glaucoma such as corticosteroid-induced glaucoma assists in establishing the correct diagnosis. This chapter will discuss those forms of secondary open-angle glaucoma associated with characteristic gonioscopic findings that aid in their diagnosis and management. Glaucomas associated with uveitis and lens-induced glaucoma where reviewed in the previous chapter as they may induce either secondary open-angle or secondary closed-angle glaucoma. Two specific forms of uveitis, however, which are complicated by open-angle glaucoma, will be further reviewed in this chapter.

Fuch's Heterochromic Cyclitis and Posner-Schlossman Syndrome

Uveitis may effect both aqueous production, and outflow resistance; as such, the net effect on the level of IOP, will be determined by a balance between the two. In uveitis with an open angle, IOP may be lowered secondary to an increase in uveo-scleral outflow and/or reduced aqueous production from an inflamed ciliary body. Conversely IOP may be increased from acute trabecular obstruction from the accumulation of inflammatory cells and fibrin, swelling or dysfunction to the trabecular endothelium, precipitates on the trabecular meshwork, and/or a positive steroid response. If the outflow compromise supersedes the reduction in inflow, increased IOP will result. Uveitis may also induce elevated IOP in the form of angle closure. This may develop secondary to ciliary body swelling, resulting in a form of malignant glaucoma, or from scarring of the outflow channels, from fibrovascular membrane development, from PAS development, or from posterior synechia—all of which have the potential to block outflow (Plates 11 and 13).

Fuch's heterochromic cyclitis and Posner-Schlossman syndrome (glaucomatocyclitic crises) are two specific forms of uveitis that are associated with open-angle glaucoma. Fuch's heterochromic cyclitis is a chronic, insidious, anterior segment inflammatory disease that frequently results in late cataract formation. Glaucoma is associated in 25% to 50% of cases (1,2). Characteristics suggesting Fuch's include unilateral disease (although it may be bilateral), a white and quiet eye with minimal aqueous cell and flare, nonpigmented stellate keratic precipitates (KPs) concentrated in the superior cornea that persist with topical steroid treatment, absence of PAS, late posterior subcapsular lens changes, and/or a moth-eaten appearance to the iris and heterochromia (2,3). It should be stressed that the observation of heterochromia is not necessary for diagnosis and may be easily overlooked in eyes with dark irides, particularly in blacks (2,4). Iris stromal atrophy, resulting in a loss of iris details and dull iris appearance, is most noticeable when compared to the fellow eye. This is a subtle but constant feature (5). Typically the anterior vitreous will have white, dotlike opacities. The involved eye is usually hypochromic; on occasion, however, it may be darker from exposure of the pigment epithelium, the result of iris stroma atrophy (3,6). The use of topical steroids rarely resolves the anterior cells, and because PAS rarely, if ever, develops, chronic steroid treatment and dilation are often unnecessary (2). In fact, chronic steroid therapy may lead to greater ocular morbidity from cataracts and glaucoma than does the inflammation itself (7). A positive aqueous cellular reduction to topical steroids should make one suspicious of Fuch's heterochromic cyclitis as the correct diagnosis (7). Chronic flare is not unusual nor is it an indication for steroid therapy. The associated glaucoma should be managed as a form of open-angle glaucoma using aqueous suppresants such as topical beta blockers and/or epinephrine compounds (topical adrenergic agonists) (5,7). Recent reports suggest an association between Fuch's heterochromic cyclitis and toxoplasmosis like chorioretinal scars (8,9).

Posner-Schlossman syndrome is characterized by recurrent unilateral spontaneous episodes of increased IOP in the range of 40 to 60 mm/Hg lasting up to a few weeks (6). Anterior chamber flare, fine white discrete nonpigmented KPs covering the entire cornea, and mild heterochromia are usually present. Because of several similar findings, some observers consider this a form of heterochromic uveitis (10). The affected eye usually has a larger pupil, unlike other forms of uveitis. Between attacks, the IOP is usually normal. The process, however, is associated with open-angle glaucoma, and patients with this syndrome have a higher incidence of positive steroid response than is normal; therefore these patients should be closely followed between crises as open-angle glaucoma suspects (11,12). Normal gonioscopic appearance during and after the crises and the lack of PAS helps differentiate this syndrome from uveitic angle closure glaucoma (13). During a crisis, tonography reveals an excessive resistance to outflow. As noted, uveitis in general may affect IOP either by lowering it from decreasing aqueous production or increasing IOP by increasing resistance to outflow. It may also increase IOP by the release of increased prostaglandins, which can raise IOP without reducing outflow. Facility aqueous prostaglandins may have a role in this disorder, and using prostaglandin inhibitors such as aspirin or nonsteroidal antiinflammatory agents for prophylaxis has been suggested (14,15).

Pigment Dispersion Syndrome and Pigmentary Glaucoma

Pigment Dispersion Syndrome (PDS)

Pigment dispersion syndrome is characterized by the liberation of pigment from the pigmented neuroepithelial layer of the posterior iris. Clinically, this may be observed by the deposition of the free pigment on the anterior and posterior chamber surfaces (16,17). The hallmark clinical finding is the spoke-like or radial transillumination of the pigment-liberated mid-peripheral iris (Plate 17). The criteria for diagnosis vary somewhat from observer to observer, some using iris transillumination and others using the presence of Krukenberg's spindle (Plate 16) and trabecular pigmentation for diagnosis (18,19, 20,21). Components of pigment dispersion have been noted following trauma or irradiation, with exfoliation syndrome, with anterior segment melanomas, with anterior segment nevi, and after ocular surgery as well as in this unique syndrome (23,24). The initial discovery of these clinical findings in PDS is often made in the third and fourth decade (19,22).

Pigmentary Glaucoma

The presence of pigment dispersion in an eye with open angles and glaucoma is called *pigmentary glaucoma*, so named by Sugar and Barbour in 1949 (Table 7.1) (25). This is a secondary form of open-angle glaucoma and is most often

TABLE 7.1
Pigmentary Glaucoma Characteristics

Secondary open-angle glaucoma
Most often bilateral
Outflow defects downstream from visible trabecular meshwork
Predominantly present in:
   Males more than females
   Caucasians
   Myopes
Onset at third to fifth decade
35% of ocular hypertensives with pigment dispersion will convert to pigment glaucoma within 15 years
Association with retinal detachments, lattice degeneration
May spontaneously revert to normal

bilateral. The obstruction to the outflow occurs from the pigment in the deeper aqueous outflow system, and it is not affected by the gonioscopically visible trabecular pigment (26) (Plates 41 and 50). In contrast to the other major forms of open-angle glaucoma, pigmentary glaucoma occurs earlier in life, usually in the third to fifth decade (19,27). Classically it is described as a disease predominantly found in young, white, male myopes, although it has been reported in older individuals, as well as in older children (18,19,25,28). The degree of myopia may be correlated to the age of onset of glaucomatous damage. The higher the myopia is, the earlier is the glaucomatous damage. The male-to-female ratios of pigment dispersion vary by study, but generally it is equal or somewhat higher for males, as is the ratio of males to females with pigmentary glaucoma (18,22). Most studies reveal a 3:2 male-to-female ratio with pigmentary glaucoma, although the likelihood of a female with pigment dispersion syndrome developing glaucoma was found to be the same as for males (18,21). Familial pigmentary glaucoma is rare (18).

The prevalence of pigment dispersion in the general population is unknown and not all cases of it result in glaucoma (26). In one study, 35% of ocular hypertensive patients with pigment dispersion converted to pigmentary glaucoma, with a majority converting within 15 years (21). It is estimated that pigmentary glaucoma accounts for 1.0% to 1.5% of the glaucomas in Western countries, and in one private practice study involving a glaucoma population of 9200 patients, they comprised 4.4% of the patients (18,29). It may take as long as 20 years for glaucoma to develop in patients with the dispersion syndrome, with conversion for females reported coming as early as age 30 and for males at age 40 (30). The incidence in females is greatest in the late fourth to early fifth decade and in men the early to mid–third decade (28).

In one study evaluating the records of a group of patients with pigmentary glaucoma and pigment dispersion, male gender, black race, severe myopia, and endothelial pigmentation were identified as risk factors for the presence and severity of pigmentary glaucoma. The number of black patients identified was small, which concurs with most other studies, but the severity of the disease was significant, as all required surgery (30); however, generally this suggests that when the disease presents in blacks, it may be severe. Another study concluded that, in eyes with pigment dispersion, the evidence of increasing pigment to the cornea and to the anterior lens capsule in the undilated pupillary zone and/or increased iris transillumination may be risk factors for increasing IOP and should be considered signs of active dispersion (31) (Plate 17). There is evidence that patients with asymmetric pigmentary glaucoma have higher pressure in the eye with greater pigment dispersion and that in patients with bilateral dispersion and unilateral glaucoma, the severity of the pigment dispersion is greater in the eye with glaucoma (16,22,31).

Pigment dispersion and pigmentary glaucoma are considered to be rare in blacks and Orientals; a recent report suggests, however, that pigment dispersion may be more common in blacks than was previously thought and that the profile in these patients is different than the classical description (26,29,32). The patients in this report tended to be older, female, and hyperopic and displayed heavy pigment deposition on the cornea and trabecular meshwork. The iris insertion was slightly below the scleral spur (Plate 22) and flat rather than the typically concave appearance in pigment dispersion, and there was a distinct absence of iris transillumination (32).

Associated Retinal Abnormalities

Pigment dispersion syndrome has been reported in two cases of retinal pigment epithelium reticular pattern dystrophy (33). In one study, retinal detachments were found in 6.4% of pigment dispersion cases and 7.6% of pigmentary glaucoma cases (18). A recent report by Weseley and colleagues may shed some light on the reason for this (34). They found an increased incidence of lattice degeneration and/or full thickness retinal breaks in eyes with pigment dispersion and/or pigmentary glaucoma. They propose that the presentation of these two findings in eyes with pigment dispersion is related to a structural abnormality of the middle third of the eye. This abnormality results in the concave peripheral iris configuration and an anterior pulling of the vitreous base. The former results in pigment dispersion, and the latter results in the retinal changes (34). The myopic predisposition of eyes with pigment dispersion and the common use of miotic therapy for pigmentary glaucoma may also be factors in the frequency and increased risk of retinal detachments in eyes with pigment dispersion and pigmentary glaucoma (35).

Pathophysiology of Pigment Release and Glaucoma

Most explanations for pigmentary glaucoma associated with pigment dispersion attempt to explain the etiology of the pigment release, as well as the resultant outflow abnormality. Most often the released pigment is implicated as the cause of the glaucoma although it has been suggested, based on familiar cases and corticosteroid response, that the glaucoma is a variant of primary open-angle glaucoma (28,29,36,37). Others believe that a genetically predetermined congenital or developmental abnormality of the iris is a cause for the pigment dispersion (16,24). Kupfer and colleagues, based on the histopathology of one eye with pigmentary glaucoma, con-

cluded that there was a congenital or developmental abnormality of the epithelial layers of the iris, with resultant pigment cell loss, and that the glaucoma that occurs is only coincidental. They also noted the poor differentiation of the dilator muscle, which they attributed to a congenital or developmental anomaly (38). Interestingly, there have been recent reports of anisocoria in unequal cases of pigment dispersion (39). Additionally, semidilated pupils have been noted in some eyes with pigment dispersion with marked iris stroma hypoplasia (40). Thus, pigment dispersion should be included in the differential of cases of anisocoria or atypical semidilated pupils. Whether this is related to a congenital defect or a later disturbance is unclear (39). Campbell believes that the hypertrophy of the dilator muscle is a late cellular reaction from mechanical rubbing of the iris against the zonules (41).

Another explanation implicating a mesodermal angle anomaly is based upon the observation of abnormal iris processes in eyes with pigment dispersion (20,24). This theory proposes a primary developmental defect to the aqueous outflow channels, with the pigmented trabecula being a secondary phenomenon and not the primary cause of outflow disturbance. Speakman has suggested that a mesodermal defect may explain the glaucoma associated with cases of only minimal pigment dispersion (22).

A recent observation by Gillies and Tangas showing the general hypovascularity of the iris by fluorescein angiography also supports a mesodermal abnormality as the explanation for pigment release (40). They showed evidence of a fine neovascularization at the pupil and peripupillary area in 11 patients with pigment dispersion. The abnormalities were also present in clinically (relatively) unaffected fellow eyes, which the authors felt was suggestive that the mesodermal and vascular changes had preceded the clinical appearance of pigment dispersion. They concluded that the pigment dispersion syndrome was the result of an abnormality of the mesodermal iris stroma support tissue and a relative iris vasculature deficiency. They theorized that the hypoplastic, poorly perfused iris stroma offers poor support for the iris pigment epithelium, which is then susceptible to degeneration and pigment release, with subsequent glaucoma developing secondary to the pigment release.

Campbell's theory that the pigment loss is mechanical is generally the most accepted one (42). He correlated the clinical and histologic appearance of eyes with attention to the relation between the anterior zonular packets and the posterior iris. In a predisposed eye, he concluded, the pigment is released in the midperipheral zone from the mechanical rubbing of the peripheral iris against the anterior packets of the zonules and that the resultant pigment release affects the outflow.

Characteristics of a Predisposed Eye

A predisposed eye is one in which the peripheral iris sags slightly posterior just prior to insertion along the angle wall, probably related to an enlarged ciliary body, which is generally found in myopic eyes (Figure 7.1). This is supported by photogrammatic studies of 37 subjects with pigment dispersion

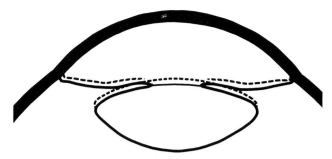

Figure 7.1 Contour of iris and position of lens in eye with pigment dispersion compared to normal (dotted lines). The midperipheral region has the greatest differences. (Reprinted with permission from Davidson JA et al. Dimensions of the anterior chamber in pigment dispersion syndrome. Arch Ophthalmol. *1983;101:81. By permission of Mayo Foundation.*

syndrome in which it was found that the anterior chamber was deeper, particularly in the midperipheral zone, and that the midperipheral iris was concave in shape (43). An iris located posteriorly can be affected by the zonules that are grouped together in packets. Gonioscopically, the iris will have a slightly concave appearance before inserting onto the ciliary body. As noted, this position of the iris may account for the anisocoria noted by Feibel and Perlmutter, who theorized that the dilator muscle, which is located posteriorly, is affected when the iris rubs against the zonules (39). The iris in blacks and Orientals, because of compactness and heavy pigmentation, may be immune from sagging, and this may explain the infrequent observation of this disorder in these groups of individuals (44). Campbell also suggests that his theory explains why pigment dispersion may not be detected until the third decade: the eyes prone to developing pigmentary dispersion do not reach their full myopic size until the second decade. The iris pigment liberation develops around that time, with the ensuing iris transillumination and secondary glaucoma following in the late second or third decades (27).

Campbell also notes that women tend to have smaller eyes than men do and that this may explain the disparity in the presentation of this disorder in men and women. He also feels it explains why pigmentary glaucoma rarely develops in the older population. He notes that in the elderly the normal increase of forward bowing to the iris lifts the iris away from the zonules, thus stopping pigment release. There are differing opinions, however, as to whether pigment dispersion and pigmentary glaucoma affect older individuals (31,41).

Karickhoff recently proposed that the presence of a reverse pupil block accounts for the peripheral iris sag. He speculated that aqueous is trapped in the anterior chamber and causes the peripheral iris to bow backwards. He feels that the iris works as a flap valve against the anterior lens, as evidenced by the frequent observation of iridodenisis associated with pigment dispersion syndrome. The flap valve is activated by eye or head movements and allows for rapid forward flow of aqueous but not for backward flow; thus the trapped anterior chamber aqueous pushes the iris posterior, creating a reverse pupil block and placing the iris in position to contact the zonular packets (45,46).

Pathophysiology of Pigmentary Glaucoma

It has been proposed by Richardsen that the development of glaucoma in individuals with pigment dispersion syndrome occurs in two stages (26,44) (Figure 7.2). First released pigment accumulates in the trabecular meshwork, and the endothelial cells that make up the trabecula phagocytize the pigment within hours. There may be an acute elevation of pressure from the sudden accumulation of pigment in the cells and spaces of the trabecular meshwork. If the onslaught of pigment is minimal, the endothelial cells retain the pigment without disruption to their function. If the process stops here, pressure elevations may be moderate and reversible because the trabecular meshwork can self-repair. When excessive pigment is released or the process continues over time, the cells digest more than they can handle, and they will disintegrate and migrate off the endothelial beams, leaving the beams bare; the beams will collapse and cease to function. If the remaining trabecular endothelial cells cannot spread over the denuded areas and the trabecular meshwork cannot self-repair, a second stage of more permanent change and irreversible damage occurs to it (26,27,41).

The pigment particles appear to cause initial obstruction to the outflow, but it is their destruction to the trabecular cells that results in a more permanent retarding of flow and the resultant long-term elevation to the IOP. This may explain the variable expression of pressure increases with pigment dispersion. The major factor in the reversibility of the disease may reside in the ability of the healthier trabecular endothelial cells to replace the defective cells (44). This theory may need further evaluation in the light of a recent histological study evaluating pigmented and nonpigmented trabecular meshwork in the same eye that revealed no differences in the cellularity or morphology of the two different cells, although it was noted that the meshwork in eyes with pigment dispersion may endure a greater pigment burden than the eyes studied (47).

Richter and colleagues suggest the possibility of four clinical groups of patients with pigment dispersion and pigmentary glaucoma:

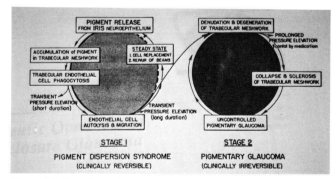

Figure 7.2 Hypothetical mechanism that may explain pathophysiology of pigmentary glaucoma. The first stage of the disease is clinically reversible and gives rise to transient rises in IOP. The second stage, characterized by irreparable damage to trabecular tissue, is irreversible and is accompanied by uncontrolled glaucoma. (Reprinted with permission from Richardson TM. Pigmentary glaucoma. In Ritch R et al, eds. The glaucomas. *St Louis: CV Mosby, 1989.)*

CHAPTER 7. OPEN-ANGLE GLAUCOMA

1. Those who have inactive pigment dispersion and have suffered dispersion at some previous time. Only residual effects from the previous dispersion may be visible in the anterior segment. They may have lessening of their trabecular pigmentation with time. An example patient is one who presents with normal IOP, glaucomatous-appearing discs and/or visual fields that do not change over time. Here, the trabecular cells have not suffered permanent damage and were able to recover.
2. Those characterized by active dispersion with normal IOP. In these cases, the trabecular meshwork still functions normally. These patients may experience transient elevations of IOP, or long-term follow-up may reveal future glaucomatous damage.
3. Those with active dispersion and progressive glaucoma with elevated IOP. Some of these patients may have remission and regression, and some may go on to further permanent damage to the trabecula and develop permanent glaucoma.
4. Those without active dispersion but progressive glaucoma. These findings can be explained as instances where the trabecula has undergone permanent changes, and although dispersion has ceased, the previous dispersion was severe enough for the eye that permanent trabecular damage occurred (31).

In general pigmentary glaucoma is progressive but it can be mild, become less severe, or actually resolve.

It may be that chronic pigment release has different etiologies in different eyes. In some cases, it may be related to the configuration of the iris and its proximity to the zonules, which results in close contact between the two and, thus, pigment release from the continued rubbing. In other cases, it may be some form of congenital mesodermal anomaly that predisposes the iris to easy pigment release, and, in addition, the congenital defect may or may not compromise the angle and outflow channels. Or it may be an abnormal iris epithelium associated with dilator muscle abnormality, resulting in pigment release and an enlarged pupil. In some eyes, it may be a combination of these factors. All or some of these may be self-limited, with pigment release ceasing. If the trabecular meshwork has not suffered permanent damage, the pressure may normalize. Clinically, this can be observed in cases where iris transillumination decreases as it becomes resurfaced by the pigment epithelium. This has been reported when miotic agents have been used (31). Thus, it may be possible in some cases to withdraw or reduce treatment (26).

Clinical Characteristics of Pigment Dispersion

Clinically, pigment dispersion is classically characterized by the deposition of the released pigment along the aqueous pathway. This is observed as endothelial corneal deposits, iris transillumination, and/or a dense pigment ring of the trabecular meshwork (Plates 16,17, and 41). Actually all surfaces contacted by the pigment-ladened aqueous can display deposits,

TABLE 7.2
Clinical Characteristics of Pigment Dispersion

Peripheral spokelike iris transillumination
Krukenberg's spindle
Pigment peppering of the iris surface
Lens pigmentation (anterior and/or posterior surface)
Pigment release in anterior chamber with excercise and/or dilation
Circumference of trabecular meshwork heavily pigmented, ringlike
Deep anterior chamber
Iris concavity at angle recess
Anterior insertion of iris
Reverse pupil block

including the lens, anterior iris zonules, and anterior vitreous face (Plate 40).

Cornea

The corneal endothelial pigment deposits, made up of phagocytosed pigment, may take a diffuse form or, more typically, present as a vertically orientated, centrally located, spindle-shaped brown pigment deposit, known as Krukenberg's spindle (28) (Table 7.2 and Plate 16). The spindle formation is related to the meeting of the aqueous convection currents, resulting in the pigment deposit within the pupil zone and adjacent endothelial phagocytosis. Occasional cases of pigment dispersion have no corneal deposits (28), and their presence is not pathognomic or predictive for pigmentary glaucoma (29), as unilateral spindles may be present in cases of trauma or inflammation (28,29,37,48). The deposits appear to have no adverse effect on the cornea. They vary in length from 1 to 6 mm and in width up to 3 mm (21). A dense spindle may cause the patient to experience rainbows around lights (21). Eyes with pigmentary glaucoma may experience increases in the spindle dimensions after exercise (49). Some patients with abundant coalesced pigment cells forming a masslike deposit at the base of the spindle.

Iris

Transillumination of the iris occurs in a number of conditions. It may be present in albinism, diabetes, pseudoexfoliation (Plate 8), chronic glaucoma, chronic recurrent uveitis, and pigment dispersion syndrome with or without glaucoma. In pigment dispersion syndrome, the transillumination is characterized by midperipheral to peripheral spokelike defects (50) (Plate 17). It is detected by observing transmitted light from the red reflex from the fundus, either with a slit lamp or by external temporal scleral transillumination. Scleral transillumination is particularly valuable in patients with a thick iris stroma. Some observers believe that iris transillumination is necessary to establish the diagnosis of pigment dispersion; however, it has been shown that transillumination defects can disappear, possibly related to pigment epithelial regeneration (19,41). The presence of transillumination offers little information regarding the presence of glaucoma or the amount of pigmentation of the trabecular meshwork (18). It is usually easier to detect in blue eyes, suggesting that pigment loss must be more advanced in dark irides before it can

TABLE 7.3
Iris Transillumination

Condition	Location
Albinism	Variable
Diabetes	Patchy/mid one-third
Pigmentary dispersion	Spokelike peripheral
Pseudoexfoliation	Pupil margin
Chronic glaucoma	Variable patchy and pupil border
Recurrent uveitis	Localized, with stroma involvement

From Donaldson D. Transillumination of the iris. *Trans Am Ophthalmol Soc.* 1974;72.

be detected (Table 7.3). IOP and iris transillumination defects have been observed to increase simultaneously in eyes with pigmentary glaucoma after exercise (49).

Careful inspection of the anterior segment may reveal pigment dusting on the iris surface. It will appear as a peppering of pigment, usually collected in the furrows. Iris color has no relationship to the disease, and heterochromia may occur in asymmetric or unilateral cases (19,28). The darker eye has the greater iris pigment release and will have the greater transillumination (20). Heterochromia and marked trabecular pigmentation have also been described with diffuse melanoma and should be included in the differential of any case of unilateral glaucoma with pigment dispersion (20).

Crystalline Lens and Posterior Chamber

The anterior lens surface will have pigment deposits. They typically coincide with the zonular fibers and frequently appear as fine bronze-colored lines located on the anterior lens periphery. On wide dilation, pigment deposition on the lens zonules and posterior lens surface located near the lens equator may be observed. This is a constant finding, either as punctate deposits or as a dense and confluent ring at the insertion of the lens zonules (Zentmayer's ring or Schie's line) (Plate 40). Pigment can also be observed on the anterior limiting membrane of the vitreous and on the zonular fibers themselves (16,18,29,51).

Anterior Chamber

Examination of the anterior chamber in a dilated eye, especially when sympathomimetics are used in an eye concurrently being treated with miotics, will often reveal released pigment floating in the anterior chamber (52) (Figure 7.3). This may be an age-related phenomenon as it was shown in one study, occur more frequently in the elderly (53). The greater the dilation the greater the pigment release (53). Occasionally the presence of significant pigment cells in the anterior chamber can be mistaken for an iritis (20). A white quiet eye, the lack of white cells, the absence of KPs, the presence of other signs of pigment dispersion, aid in the differential.

Pigment may also be released during exercise. Exercise and dilation-related pigmentary cascades may result in acute clogging of the trabecular meshwork with resultant increase in IOP. The patient may experience symptoms of blurred vsion and or halos after either of these activities (20,27). According to Speakman, this tends to occur early in the PDS process and stops after several years (22). It has been suggested that

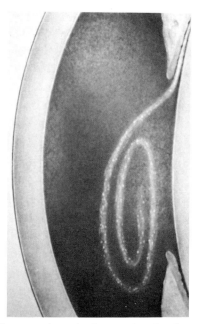

Figure 7.3 Pigment release in the anterior chamber. The pigment granules can appear to be embedded in a gelatinous matrix. (Reprinted with permission from Gorin G, Posner A. Slit lamp gonioscopy, *3d ed. Baltimore: Williams & Wilkins, 1967.)*

most patients who experience the elevation of IOP with this phenomenon already have glaucoma. Kristenson showed that, with repeated mydriasis, the pigment showers in the anterior chamber were less dense; if he waited two weeks before repeating mydriasis, however, the amount of dispersed pigmentation was similar to the first mydriasis (54). The elevation of the IOP from mydriatic-induced acute pigment dispersion occurs about 1-1/2 to 2 hours after dilation and usually starts to fall within 4 to 6 hours (53). The pigment can be so dense that it appears suspended within a clear, gelatinous substance, similar in appearance to a plastic iritis (54). When the pigment acutely obstructs the outflow channels, the IOP may increase to very high levels, as high as 40 to 60 mm/Hg. Once the pigment is phagocytized and purged, the IOP may return to normal levels over 24 hours. In exercise-induced pigment release, IOP may be elevated within 15 minutes and return to preexercise levels within a half hour or remain elevated for extended periods (49). Some investigators recommend the use of prophylactic low-strength pilocarpine (0.5%) 30 minutes prior to exercise to prevent pigment showering and associated elevated IOP (55,56).

It is unusual for patients to experience pain from the acute, excessively elevated IOP; however, at least one patient presented with bilateral acute extreme elevation of IOP, greater than 60 mm/Hg in each eye and with a complaint of a foreign body sensation in both eyes. The symptoms developed after this patient had experienced mild blunt trauma to only one eye. The elevated IOP resulted in a pressure-induced bilateral corneal microcystic edema with small bullae, some of which had become exposed, causing the patient's symptoms. The edema and symptoms resolved once the IOP was medically lowered. In one case reported, emotional stress and dim illumination were implicated for the pigment release and IOP elevation (57). Emotional stress from the trauma may have had a role in the bilateral pigment release in the first patient.

Gonioscopic Appearance

As noted, the anterior chamber depth has been found to be deeper in eyes with pigment dispersion syndrome when matched against controls. It has also been found to be deeper in the more affected eye, suggesting that the angles in these patients will be somewhat wider than normal (58). Careful slit lamp observation may detect a slight concavity to the iris in the midperipheral zone. Rarely, pigment dispersion syndrome has been reported in eyes with narrow angles (Table 7.4) (20).

Gonioscopically, normal pigmentation occurs in varying amounts. It is detectable in 40% to 50% of adult eyes and is present in all eyes after age 80 (28). Typically, the normal increased pigmentation is heavier in the inferior or nasal quadrants (28,59). With pigmentary dispersion syndrome and pigmentary glaucoma the posterior half of the trabecula overlying Schlemm's canal is heavily pigmented in all quadrants and may involve the total width of the trabecula. It can be so dense that it appears as a ring (18,19,28) (Plate 41). A large quantity of aqueous pigment, made available for extended periods of time, is required for the pigment ring to develop. Occasional dilation-induced pigment release will not cause the trabecular meshwork to appear abnormally pigmented. In the 799 eyes with pigment dispersion reported by Schie and Cameron, most had grade III or greater pigmentation. The authors did note that heavy pigmentation can be present without elevated IOP, suggesting that other factors may be responsible for the glaucoma in pigmentary glaucoma (18). The degree of pigmentation at initial presentation is not helpful for predicting which eyes will develop glaucoma; however, once there is a diagnosis of glaucoma, the degree of trabecular pigmentation correlates with the severity of the glaucoma (16,18,21).

Any variation in trabecular pigmentation may express an equilibrium between the pigment released and the pigment phagocytized and also may indicate variations in the outflow capacity of various meshwork regions in an individual eye (47). The greater the pigmentation is, the more pigment released and the less being phagocytized. The lighter the pigmentation is, the less pigment is being released and the more it is phagocytized.

TABLE 7.4

Conditions with Pigmented Trabecular Meshwork

Condition	Pigmented Meshwork Characteristics
Pigment dispersion	All quadrants, dense, bilateral, heavy in filtration portion
Exfoliation	Variable, unilateral first, patchy, Sampaolesi line inferior angle
Narrow angles	Superior angle heaviest
Inflammatory	Usually inferior, unilateral, diffuse, coarse, scattered
Nevus, melanoma	Localized, unilateral
Postoperative	Variable, unilateral, coarse

Adapted from Stewart C. *Clinical practice of glaucoma*. (Thorofare, NJ: Slack Inc., 1990.)

Patchy pigmentation circumferentially may be an indication of irregular alterations of the aqueous outflow (Plate 6). Pigment collects where normal flow exists; no pigment or less pigment collects where resistance to outflow exists (47,59).

Speakman observed that where pigment dispersion decreased, corneal pigmentation decreased and the trabecular pigmentation did not (22). This suggests that evidence of pigmented trabecular meshwork may persist after other evidence of dispersion has resolved.

Gonioscopically, one may observe a wavy pigmented band just above Schwalbe's line in the inferior angle (Plate 33). This is characteristically described with the exfoliation syndrome (19). In eyes with exfoliation, pigment may deposit in the trabecular meshwork as well, but this tends to be more patchy, less localized, and denser in the inferior angle and to take more time to develop into a pigmented ring around the meshwork than the ring in the pigment dispersion syndrome (Plate 18) (28).

Most often, pigmented deposits in the angle associated with inflammation, surgery, and trauma collect in the inferior angle (Plates 15 and 24). This is probably related to gravity and aqueous currents. The presence of a pigmented trabecular band involving the superior angle should be considered a sign of abnormal pigment dispersion, especially if the entire circumference of the meshwork is involved. An exception may be found in eyes with narrow angles where the pigment may collect in the superior angle, producing a paradoxical pigment inversion (Plate 15). Desjardins and Parrish reported this finding and theorized that this inversion may be the result of prolonged contact between the peripheral iris and the trabecular meshwork, causing rubbing of the iris against the trabeculum. This releases iris stromal pigment, which remains trapped in the narrow angle and unable to fall to the inferior angle, thereby producing this appearance (60).

Lichter and Shaffer reported an increased incidence of iris processes in eyes with pigmentary glaucoma and recommend transillumination to observe them (20). They believe their presence is a diagnostic characteristic of pigmentary glaucoma; however, their findings were not confirmed by other investigators (18).

Eyes with pigment dispersion may have a gonioscopically concave appearance to the peripheral iris as it inserts along the anterior chamber wall (Plate 22). The root of the iris appears to project or bow posterior (19,41). The iris may appear to sweep anterior just before insertion and actually insert more anterior than usual, possibly as high as the posterior edge of the filtering trabecular meshwork, resembling eyes with congenital glaucoma (61). This will not be obvious on slit lamp inspection. Iridodonesis is frequently present, and gonioscopic evaluation of the dilated eye will reveal pigment on the posterior lens where the anterior hyaloid face inserts into the posterior lens periphery, on the posterior zonules, and on the anterior vitreous face (16,17,27).

Reversal of Pigment Dispersion

Pigment dispersion has been shown to decrease over time (21, 22). In some cases when it ceases, the pigmented trabeculum may lighten in association with the healing of the iris transillumination (27). This is consistent with the theory that pigment dispersion may be a self-limited disease. Possibly, the primary pigment dispersion occurs in a short time span and then takes many years to resolve. Speakman, measuring pigment on the cornea, pigment in the angle, and transillumination of the iris, found that after 5 years, eight out of nine patients he followed either had dispersion that remained the same or decreased, with most showing decreases after 10 years (22). If the trabecular meshwork does not suffer permanent damage, it may regain normal function once dispersion stops, and the glaucoma will go into remission. Thus, in older patients with evidence of glaucomatous disc damage, mild evidence of pigment dispersion and normal IOP, and no progression of disc damage, suspicion of previous pigmentary glaucoma in remission should be included in the differential diagnosis of "low-tension" glaucoma. As Campbell suggests, this may be the result of age-related increasing lens diameter with decreasing pupil size combining to lift the iris. away from the zonules. This reduces or eliminates the pigment dispersion and allows for the recovery of the meshwork function (19,41). On successive visits, observing whether the iris transillumination is increasing or decreasing and grading trabecular pigmentation with gonioscopy will allow the clinician to judge whether the disease process is stable, regressing, or progressing (31,41). This reversal can also be induced by long-term miotic therapy (41).

Pigment dispersion associated with implantation of anterior chamber, iris-supported, and posterior chamber intraocular lenses has been reported (41,48,62). Sometimes the pigment dispersion may exacerbate a preexisting glaucoma, and sometimes it may be the cause. This can occur early in the postoperative course from surgical difficulties, resulting from unusual manipulation of the lens against the iris, or as late as two years from chronic lens-iris touch because of poor lens edges, or continued iris-lens movement. Preoperative evaluation, including gonioscopy, should reveal eyes already suffering pigment dispersion that may be more inclined to suffer from any postoperative pigment dispersion trabecular damage.

Treatment

Pigmentary glaucoma is treated as an open-angle glaucoma. Medical management is the initial therapeutic choice. If it is unsuccessful, anterior laser trabeculoplasty is often the second level of treatment, with filtering surgery following if the other therapies fail. Compared to patients with primary open-angle glaucoma, a higher percentage of patients with pigmentary glaucoma require filtering surgery.

Theoretically, miotic therapy based on Campbell's theory, is an excellent choice since miotic agents will result in pulling the iris away from the zonules and reduce rubbing and, thus, the pigment dispersion. Younger patients with this disease, however, often will not tolerate miotic therapy. Care should be used in prescribing miotic agents in this group of patients in the light of the reported high incidence of retinal detachments and lattice degeneration associated with PDS and

pigmentary glaucoma. The theoretical value of miotics as a prophylactic treatment was not borne out in Migliazzo's report where 38% of his patients treated with miotics continued to show glaucomatous damage (21).

Epinephrine and beta blockers have had success; pigment release secondary to adrenergic agonists, however, should be considered as a potential negative side effect, particularly in older individuals receiving concomitant miotic therapy. Alpha adrenergic agonists such as thymoxamine or dapiprazole have potential therapeutic value as they cause miosis without affecting accommodation; in one recent case report, however, thymoxamine was found to be ineffective where low-strength pilocarpine was effective (18,55). In another report, dapiprazole was found to increase flaccidity to the mid-peripheral iris, increasing the posterior iris bowing (46). It should also be remembered that some cases of pigmentary glaucoma may terminate on their own and some may require therapy only when the IOP is acutely elevated. Thus the potential for overtreating patients should be balanced with the potential for glaucoma and elevated IOP to be self-limited (19,31,41).

Exfoliation Syndrome

The exfoliative syndrome was first described by the Finnish ophthalmologist Lindberg in 1917 when he noticed bluish gray flakes located on the pupillary border in a number of his patients with glaucoma (63,64,65). Over the years, this syndrome has been given numerous names including *senile exfoliation, pseudoexfoliation syndrome, the basement membrane exfoliation syndrome*, and *exfoliation syndrome* (63,66). In 1954, the term *pseudoexfoliation* was proposed by Dvorak-Theobold in an attempt to distinguish the associated lens deposits from true lens exfoliation, but current evidence suggests that the material is in fact partially from the lens so the term *exfoliation syndrome* is now suggested (67,68). When glaucoma is associated with exfoliation, the condition is often referred to as *capsular glaucoma*, and it is considered a form of secondary open-angle glaucoma (69). The term *exfoliative syndrome* is preferable because it indicates the broad nature of this process, and cases should be further distinguished by noting whether glaucoma is present or absent rather than using the term *capsular glaucoma*.

Prevalence

The prevalence of exfoliation varies in different parts of the world, occurring in 3% to 8% of the adult population, but it is generally thought to be most common in Scandinavia, where it appears in 18% to 20% of patients over the age of 60 (63,64). There are similar prevalence figures in isolated areas of Russia and Spain (70,71). There is also a high prevalence among the Navajo Indians (35%), and in the Framingham study, it was found in 5% of patients age 75 to 85 (72,73). In southern Louisiana its prevalence was found to be 2% in whites and 0.3% in Blacks within a group of glaucoma patients over the age of 50 (74). In another study, it was found in no Eskimos over age 60 (70). The variation in study results may have something to do with actual prevalence differences in different world religions. Inconsistent definitions of the disease, population biases, ethnic and racial composition, and variation of examination techniques may also bias study results (69,70,75). Although the rate of occurrence varies from study to study, in all studies its prevalence increases with age. It rarely presents before the middle of the fourth decade and increases in incidence with each succeeding decade (63,65,76,77). Its association with glaucoma also varies, depending on the study, but there does appear to be an association with open-angle glaucoma. More recently, it has been noted that patients with exfoliation also have a high frequency of narrow angles (78). In the initial presentation, it is usually found unilaterally with 6.8% of fellow eyes developing clinical signs within five years. The prevalence of bilaterality increases with age (64,79).

Patients with exfoliation have a high incidence of cataracts and common findings of inferior crystalline lens displacement (78). They suffer a higher rate of complications when they undergo cataract surgery as the eyes typically dilate poorly and suffer zonular dialysis, vitreous loss, and fibrin reaction in the anterior chamber and posterior synechia (63,64,75, 80). Ciliary sulcus fixation of intraocular lenses with large-diameter haptics is one recommendation for use in eyes with the exfoliative syndrome (75).

Clinical Characteristics

Clinically the diagnosis of exfoliation syndrome is made by careful observation of the deposition of dandrufflike flakes of exfoliative material on the pupil margin (frill) (Plate 26). This can be observed on routine undilated examination by direct slit lamp examination. Gonioscopy can enhance detection by providing a direct view of the medial aspect of the pupil frill (Figure 7.4). The material may also be observed on the anterior lens surface in an undilated eye by using minimal slit lamp illumination or a blue slit lamp filter. This allows the pupil to enlarge, offering a glimpse of the lens deposits. When the eye is dilated, the presence of characteristic anterior lens

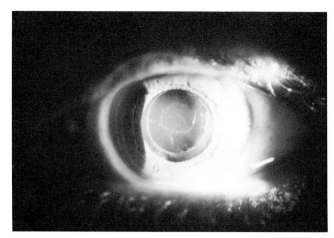

Figure 7.5 Exfoliation on the lens. This illustration shows a characteristic double ring formation with a clear zone between the two rings.

capsule changes is usually quite obvious, and the lens capsule will often have a characteristic double ring of exfoliative material (Figure 7.5). The central zone corresponds to the location of the pupil at its normal resting position. The peripheral zone has a circular deposit of exfoliative material that appears gray and granular and sometimes extends to the lens equator. The area between the two zones is usually without exfoliative material or with occasional exfoliative bands connecting the two zones, probably as a result of iris movement across the lens (63). The edges of the sheets of material may be slightly raised and folded (Figure 7.6), appearing detached from the lens capsule and yielding an appearance similar to infrared radiation-induced lens exfoliation. Failure to dilate patients will limit detection of the characteristic lens changes and recognition of the condition (78).

There are two theories explaining this characteristic lens appearance. One proposes that the material is a deposition from structures elsewhere in the eye and that it then becomes deposited from the aqueous on the lens capsule. This theory was originally proposed in the 1930s. Evidence of exfoliation

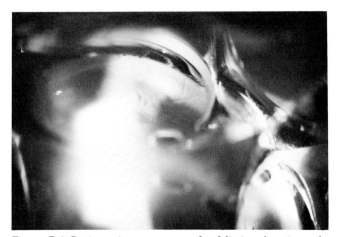

Figure 7.4 Gonioscopic appearance of exfoliation deposit on the medial aspect of the pupil.

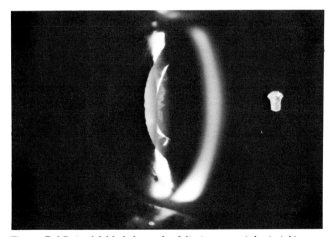

Figure 7.6 Raised folded sheet of exfoliation material mimicking exfoliation from infrared radiation.

after intracapsular cataract extraction supports this theory (81). The other theory, proposed in the 1920s, suggests that the exfoliative material originates from the lens capsule. Recent evidence reveals exfoliative material originating from the lens epithelium and migrating through the lens capsule to the surface, which supports this latter theory (82). It is likely that both processes take place and that a combination of the two accounts for the clinical picture (83). Flakes of coalesced exfoliative material may be observed on the posterior cornea (Figure 7.7). This is probably deposition of material originating from the lens or from another source, carried by the aqueous, and deposited on the endothelium. There does not appear to be a relationship between exfoliative material production and the cornea.

Other clinical signs associated with dispersion of pigment from the iris pigment epithelium include loss of the pupillary ruff (Plate 8), peppering of pigment deposits on the iris in the sphincter region, transillumination of the iris in the area of the sphincter, the presence of pigment cells in the anterior chamber after dilation, and moderate-to-dense trabecular pigmentation (80) (Plate 18). The pigment floating in the anterior chamber may be sufficiently dense to appear to be in a gelatinous material that can be misconstrued as vitreous (84). All these findings are consistent with an aging eye. They appear more increased, however, in an eye with exfoliation. Thus the presence of these findings out of proportion to the norm is suggestive of abnormal pigment dispersion and may be a precursor to the clinical observation of exfoliative material. It has been shown that exfoliative material is present in conjunctival biopsies before there is clinical evidence of the material (85).

Postdilation IOP measurements should be done in all cases of exfoliative syndrome with and without glaucoma as some eyes may experience large postdilation IOP spikes. In a glaucomatous eye with a fragile nerve, it is important to have the IOP return to baseline as quickly as possible to prevent further nerve damage and to reduce the risk for central retinal vein occlusion. (By histological examination, exfoliation was shown to be a frequent finding in eyes previously suffering central retinal vein occlusions [86]). Patients may also experience blurred vision and colored halos from IOP-induced corneal edema.

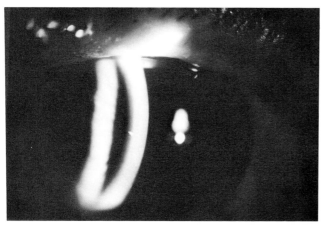

Figure 7.7 Deposit of exfoliation material on the corneal endothelium.

Gonioscopically the trabecular meshwork will often show increased pigmentation in cases of exfoliation; it is rare, however, to visualize the exfoliative material in the angle. If it is present, the material may appear white to bluish (Plate 46) and may be noticed on the trabecular surface mixed with the pigment. It may also be observed on the iris root, the ciliary body, or the posterior cornea; usually only the larger flakes are observable. The area just above Schwalbe's line will have a characteristic irregular pigment dusting, particularly in the inferior angle known as *Sampaolesi's line,* described as waves of pigment lines parallel to each other and located in the lower chamber angle between four and eight o'clock (Plate 33). This line is considered by some to be the earliest sign of the exfoliative syndrome (87). Pigment dispersion in the exfoliation syndrome probably results from mechanical rubbing of the iris against the roughened lens surface. The pigmentation to the trabecular meshwork is slower to develop into a complete ring when compared to the pigment dispersion syndrome and generally remains scattered rather than ringlike. In one study, the observation of heavy pigmentation in the superior angle was suggested as an early sign for the exfoliation syndrome and interestingly was observed more frequently than pupil frill deposits in eyes with lens changes. There was a high incidence of PAS and narrow angles in the same group of eyes, which may have influenced the pigment deposit in the superior angle (60,78).

The pigment dispersion syndrome and the exfoliation syndrome are two separate clinical conditions with similarities related primarily to the pigment liberation from the posterior iris (Table 7.5). Their clinical presentations in most cases, are sufficiently dissimilar to allow for clear differentiation. The pigment release in each condition appears mechanically related but in different iris locations. In the exfoliation syndrome, the constant movement of the iris over the roughened anterior central lens surface probably accounts for the more patchy, pupil margin iris transillumination located in the sphincter area. In contrast to the pigment dispersion syndrome, the exfoliative syndrome typically presents unilaterally in older patients with no consistent pattern to corneal endothelial pigment deposits and is unrelated to gender, refractive error, or race. The two syndromes have been reported to occur in the same eye, their simultaneous presentation resulting in a difficult-to-control glaucoma (88).

A fine neovascular change, *microneovascularization of the iris,* detectable by fluorescein angiography, has been described in the exfoliation syndrome. The microneovascularization is secondary to iris hypoperfusion and is not associated with neovascularization of the angle and or iris fibrovascular membrane formation. It is probably a secondary change resulting from exfoliation rather than a cause (89).

Jerndal recently described a two-stage clinical presentation of exfoliation associated with glaucoma. He described stage I as the *brown* stage. This affects primarily the uveal tissue, expressed as atrophy and liberation of pigment. Clinically, this manifests as a granular pigment ring adjacent to the pupillary iris surface heaviest in the 5:30 to 6:30 area with a

TABLE 7.5
Exfoliation Syndrome vs. Pigment Dispersion Syndrome

	Exfoliation Syndrome	Pigment Dispersion Syndrome
Age of onset	>60	35 to 50
Race	Varies	White
Sex	M = F	M > F
Initial presentation	Unilateral	Bilateral
Iris transillumination	Pupil/sphincter area	Midperipheral
Trabecular pigmentation	Patchy	Concentric ring
Pigment release on dilation	Yes	Yes
Sampaolesi line	Yes	Variable
Pupil dandruff	Yes	No
Lens granulation	Yes	No
Anterior chamber	Shallow	Deep

corresponding iris transillumination. The cornea has scattered pigment concentrated centrally and inferior. The angle has a line with increased pigmentation to the inferior angle and isolated patches elsewhere, possibly indicating the location of angle sites with the greatest outflow. On dilation, the peripheral lens surface may display a radial pattern of spotty pigmentation that later demonstrates the granular lens changes associated with exfoliation. In addition, a microscopic pigment deposition at the insertion of the zonules onto the lens capsule may be observed. Stage II, the gray stage, may take several years to develop and consists of the observation of the gray exfoliative material on different anterior segment structures (75).

Nature of the Material

The exfoliative material itself probably originates from basement membrane-secreting cells, including the epithelial cells of the anterior lens equator, iris pigment epithelium, and ciliary body, and then becomes deposited on the surfaces of the anterior and posterior chambers (66,81,86). Electron microscopy studies have shown that the material can be found deposited on and in the trabecular meshwork, on the posterior cornea, in the iris, and on the ciliary processes, lens zonules, and vitreous body (81). Electron microscopy studies have also shown the material in the stroma of the bulbar and palpebral conjunctiva of both eyes in cases clinically involving one eye and in the wall of the short ciliary artery, indicating that the material is not limited to the lens or ocular tissues (64,66,76, 90). Thus the presence of the crystalline lens is not necessary for this condition to manifest clinically (29). The exact nature and cause of the material is still uncertain, with proposals suggesting it is amyloid, elastin, or glycosaminoglycans, the result of a metabolic disorder related to aging (63,86,92).

Pathogenesis of Exfoliative Glaucoma and Treatment

In one study, scanning electromicroscopy of the trabecular meshwork in exfoliation syndrome revealed it to be similar to the meshwork in chronic open-angle glaucoma except that it appeared "dirtier". Three distinct characteristics in exfoliation

were noted: (1) a gray appearance to the trabecular meshwork with white exfoliation deposits, (2) pigment granules remaining on the chamber aspect of the trabeculum (this is different from pigmentary dispersion where most pigment passes through the intertrabecular spaces), and (3) collar arrangements of pigment granules around the trabeculum (87). Apparently, the pigment granule exfoliation complex, because of its size, has a more difficult time passing through the entire meshwork and may remain on the superficial layers. In another study, light microscopy showed the exfoliative material on the trabecular meshwork, in the intertrabecular spaces, and in Schlemm's canal (93). Material has also been found within the endothelial cell vacuoles, suggesting local production within the trabeculum.

The glaucoma associated with the exfoliation syndrome probably results from deposition of pigment and exfoliative material within the endothelial cells of the trabecular beams. The trabecular tissue swells, compacts the intertrabecular spaces, and increased resistance to outflow results. Jerndel has proposed the presence of a dysgenic cellular membrane as evidence of a congenital goniodysgenesis, which he feels contributes to outflow disturbances in this syndrome (75,94). Tarkkanen has proposed that exfoliative glaucoma results from an overload from pigment and exfoliative material in an already impaired outflow system and that eyes that develop glaucoma with exfoliation already have an underlying predisposition to open-angle glaucoma (86).

The reports of glaucoma associated with exfoliation are quite variable, probably owing to population bias and criteria for defining glaucoma. Looking at subjects reporting for routine examinations, one study found an incidence of glaucoma in 7% of eyes with exfoliation. Ocular hypertension was observed in 13% of the eyes (95). In another study of the long-term follow-up of exfoliative patients, the cumulative probability of developing elevated IOP was 5.3% in 5 years and 15.4% in 10 years, leading the authors to conclude that patients with exfoliation have a higher incidence of developing elevated IOP than is expected of patients in the same age category without exfoliation (79). These studies yield a lower incidence of elevated IOP associated with exfoliation than is generally perceived.

In comparison to open-angle glaucoma, glaucoma with exfoliation is characterized by lack of steroid responsiveness, unilateral presentation, higher IOP, more severe visual field loss, more frequent need for multiple medications and drainage surgery to control IOP, and good initial IOP response to ALT (although visual field loss may continue) (78,80,96,97,98,99). As with pigmentary glaucoma, an eye with heavier angle pigmentation appears to suffer more severe glaucoma. The presence of an underlying predisposition for chronic open-angle glaucoma may tip the scales toward glaucoma production and may explain why not all eyes with exfoliation develop glaucoma (85).

Medical management consists of agents typically used for treating chronic open-angle glaucoma. Care should be used with miotic and epinephrine agents. Miotics may induce posterior synechia and or increase pupil block in eyes with associated narrow angles and shallow chambers. Cataracts are common in eyes with exfoliation syndrome, and miosis may reduce vision. Epinephrine compounds (adrenergic agonists) may create a paradoxical pressure increase from pigment and exfoliation dispersion (100).

Hemosiderotic, Hemolytic, and Ghost Cell Glaucoma

Hemosiderotic, hemolytic, and ghost cell glaucoma are three rare forms of secondary open-angle glaucoma associated with intraocular hemorrhage. Confusion exists because the three entitites are at times all referred to as *hemolytic glaucoma* although their clinical presentations and pathogenesis for glaucoma are different. Questions have also been raised about whether there is actually a separate form of hemolytic glaucoma.

Hemosiderotic Glaucoma

Hemosiderotic glaucoma is associated with recurrent long-standing intraocular hemorrhage. Hemoglobin, hemosiderin, and macrophages combine to block the meshwork and obstruct the aqueous outflow (101). The glaucoma develops many years after the original hemorrhage (102). It presents in an eye with other signs of siderosis including retinal degeneration, cataract, iris discoloration, and iron staining of the cornea (103).

Hemolytic Glaucoma

In hemolytic glaucoma, macrophages phagocytize the contents of red blood cells and, along with pigment, accumulate in the trabecular meshwork, causing temporary outflow obstruction resulting in an acute open-angle glaucoma (102,104). The anterior chamber will have reddish cells and a pigmented fawn-colored meshwork will be detectable on gonioscopy (103). The glaucoma is usually self-limited and responds to medical therapy but in some instances requires an anterior chamber washout (29,69). Invariably hemolytic glaucoma results from vitreous hemorrhage in eyes without an intact vitreous face although there was one case reported that was associated with a traumatic anterior chamber hemorrhage (105).

Ghost Cell Glaucoma

Ghost cell glaucoma was originally described by Campbell and colleagues in 1976 (106). This glaucoma is often transient and results from obstruction of the trabecular meshwork by degenerated erythrocytes that have moved from the vitreous into the anterior chamber.

Typically, within one to three weeks after a vitreous hemorrhage, the normal erythrocytes degenerate to a tan- or khaki-colored spherical hollow ghost cell. The intracellular hemoglobin leaves the cells and becomes enmeshed within the vitreous strands. The ghost cells normally remain free within the vitreous for many months following the hemorrhage and are eventually ingested by macrophages (107). If the anterior vitreous face is broken, the ghost cells have the ability to pass forward into the anterior chamber. The ghost cells are less pliant than are normal erythrocytes, and because of this inflexibility, they clog the trabecular meshwork. Breaks in the vitreous face in association with vitreous hemorrhage occur with trauma or surgery, or in some uncommon cases, they are presumed to occur spontaneously from vitreous liquification and degeneration or from a functional defect of the anterior hyaloid face (102,103,108). Most cases of ghost cell glaucoma have been reported after vitrectomy, cataract extraction, or trauma. Ghost cell glaucoma has also been reported in an eye with vitreous hemorrhage secondary to choroidal neovascular membrane associated with age-related macular degeneration (109). Typically the elevation in pressure occurs within three to four weeks of the vitreous hemorrhage although late-developing cases in phakic nontraumatized eyes have been reported (103). The presentation of the glaucoma may be dependent on the time of the hemorrhage, the presence of ghost cells, their ability to pass forward, and the load of ghost cells reaching the meshwork. If there are only scattered ghost cells, then pressure may remain normal. It is possible for the IOP to become elevated within days of vitreous hemorrhage with associated vitreous face disruption.

Ghost cell glaucoma does not occur after pure anterior chamber hemorrhage. The reason for this, according to Campbell, is that the higher levels of oxygen, rapid circulation of fluid, and decreased volume in the anterior chamber in comparison to the vitreous compartment account for many fewer ghost cells being present after anterior chamber hemorrhage (107).

Gonioscopically the trabecular meshwork has been described as having either a normal appearance or a tan coloration (107). When the ghost cells are numerous, the posterior portion of the trabecular meshwork looks like it has a layer of butter overlying it (59). A pseudohypopyon, khaki in color, may develop when there are large numbers of ghost cells (Plate 42). The tan or khaki color differentiates this from a true hypopion. If the ghost cells are numerous in the anterior chamber, they can be mistaken for inflammatory cells. The lack of keratic precipitates, a relatively quiet conjunctiva, and a history of a recent vitreous hemorrhage with disruption of the hyaloid face, however, would make the differentiation easier (102). Phase-contrast examination of aspirated aqueous humor from the anterior chamber will confirm the diagnosis (110).

Glaucoma treatment consists of the standard medical management for open-angle glaucoma. Once the anterior chamber is gradually cleared and there is no longer a ghost cell supply, the pressure will normalize. This may take months and is often dependent on the severity of the hemorrhage and the numbers and persistence of the ghost cells. If the IOP is severely elevated to the 60 to 70 mm/Hg level or if it persists for a number of weeks in the 40 to 50 mm/Hg level, surgical intervention is necessary. This consists of draining the anterior chamber and washing it out with physiological saline (59). Some nonresponsive cases may require trabeculectomy and/or vitrectomy (103,107).

Campbell and colleagues question the existence of hemolytic glaucoma from only red cell debris and macrophages, noting that they have never observed such a case. They feel that all cases of hemolytic glaucoma involve ghost cells (102,107). Ghost cell glaucoma and hemosiderotic glaucoma have been described in the same eye (103).

Blunt Trauma-Induced Angle Abnormalities

Blunt trauma to the eye may cause local injury at the point of impact to the cornea or conjunctiva, resulting in corneal abrasions or subconjunctival hemorrhages. The more serious damage tends to take place elsewhere, secondary to the shock waves coursing through the interior portion of the globe, a contrecoup injury (Figure 7.8) (111). The internal fluids of the eye cannot compress, and, thus, according to Campbell, the rings of tissue inside the eye expand and may undergo separation or tearing (112). This includes the pupil sphincter, the iris base (iridodialysis), anterior ciliary body (angle recession), the site of ciliary-scleral spur attachment (cyclodialysis), trabecular meshwork, zonules, and attachment of the retina to the ora serrata (Figure 7.9). In addition to the obvious presentation of iridocyclitis and hyphema, these tears may clinically manifest as iris sphincter splits, lens subluxation, phacodonesis, retinal tears or dialysis, retinal detachments, vitreous hemorrhage, choroidal rupture and an angle recession (ciliary body tear), iridodialysis, or cyclodialysis. In any eye suffering blunt trauma, a combination of these findings may be present. Observation of at least one of these findings should alert the examiner to search for signs of the others.

Histologically, angle recession represents a tear between the longitudinal and circular muscles of the ciliary body, resulting in the posterior displacement of the ciliary body along the iris root (Figure 7.10). It is the most common angle

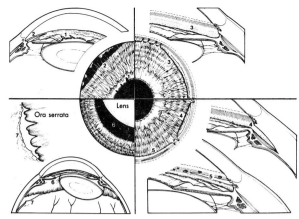

Figure 7.9 Locations of anterior globe tears following blunt ocular trauma. (1) Pupillary tears, (2) iridodialysis, (3) angle recession, (4) cyclodialysis, (5) trabecular meshwork tears, (6) ruptured zonules, (7) retinal dialysis. (Reprinted with permission from Campbell D. Traumatic glaucoma. In Shingleton BJ et al, eds. Eye trauma. St Louis: Mosby-Yearbook, 1991.)

change from blunt trauma (Table 7.6) and requires gonioscopic evaluation for detection (112,113). An *iridodialysis* is a tear in the root of the iris (Plates 14 and 43A), and a *cyclodialysis* is separation of the ciliary body from the scleral spur. They occur less frequently than does angle recession and can be observed by slit lamp examination, as well as gonioscopically. Contusion injuries result from small objects, such as BBs, stones, paper clips, or rubber bands, and large objects, such

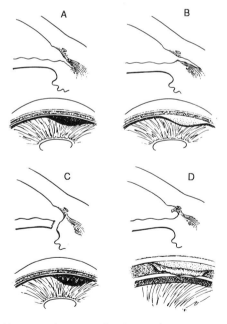

Figure 7.10 Forms of anterior chamber angle injury associated with blunt trauma showing cross-sectional and corresponding gonioscopic appearance. (A) Angle recession (tear between longitudinal and circular muscles of ciliary body). (B) Cyclodialysis (separation of ciliary body from scleral spur, with widening of the suprachoroidal space. (C) Iridodialysis (tear in root of iris). (D) Trabecular damage (tear in anterior portion of meshwork, creating flap that is hinged. (Reprinted with permission from Shizlo MB. Textbook of glaucoma, 3d ed. Baltimore: Williams & Wilkins, 1992.)

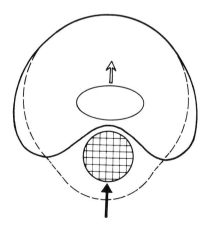

Figure 7.8 Momentary changes occurring after blunt trauma. The cornea and sclera are displaced posteriorly, and there is a compensatory expansion of the eye at the equator. This may result in tissue separation at a number of sites within the eye, including the angle. (Reprinted with permission from Campbell DG. Traumatic glaucoma. In Shingleton BJ et al, eds. Eye trauma. St Louis: Mosby-Yearbook, 1991.)

TABLE 7.6

Angle recession	Tear between the longitudinal and circular muscles of the ciliary body
Iridodialysis	Tear in the root of the iris
Cyclodialysis	Ciliary body separation from the scleral spur

as soccer balls or fists (113,114). Most contusion injuries are related to domestic or athletic accidents, and they occur predominantly in children and young adults (111).

Traumatic Hyphema

Hyphema is a common presenting condition with blunt trauma, with ciliary body tears being the most common reason for it (Table 7.7) (111, 115). This results from embarrassment to the major arterial circle and its small branches. Ruptured iris blood vessels may also cause a hyphema (115).

Hyphemas are graded based on the amount of layered blood occupying the anterior chamber (44):

Grade 1, less than one-third.
Grade 11, one-third to one-half.
Grade III, one-half to almost total.
Grade IV, total or "eight-ball" hyphema.

When only microscopic circulating blood cells are present without any layered blood, the hyphema is called a *microscopic hyphema* (115). Glaucoma results from hyphema when there is an initial clogging of the trabecular meshwork with red blood cells, plasma, fibrin, and debris. If the patient suffers a rebleed, usually within the first two to four days after the original bleed, pressure may become elevated from a clot formation that blocks aqueous outflow.

The prevalence of angle recession in eyes with traumatic

TABLE 7.7
Blood in the Angle

Conditions	Findings
Fresh blood	Bright red clot
Old, degenerated blood	Clumped black particles and balls scattered in the angle
Organized persistent clot	Synechia filling the angle
Spontaneous hyphema	From new vessels in angle or iris associated with neovascular glaucoma
	From microhemangiomas of pupil frill
	From blood in Schlemm's canal
	From tumor
	From intraocular lens foot plates
Hyphema from sudden hypotony	From new vessels in the angle in heterochromic cyclitis
	From blood in Schlemm's canal
Hyphema from blunt trauma	From rupture of vessels in angle or iris

(From Epstein DL. *Chandler and Grant's glaucoma.* 3d ed. Phildelphia: Lea & Febiger, 1986.)

hyphema ranges from 60% to 100%, and it is rare to have a recession in an eye that has not experienced some hyphema (112,116–121). Gonioscopic examination within 48 hours after blunt trauma to an eye with even mild hyphema, consistently reveals damage to the meshwork, the inner wall of Schlemm's canal, and angle recession (Figure 7.11). Evidence of trabecular damage consists of hemorrhage into Schlemm's canal from branches of vessels near the canal and/or rupture of the entire meshwork either focally or in an entire quadrant (Plate 44). This results in the appearance of a flap extending posterior from Schwalbe's line to its attachment at the scleral spur (118) (Plate 44). The appearance of angle recession changes rapidly within the first week, with a tendency toward scarring and closure of the tear by means of ciliary peripheral anterior synechia (PAS) (114,118) (Figure 7.11). Trabecular lesions also scar and become more difficult to detect. Dark ovallike deposits may be observed in the

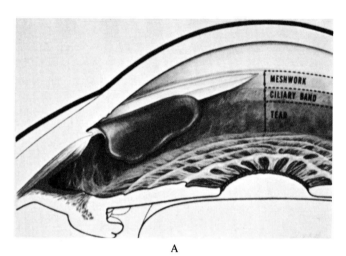

A

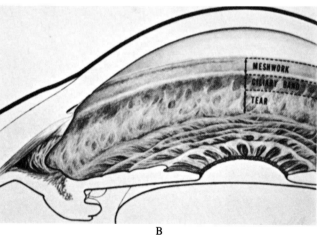

B

Figure 7.11 (A) Artist's rendition of the appearance of the angle within 24 hours of blunt trauma to the eye. There is a blood clot hanging from the torn trabecular meshwork and a deep-angle recession grade 2 to 3. (B) The same eye eight days later. The blood has cleared, and the flap has healed. A ciliary PAS has developed and narrowed the recession. (Published courtesy of Herschler J. Trabecular damage due to blunt anterior segment injury and its relationship to traumatic glaucoma. Trans Am Acad Otolaryngol. *1977;83: OP239-248.*

angle after a hemorrhage has resolved and serve as evidence of previous hemorrhage (Plates 3 and 45) (112).

Gonioscopy during the acute stages is generally contraindicated in eyes with hyphema because it could traumatize the eye and cause rebleeding. If necessary for localization of the bleeding site, quick screening examinations, without any pressure against the globe, may be performed. A flat-base-curve four-mirror gonioscopy lens is preferable. The examination requires a gentle, steady technique, without compression against the cornea, to avoid posterior iris movement. Once the blood is cleared and the eye is quiet, gonioscopy will reveal that the blunt trauma has caused a tear to the structures in the anterior chamber (14) (Plate 5). Gonioscopy should be performed about six weeks after the injury. The observation of an angle recession of greater than 180 degrees at that time implies a 10% likelihood of future glaucoma (112). Over time, deep recessions may become obscured by late-developing adhesions between the iris root and the longitudinal muscle (118). Therefore, the sooner gonioscopy can be performed, the more evident the angle damage will be.

Angle Recession

The force from a contusion injury will cause displacement of the outer limits of the angle laterally and peripherally, resulting in an angle recession, iridodialysis, or cyclodialysis (119). If an angle recession is greater than 180 degrees, the depth of the chamber may be altered sufficiently to be evident on slit lamp examination when compared with the other eye (119).

In normal eyes, the ciliary body band appears even throughout its circumference and is symmetrical between eyes. Gonioscopically, an angle recession appears as either a small, localized or a diffuse, irregular widening of the ciliary body band, increasing the visibility of this structure (Table 7.8). According to Campbell, the ciliary body band is usually not wider than the trabecular meshwork; observation of unevenness greater than the width of one trabecular meshwork width is evidence of recession (114) (Plate 21). In addition to depth and width changes, color and texture changes can also be observed. Any of these permutations may be variable in depth and extent along the circumference of the angle (Plate 14).

At the time of injury, the recession may be more extensive in appearance, with the ensuing scarring making it less obvious; thus, an older contusion injury will have less obvious signs in the anterior chamber angle (114,118). As healing takes place, the tears become less distinct, and any color difference between the normal and traumatized tissue disappears (117). In most cases, however, late signs of recession are still obvious. In one study, 80% of patients suffering blunt trauma still had gonioscopic evidence of angle recession 1 to 14 years after the trauma (111).

In addition to the generally obvious widening of the visible ciliary body band and posterior displacement of the iris root, other subtle, early gonioscopic clues include the absence of iris processes or evidence of torn iris processes with an abnormally prominent Schwalbe's line, or scleral spur, in the same area as the torn processes (118) (Plate 14).

TABLE 7.8
Gonioscopic Appearance of Angle Recession

Early	Late
Localized or diffuse widening of ciliary body band; color and texture changes	Localized or diffuse widening of ciliary body band; color and texture changes
Absence of, or evidence of, torn iris processes, abnormally prominent scleral spur or Schwalbe's line in the same area as the torn processes	Increased whiteness of the scleral spur; dense pigmentation, PAS, and fibrous grayish tissue may mask recession; anterior ciliary arteries may be visible in a moderate angle tear
Flap tear of the trabecular meshwork extending posterior to its attachment at the scleral spur	Mother-of-pearl gray-white membrane covering angle recess
	Dark, oval pigment balls suggestive of old hyphema

The tags of iris processes may be visible as attachments to the surface of the iris, scleral spur, ciliary body, or trabecular meshwork and have been detected within two to three weeks after blunt trauma (114). Also, tags of actual iris tissue may remain attached to the angle wall. Later, the subtle, more prominent appearance of the scleral spur, characterized by its increased whiteness, may be the only visible gonioscopic sign. Dense pigmentation, PAS, and fibrous tissue at the iris root may also be visible, and all may mask early or late evidence of recession (111,117). Peripheral iridodonesis may be discernable on gonioscopy without evidence on slit lamp examination. This is most likely related to the iris root detachment from its base, resulting in flaccidity of the root (114).

Gonioscopically some deep chambered, darkly pigmented eyes and eyes with pigment dispersion syndrome may have a ciliary body band that appears as a mottled gray-brown tissue with a significant mixture of white, suggestive of the white band of sclera. Older patients with deep chambers may have a gray mottled appearance to the ciliary body band. These normal appearances can be confused for an angle recession or cyclodialysis (116). The lack of history and signs of trauma, such as localized lens opacities, lens subluxation phacodonesis, iris sphincter tears, and posterior segment changes, and a bilateral presentation should reinforce the normality of these anomalous appearances.

In his series of patients, Alper described "a mother of pearl grayish white membrane" covering the whole angle recess many years after the trauma (122). This needs to be differentiated from a cyclodialysis, where the ciliary body is detached from the scleral spur and sclera is directly observed.

In suspected cases of angle recession, gonioscopy should always be performed bilaterally, with the nonsuspect eye used for comparison. Comparison is especially helpful when a shallow 360-degree angle recession is present. It will also prevent misdiagnosis in the presence of a bilateral nonpathological posterior iris insertion. Some observers recommend using the Koeppe system since lenses can be placed simultaneously on both eyes and the examiner can move from one eye to the other, quickly comparing the angles (116). In cases where angle recession is suspected, compression gonioscopy may be a valuable technique. The compression causes maximum deepening of the angle recess and thus will provide more exact localization of the iris insertion and width of the ciliary body band. Examining the entire circumference of the angle with this technique will highlight any areas of recession and trauma-induced PAS. This should be done for both eyes, looking for abnormal areas of increased ciliary body visibility within an eye and between eyes.

Pupil Abnormalities

Pupil abnormalities in eyes suffering blunt trauma are not unusual. They may the result of damage to the nerve fibers, the sphincter muscle, or both. In his evaluation of 53 eyes suffering traumatic hyphema, Tonjum noted a correlation between pupil appearance, reactions, and gonioscopy (117). Pupil involvement, consisting of flattening of the pupil border, was located in the same sector as the angle recession. Usually, pupil reaction recovers as the nerve fibers regenerate or anastomosing fibers assume the function for the damaged fibers, but when a deep recession of at least 270 degrees occurs, pupil mydriasis may persist. In addition to obvious pupil abnormalities of size and reaction, the pupil margin is particularly vulnerable to blunt trauma. Small iris notches are visible in most eyes after blunt trauma (111). Evidence of this on slit lamp examination should direct the clinician toward the angle, looking for any signs of angle recession.

Classification of Angle Recessions

Angle recession can be classified as shallow, moderate, or deep (114,120). A *shallow angle tear* is characterized by a darker, wider ciliary band and a whiter, more obvious scleral spur when compared to the other eye. There is no visible cleft in the face of the ciliary muscle. In a shallow tear, angle recession may be noted to involve up to 360 degrees of the angle circumference, but usually it involves less than 100 degrees. Mooney noted that in some eyes, it is difficult to discriminate between tears of the uveal meshwork overlying the ciliary muscle and an actual tear into the ciliary muscle itself (Plate 21) (120).

A *moderate angle tear* (Plate 5) is characterized by a definite, actual cleft of the ciliary body band. Fibrous strands, pigment granules, and normal blood vessel anastomosis of the anterior ciliary arteries become visible, and in old injuries, a grayish membrane may be seen (117). The angle appears deeper than in the fellow eye (Plate 14).

A *deep angle recession* is characterized by a profound fissure into the ciliary body, but the apex of the tear is not visible gonioscopically (111,114,120). Eyes with deep recessions often have shallow or moderate tears in other areas of the angle (Plates 3 and 14).

Glaucoma

During the acute phase of angle trauma, patients may experience a transient posttraumatic decrease in IOP secondary to reduced aqueous production or temporary increase in outflow from the disrupted structures, especially if a cyclodialysis is present (122). When IOP is lower than 9 to 10 mm/Hg, small, one-quarter in circumference cyclodialysis clefts should be explored for (112).

Other patients may suffer transient IOP elevations from obvious causes, such as hyphema and/or uveitic clogging of the outflow areas. Uveal effusion or vitreous filling of the anterior chamber may also increase IOP (123). Other instances may have no obvious etiology, and gonioscopy will be normal as well. This may be the result of angle edema (124). The most frequent reason for raised IOP during the early posttraumatic interval is mechanical insult to the trabecular meshwork. This is usually self-limited as healing of the meshwork ensues (125). Campbell recommends the vigorous use of topical steroids four to six times daily for up to six weeks following blunt trauma to reduce cellular infiltration of the meshwork and to reduce the potential for scarring and fibrosis of the meshwork, which has a role in late-onset angle recession glaucoma (Table 7.9) (112).

Elevated IOP may result as a late consequence of blunt trauma with or without hyphema (112). These eyes typically suffer higher IOP than does an eye with primary open-angle glaucoma (124). In cases of unilateral glaucoma, the clinician is obligated to perform careful gonioscopy in both eyes, looking for signs of neovascularization (Plates 20 and 27), exfoliation (Plates 18 and 33), pigment dispersion (Plate 50), PAS (Plate 4), and angle recession. In unilateral glaucomatous eyes with evidence of retinal detachments, traumatic corneal scars, subluxated lenses, cataracts, traumatic chorioretinal scars, and/or iris sphincter tears, angle recession should be suspected. Gonioscopic evidence of previous angle damage will clarify the etiology of the glaucoma.

It is important for patients suffering blunt trauma with evidence of angle recession to be followed closely and be advised of the potential for developing glaucoma since anywhere from 4% to 9% of eyes with angle recession greater than 150 degrees develop chronic angle recession glaucoma (69,119,121,122,126). This is more frequent with angle recession involving 180 degrees or more (121,122). The glaucoma may take as long as 14 years to develop. In one case, it was reported 47 years and in another 64 years after trauma (119,120,121,122,127). Blanton, in his study of 130 cases, found two peak incidences of glaucoma after angle recession. One occurred early, within the first 1 to 3 years, and was transient and difficult to control; the other occurred 10 or more years later (119). In both groups, there was no association between the amount (circumference) of angle recession and the development of glaucoma. Alper also noted

TABLE 7.9
Characteristics of Glaucoma in angle recession

Early or late
More common with 180-degree recession
Miotics and argon laser trabeculoplasty (ALT) usually not effective
Usually an underlying defect present; follow fellow eye carefully

two temporal incidences of glaucoma—one early, within 4 years, and one as late as 14 years (122).

The gonioscopic appearance of angle recession changes with time. This makes scrupulous gonioscopic examination important to detect this as an etiology especially for late-developing cases. In these late-onset glaucoma cases, the angle recession itself is probably not the total cause of the elevated IOP; rather, it is a sign that the trauma was probably significant enough to result in fibrosis and hyalinization to the meshwork, with possible formation of a cuticular membrane (113,114). In some eyes, these changes may be sufficient to eventually decrease the meshwork's filtering ability, resulting in glaucoma. In other eyes, they may be additive to the decrease in outflow in an already vulnerable eye. This vulnerability may be from decreased outflow secondary to aging or some other underlying defect (113,119,127).

The information that traumatized eyes with angle recession and fellow eyes of patients suffering angle recession are positive responders to steroid testing suggests that eyes suffering angle recession may be predisposed to glaucoma from other factors associated with primary open-angle glaucoma (116). The trabecular damage suffered at the time of the trauma is probably just tipping the scales. Observation that fellow eyes of patients with unilateral angle recession glaucoma are at risk for open-angle glaucoma also supports this underlying-mechanism theory (127). Telsuk and Spaeth have suggested that the underlying predisposition facilitates the resulting glaucoma in the traumatized eye. Their observation points to the need to follow the fellow eyes of patients with unilateral angle recession glaucoma because the underlying defect implies a significant risk for glaucoma to the fellow eye. In their series, they found a 50% risk to the fellow eye (127).

It is thus possible to have cases of asymmetric glaucoma, especially if the pressures are asymmetric, where the worse eye may have suffered an angle recession (125). Careful, detailed comparative gonioscopy is imperative to reveal evidence of the recession, particularly with the knowledge that late angle recession may be very subtle because of healing and fibrosis. The presence of angle recession may limit treatment options because the therapy for this glaucoma should be directed toward lowering the aqueous production by means of beta-blockers, epinephrine compounds, and carbonic anhydrase

TABLE 7.10
Particles in the Angle

Findings	Conditions
Brown chunks	Tissue remnants from surgery
Black balls	Old blood
Gray flakes or particles	Exfoliation
Refractile scrolls	Descemet's membrane
Refractile solid particles	Glass, plastic, cortex
Light gray fibers	Cotton fibers
Bright red specks	Rubber
Silvery particles	Aluminum
Chalk-white particles	Congenital cataract remnants
Blue	Sutures

From Epstein DL. *Chandler and Grant's glaucoma*, 3d ed. Philadelphia: Lea & Febiger, 1986.

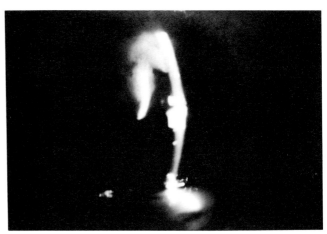
Figure 7.12 Retained lens cortex material.

inhibitors (128). Attempts to increase outflow through the damaged and scarred trabecular meshwork are unlikely to be successful, and the detached ciliary muscle may no longer be able to open the meshwork (113,129). Additionally, laser trabeculoplasty is not very successful in this form of glaucoma, possibly because of the angle scarring and of the difficulty in localizing the exact structure for laser application.

Retained Anterior Chamber Foreign Bodies

Evidence of a healed corneal perforation, especially without lens or iris damage, indicates the need for a gonioscopic evaluation (130,131). Steel, iron, brass, and copper usually cause irritation to the eye (Table 7.10 and Plate 36). Glass is inert and usually causes no irritation; however, even small slivers of glass, if localized to the anterior chamber and in contact with the endothelium, can cause a severe late-onset corneal edema resembling bullous keratitis (132). This should not be confused with endothelial damage from the trauma, as removal of the retained particles has resulted in complete resolution of signs and symptoms in these cases. It is important that a thorough gonioscopic examination be performed on any patient who presents with unexplained corneal edema with a history of an accident involving broken glass (132). Other particles may be observed in the angle. After surgery, strands of iris tissue; refractile, glassy, loose plastic scrolls of Descemet's membrane or similar-appearing remnants of lens capsule; and small black balls of degenerated blood, which remain for many years after a hyphema (23) (Figure 7.12).

References

1. Huber A. Glaucoma as a complication in heterochromia of Fuch's heterochromatic cyclitis. *Ophthalmologica*. 1961;66:142.
2. La Hey E et al. Clinical analysis of Fuch's heterochromic cyclitis. *Doc Ophthalmol*. 1991;78:225–235.
3. Lightman S, Towler H. Editorial. Fuch's heterochromic cyclitis. *Eye*. 1991;5:648.
4. Tesler HH, Williams D. Fuch's heterochromic iridocyclitis in blacks. *Arch Ophthalmol*. 1988;106:1688–1690.

5. Day KA. Fuch's syndrome. *N Engl J Optom*. 1992;44:9–13.
6. Krupin T. Glaucoma associated with uveitis. In Ritch R, Shields BM, eds. *The secondary glaucomas*. St. Louis: CV Mosby, 1982.
7. Smith RE, Nozik RA. Uveitis: A clinical approach to diagnosis and management, 2d ed. Baltimore: Williams & Wilkins, 1989.
8. Schwalb IR. The epidemiologic association of heterochromic iridocyclitis and ocular toxoplasmosis. *Am J Ophthalmol*. 1991;11:356–362.
9. Arffa RC, Schlaegel TF Jr. Chorioretinal scars in Fuch's heterochromic iridocyclitis. *Arch Ophthalmol*. 1984;102:1153–1155.
10. Hollwich F. Clinical aspects and therapy of the Posner-Schlossmann syndrome (authors abstract in English). *Klin Monatsbi Augenheilkd*. 1978;172:726–744.
11. Raitta C, Vannas A. Glaucomatocyclitic crisis. *Arch Ophthalmol*. 1977;95:608.
12. Kass MA, Becker B, Kolker A. Glaucomatocyclitic crises and primary open angle glaucoma. *Am J Ophthalmol*. 1973;75:668.
13. Hart CT, Weatherill JR. Gonioscopy and tonography in glaucomatocyclitic crises. *Br J Ophthalmol*. 1968;52:682.
14. Spivey BB, Armaly MF. Tonographic findings in glaucomatocyclitic crises. *Am J Ophthalmol*. 1963;55:47.
15. Krupin T et al. Secondary glaucoma associated with uveitis. *Glaucoma*. 1988;10:85–90.
16. Schie HG, Fleischhauer HW. Idiopathic atrophy of the epithelial layers of the iris and ciliary body. *Arch Ophthalmol*. 1958;59:216–228.
17. Zentmayer W. Association of an annular band of pigment on posterior capsule of lens with a Krukenberg spindle. *Arch Ophthalmol*. 1938;20:52.
18. Schie HG, Cameron JD. Pigment dispersion syndrome: A clinical study. *Br J Ophthalmol*. 1981;65:264–269.
19. Ritch R. Nonprogressive low-tension glaucoma with pigmentary dispersion. *Am J Ophthalmol*. 1982;94:190–196.
20. Lichter PR, Shaffer RM. Diagnostic and prognostic signs in pigmentary glaucoma. *Trans Am Acad Ophthal Otol*. 1970;74:984.
21. Migliazzo C et al. Long-term analysis of pigmentary dispersion syndrome and pigmentary glaucoma. *Ophthalmology*. 1986;93:1528–1536.
22. Speakman JS. Pigmentary dispersion. *Br J Ophthalmol*. 1981;65:249–251.
23. Iwamoto T, Witmer R. Light and electron microscopy in absolute glaucoma with pigment dispersion phenomena and contusion angle deformity. *Am J Ophthalmol*. 1971;72:420.
24. Rodrigues MM et al. Spectrum of trabecular pigmentation in open-angle glaucoma: A clinicopathologic study. *Am Acad Ophthalmol Otol*. 1976;81:258.
25. Sugar HS, Barbour FA. Pigmentary glaucoma: A rare clinical entity. *Am J Ophthalmol*. 1949;32:90.
26. Richardson T. Pigmentary glaucoma. In Ritch R et al, eds. *The glaucomas*. St. Louis: CV Mosby, 1989.
27. Campbell D. Advances in the understanding of the secondary glaucomas. In McAllister JA, Wilson RP, eds. *Glaucoma*. Boston: Butterworth-Heinemann, 1986.
28. Sugar HS. Pigmentary glaucoma: A 25-year review. *Am J Ophthalmol*. 1966;62(3):499–507.
29. Hoskins HD Jr, Kass MA. *Becker-Shaffer's diagnosis and therapy of the glaucomas*. St Louis: CV Mosby, 1989.
30. Farrar S et al. Glaucoma in the pigment dispersion syndrome. Risk factors for the development and severity of glaucoma in the pigment dispersion syndrome. *Am J Ophthalmol*. 1989;108:223.
31. Richter C et al. Pigmentary dispersion syndrome and pigmentary glaucoma. *Arch Ophthamol*. 1986;104:211–215.
32. Semple HC, Ball SF. Pigmentary glaucoma in the black population. *Am J Ophthalmol*. 1990;109:518.
33. Chew EV, Deutman AF. Pigment dispersion syndrome and pigment pattern dystrophy of retinal pigment epithelium. *Br J Ophthalmol*. 1983;67:538–541.
34. Weseley P et al. Lattice degeneration of the retina and the pigment dispersion syndrome. *Am J Ophthalmol*. 1992;114:539.
35. Robinson A, Savir H. Glaucomatocyclitic crisis and pigmentary glaucoma; A case report. *Glaucoma*. 1991;13:48–50.
36. Becker B, Podos SM. Krukenberg's spindles and primary open-angle glaucoma. *Arch Ophthalmol*. 1966;76:635.
37. Wilensky JT, Buerk KM, Podos SM. Krukenberg's spindles. *Am J Ophthalmol*. 1975;79:220.
38. Kupfer C et al. The histopathology of pigment dispersion syndrome with glaucoma. *Am J Ophthalmol*. 1975;80:857.
39. Feibel RM, Perlmutter JC. Anisicoria in the pigmentary dispersion syndrome. *Am J Ophthalmol*. 1990;110:657–660.
40. Gillies WE, Tangas C. Fluorescein angiography of the iris in anterior segment pigment dispersal syndrome. *Br J Ophthalmol*. 1986;70:284–289.
41. Campbell DG, Boys-Smith JW. Pigmentary glaucoma. *Trans New Orleans Acad Ophthalmol*. 1985;33:102–110.
42. Campbell D. Pigment dispersion and glaucoma. *Arch Ophthalmol*. 1979;97:1667.
43. Davidson JA et al. Dimensions of the anterior chamber in pigment dispersion syndrome. *Arch Ophthalmol*. 1983;101:81.
44. Richardson T. Pigmentary glaucoma. In Ritch R, Shields MB, eds. *Secondary glaucomas*. St Louis: CV Mosby, 1982.
45. Karickhoff JR. New ideas. Pigmentary dispersion syndrome and pigmentary glaucoma: A new mechanism concept, a new treatment, and a new technique. *Ophthalmic Surg*. 1992;23:269.
46. Karickhoff JR. Pigmentary glaucoma: The theory on a new mechanism and results of new treatment. *Ocular Surg News*. 1992;(10)17:43.
47. Johnson D. Does pigmentation affect trabecular meshwork? *Arch Ophthalmol*. 1989;107:250.
48. Vanoff M, Fine BS. Ocular pathology. A text and atlas, 3d ed. Philadelphia: Lippincott, 1989.
49. Smith DL et al. The effects of exercise on intraocular pressure in pigmentary glaucoma patients. *Ophthalmic Surg*. 1989;20:561.
50. Donaldson D. Transillumination of the iris. *Trans Am Ophthalmol Soc*. 1974;72:89.
51. Cassin M. Pigmentary dispersion syndrome. *Clin Eye Vison Care*. 1989;1:196.
52. Mapstone R. Pigment release. *Br J Ophthalmol*. 1981;65:258.
53. Kristenson P. Pigment liberation test in open-angle glaucoma. *Act Ophthalmol*. 1968;46:586.
54. Kristensen P. Mydriasis-induced pigment liberation in the anterior chamber associated with acute rise in intraocular pressure in open-angle glaucoma. *Act Ophthalmol*. 1965;43:714.
55. Haynes WL et al. Inhibition of excercise-induced pigment dispersion in a patient with the pigmentary dispersion syndrome. *Am J Ophthalmol*. 1991;109:601.
56. Haynes et al. Effects of jogging excercise on patients with the pigmentary dispersion syndrome and pigmentary glaucoma. *Ophthalmology*. 1992;99:1096–1103.
57. Shenker HI et al. Exercise-induced increase of intraocular pressure in the pigmentary dispersion syndrome. *Am J Ophthalmol*. 1980;89:598.
58. Kaiser-Kupfer MI et al. Asymmetric pigment dispersion syndrome. *Trans Am Ophthamol Soc*. 1983;83:310.
59. Epstein DL. *Chandler and Grant's glaucoma*, 3d ed. Philadelphia: Lea & Febiger, 1986.
60. Desjardins D, Parrish RK. Inversion of anterior chamber pigment as a possible prognostic sign in narrow angles. Letter to the *Am J Ophthalmol*. 1985;100:480–481.
61. Sampaolesi R. New gonioscopic signs in congenital glaucoma of late onset. *Mod Prob Ophthalmol*. 1966;6:106.
62. Caplan M et al. Pseudophakic pigmentary glaucoma. *Am J Ophthalmol*. 1988;105(3):320–321.

CHAPTER 7. OPEN-ANGLE GLAUCOMA

63. Morrison JC, Green WR. Light microscopy of the exfoliation syndrome. *Act Ophthamol.* 1988(Suppl);66(184):5–27.

64. Rouhianen H, Terasvirta M. Presence of pseudoexfoliation on clear and opacified crystalline lenses in an aged population. *Ophthalmologica.* 1992;204:67–70.

65. Gutner R. Pseudoexfoliation syndrome. *Clin Eye Vision Care.* 1988;1:48.

66. Eagle RC et al. The basement membrane exfoliation syndrome. *Arch Ophthalmol.* 1979;79:510.

67. Dvorak-Theobald T. Pseudo-exfoliation of the lens capsule. *Am J Ophthalmol.* 1954;37:1.

68. Sunde OA. Senile exfoliation of the anterior lens capsule. *Act Ophthalmol.* 1956(Suppl);45:1.

69. Shields MB. *Textbook of glaucoma*, 3d ed. Baltimore: Williams & Wilkins, 1992.

70. Forsius H. Exfoliation syndrome in various ethnic populations. *Act Ophthalmol.* 1988(Suppl);66(184):71–85.

71. Montanes JM et al. Prevalence of pseudoexfoliation syndrome in the northwest of Spain. *Act Ophthalmol.* 1989;67:383–386.

72. Faulkner HW. Pseudo-exfoliation of the lens among Navajo indians. *Am J Ophthalmol.* 1971;72:206–207.

73. Hiller R et al. Pseudoexfoliation, intraocular pressure, and senile lens changes in a population-based survey. *Arch Ophthalmol.* 1982;100:1080.

74. Ball SF, Graham S, Thompson H. The racial prevalence and biomicroscopic signs of exfoliation syndrome in the glaucoma population of southern Louisiana. *Glaucoma* 1989;11:169–180.

75. Jerndal T. New perspective on exfoliation syndrome and associated glaucoma. *Seminars Ophthalmol.* 1989;4:41–45.

76. Aasved H. The frequency of epitheliocapsularis. *Act Ophthalmol.* 1971;49:194–210.

77. Tarkkanen AHA. Pseudoexfoliation of the lens capsule. A clinical study of 418 patients with special reference to glaucoma, cataracts and changes of the vitreous. *Act Ophthalmol.* 1962(Suppl);71:1–98.

78. Wishart P et al. Anterior chamber angle in the exfoliation syndrome. *Br J Ophthalmol.* 1985;69:103–107.

79. Henry JC et al. Long-term follow-up of pseudoexfoliation and the development of elevated intraocular pressure. *Ophthalmology.* 1987;94:545–552.

80. Prince A et al. Preclinical diagnosis of pseudoexfoliation syndrome. *Arch Ophthalmol.* 1987;105:1076–1082.

81. Gosh M, Speakman JS. The origin of senile lens exfoliation. *Can J Ophthalmol.* 1972;18:34.

82. Betelsen TI, Ehlers JH. Morphological and histochemical studies on fibrillopathia epitheliocapsularis. *Act Ophthalmol.* 1969;47:476.

83. Sugar HS et al. The exfoliative syndrome: Source of the fibrillar material on the capsule. *Surv Ophthalmol.* 1976;21:59–64.

84. Gorin G, Posner A. *Slit lamp gonioscopy*, 3d ed. Baltimore: Williams & Wilkins, 1967.

85. Speakman JS, Ghosh M. The conjunctiva in senile lens exfoliation. *Arch Ophthalmol.* 1976;94:1757–1761.

86. Tarkkanen AHA. Exfoliation syndrome. *Trans Ophthalmol Soc UK.* 1986;105:233.

87. Sampaolesi R, Zarate J, Croxato O. The chamber angle in exfoliation syndrome. Clinical and pathological findings. *Act Ophthalmol.* 1988(Suppl):66:48–53.

88. Layden W et al. Combined exfoliation and pigment dispersion syndrome. *Ophthalmology.* 1990;109:530–534.

89. Brooks AM et al. The development of microvascular changes in the iris in pseudoexfoliation of the lens capsule. *Ophthalmology.* 1987;94:1090–1097.

90. Speakman JS, Ghosh M. The conjunctiva in senile exfoliation. *Arch Ophthalmol.* 1976;94:1757.

91. Chen V, Blumenthal M. Exfoliation syndrome after cataract extraction. *Ophthalmology.* 1992;99:445–447.

92. Ringvold A, Husby G. Pseudo-exfoliation material—an amyloid-like substance. *Exp Eye Res.* 1974;17:289. Davcanger M. Studies on the pseudoexfoliation material v Graefes. *Arch Klin Exp Ophthalmol.* 1978;208:65.

93. Ringvold A, Veggie T. Electron microscopy of the trabecular meshwork in eyes with exfoliation syndrome. *Virchows Arch A Pathel Anat Histopathel.* 1971;353:110.

94. Jerndal T, Svedbergh B. Goniodysgenesis in exfoliation glaucoma. *Adv Ophthalmol.* 1978;35:45–64.

95. Kozart DM, Yanoff M. Intraocular pressure status in 100 consecutive patients with exfoliation syndrome. *Ophthalmology.* 1982;89:214–218.

96. Gillies WE. Corticosteroid-induced ocular hypertension in pseudoexfoliation of lens capsule. *Am J Ophthalmol.* 1970;70:90.

97. Layden WE. Exfoliation syndrome in secondary glaucomas. In Ritch R, Shields MB, eds. *The secondary glaucomas.* St Louis: CV Mosby, 1982; chapter 8.

98. Crittendon JJ, Shields MB. Exfoliation syndrome in the southeastern United States. II. Characteristics of patient population and clinical course. *Act Ophthalmol.* 1988(Suppl);66:103–106.

99. Bruni P. Argon laser trabeculoplasty in pseudoexfoliation glaucoma: A long-term follow-up. *Glaucoma.* 1990;12:180.

100. Wandel T. Synopsis: Disease of the internal eye. Exfoliation syndrome. In Henkind P, ed. *Clinical signs of ophthalmology*, Vol II, No 6. St. Louis: CV Mosby, 1986.

101. Fenten R, Zimmerman LZ. Hemolytic glaucoma an unusual cause of acute open-angle secondary glaucoma. *Arch Ophthalmol.* 1963;70:236.

102. Campbell DG et al. Ghost cell glaucoma. In Ritch R et al, eds. *The glaucomas.* St Louis: CV Mosby, 1989.

103. Brooks et al. Haemolytic glaucoma occurring in phakic eye. *Br J Ophthalmol.* 1986;70:603–606.

104. Fenton RB, Hunter WS. Hemolytic glaucoma. *Clin Path Conf Surv of Ophthalmol.* 1965;10:355–361.

105. Phelps CD, Watzke RC. Hemolytic glaucoma. *Am J Ophthalmol.* 1973;80:690–695.

106. Campbell DG, Simmons RJ, Grant WM. Ghost cells as a cause of glaucoma. *Am J Ophthalmol.* 1976;81:441–450.

107. Campbell D. Ghost cell glaucoma following trauma. *Ophthalmology.* 1981;88:1151.

108. Campbell DG. Ghost cell glaucoma. In Ritch R, Shields MB, eds. *Secondary glaucomas.* St Louis: CV Mosby, 1982.

109. Rodriguez FJ et al. Age related macular degeneration and ghost cell glaucoma. *Arch Ophthalmol.* 1991;109:1304.

110. Summers CG et al. Phase contrast microscopy; Diagnosis of ghost cell glaucoma following cataract extraction. *Surv Ophthalmol.* 1984;28:342.

111. Canavan VM, Archer DB. Anterior segment consequences of blunt ocular injury. *Br J Ophthalmol.* 1982;66:549–555.

112. Campbell D. Traumatic glaucoma. In Shingleton BJ et al, eds. *Eye trauma.* St Louis: Mosby-Yearbook, 1991.

113. Wolff SM, Zimmerman LZ. Chronic secondary glaucoma. *Am J Ophthalmol.* 1962;54:547.

114. Howard GM. Hyphema resulting from blunt trauma. *Trans Am Acad Ophthalmol Otol.* 1965;69:294.

115. Shingleton BJ, Hersh PS. Traumatic hyphema. In Shingleton BJ et al, eds. *Eye trauma.* St Louis: Mosby-Yearbook, 1991.

116. Spaeth GL. Traumatic hyphema, angle recession. *Arch Ophthalmol.* 1967;78:714.

117. Tonjum AM. Gonioscopy in traumatic hyphema. *Act Ophthalmol.* 1966;44:650.

118. Herschler J. Trabecular damage due to blunt anterior segment injury and its relationship to traumatic glaucoma. *Trans Am Acad Ophthalmol.* 1977;83:239.

119. Blanton FM. Anterior chamber angle recession and secondary glaucoma. *Arch Ophthalmol.* 1964;72:39.

120. Mooney D. Anterior chamber angle tears after non-perforating injury. *Br J Ophthalmol.* 1972;56:418.

121. Mooney D. Angle recession and secondary glaucoma. *Br J Ophthalmol.* 1973;57:608.

122. Alper MG. Contusion angle deformity and glaucoma. *Arch Ophthalmol.* 1963;69:455–467.

123. Suson EB et al. Angle recession with loss of anterior chamber. *Am J Ophthalmol.* 1969;68:516.

124. Hadar-Hundert I, David R. Diagnosis and treatment of angle-recession glaucoma. *Glaucoma.* 1991;13:91–93.

125. Herschler J, Cobo M. Trauma and elevated intraocular pressure. In Ritch R et al, eds. *The glaucomas.* St Louis: CV Mosby, 1989.

126. Kaufman JH, Tolpin DW. Glaucoma after traumatic angle recession: A ten-year prospective study. *Am J Ophthalmol.* 1974;78:648–654.

127. Telsuk GC, Spaeth GL. The occurrence of primary open-angle glaucoma in the fellow eye of patients with unilateral angle-cleavage. *Ophthalmology.* 1985;92:904.

128. Aminlari A. Late-onset glaucoma in traumatic angle recession. *Glaucoma.* 1988;10:62–64.

129. Chandler PA. Secondary glaucoma. *Trans Ophthalmol Soc Aust.* 1960;20:17–24. In Wolf SM, Zimmerman LZ, eds. Chronic secondary glaucoma. *Am J Ophthalmol.* 1962;54:547.

130. Thorpe H. Foreign bodies in the anterior chamber angle. *Am J Ophthalmol.* 1966;61:1339.

131. McDonald DB, Ashodian MJ. Retained glass foreign bodies in the anterior chamber. *Am J Ophthalmol.* 1959;48:747.

132. Archer DB et al. Non-metallic foreign bodies in the anterior chamber. *Br J Ophthalmol.* 1969;53:453.

Chapter 8

Congenital Anomalies

Childhood Glaucoma

The classifications used for childhood glaucoma are variable and perplexing (1). They include terms such as *primary congenital glaucoma, infantile glaucoma, developmental glaucoma, primary* or *secondary developmental glaucoma, trabeculodysgenesis,* and *juvenile glaucoma* (2–6). Other classifications have also been used, reflecting structural changes, inheritance patterns, and etiologic factors, and sometimes the same term will be used to refer to different types of glaucoma (7). Common to all primary forms is the abnormal development of the anterior chamber, resulting in a glaucoma usually present in childhood, although it may not manifest until early adulthood (3).

The Shields and the Shaffer-Weiss classifications consist of three categories (2,3–5): primary congenital, developmental, and secondary glaucomas.

Primary Congenital Glaucomas

Primary congenital glaucomas (primary infantile glaucomas) are the result of a developmental abnormality of the anterior chamber angle, resulting in aqueous outflow obstruction. There is an absence of other ocular or systemic developmental abnormalities. This is the most common form of glaucoma in infancy, occurring in 1 in 30,000 live births (8).

Developmental Glaucomas

Developmental glaucoma refers to glaucoma occurring in infants with associated ocular or systemic anomalies. The glaucoma results from developmental abnormalities of the anterior chamber as in primary congenital glaucoma, but additionally, these patients have other ocular or systemic developmental anomalies. Included within this category are the anterior chamber anomalies of the Axenfeld's or Reiger's syndromes as well as glaucomas associated with aniridia,

neurofibromatosis, Sturge-Weber syndrome, Marfan's syndrome, as well as other disorders (Table 8.1).

Marfan's syndrome was reviewed in the section on lens-induced glaucomas, and the Axenfeld's and Reiger's anomalies/syndromes will be reviewed later in this chapter. Neurofibromatosis is one of the phakomatoses. It is a genetic disease characterized by harmatomas of the skin, eyes, and central nervous system (CNS). *Iris lesions*, known as *Lisch nodules*, are considered diagnostic of the peripheral nervous system form. Electron microscopic examination demonstrates the lesions to be melanocytic harmatomas. Clinically they appear as tan-to-brown dome-shaped lesions sitting on and within the iris surface. They tend to be bilateral and to increase in size and number with age and severity of the neurofibromatosis skin-related manifestations. In one study, they were observed in 92% of patients with neurofibromatosis over the age of six (9,10). Glaucoma associated with neurofibromatosis is usually unilateral and associated with an upper lid neurofibroma and bupthalmos. Most often it manifests around the time of birth. The glaucoma may develop from neurofibroma infiltration to the angle, from closure of the angle by neurofibroma thickening of the choroid or ciliary body, or by secondary synechia from fibrovascular formation. Gonioscopically neurofibroma infiltration of the angle, large numbers of iris processes, and anomalous angle vessels have been observed in eyes with neurofibromatosis (11). Glaucoma may develop in adulthood, but its association with neurofibromatosis in adult cases is unclear.

The angle in Sturge-Weber syndrome has been reported to have similar anomalies as those seen in other forms of congenital glaucoma (12,13). This syndrome consists of a hemangioma to the lid (port wine stain or nevus flammeus), considered the hallmark of this syndrome and intracranial meningeal hemangioma. The associated glaucoma is classified as one of the glaucomas secondary to increased episcleral venous pressure. Glaucoma in this class of disorders result from obstruction to venous flow, arteriovenous fistula, or

TABLE 8.1
Syndrome Classification of Congenital Glaucoma,
as Modified from Shaffer and Weiss

Primary congenital glaucoma (primary infantile glaucoma)
Glaucoma associated with other congenital anomalies
    Familial hypoplasia of the iris with glaucoma
    Developmental glaucoma with anomalous superficial iris vessels
    Aniridia
    Sturge-Weber syndrome
    Neurofibromatosis
    Marfan's syndrome
    Pierre Robin syndrome
    Homocystinuria
    Goniodysgenesis (iridocorneal mesodermal dysgenesis: Rieger's
      anomaly and syndrome, Axenfeld's anomaly, Peter's anomaly)
    Lowe's syndrome
    Microcornea
    Microspherophakia
    Rubella
    Chromosome abnormalities
    Broad thumb syndrome
Secondary glaucoma in infants
    Persistent hyperplastic primary vitreous
    Retinopathy of prematurity
    Tumors
      Retinoblastoma
      Juvenile xanthogranuloma
    Inflammation
    Trauma

Reprinted with permission from Hoskins JD Jr, Kass MA. *Becker-Shaffer's diagnosis and therapy of the glaucomas,* 6th ed. St. Louis: CV Mosby, 1989.

from an idiopathic increased episcleral venous pressure. In addition to the Sturge-Weber syndrome increased episcleral venous presssure, it is found in association with thyroid exophthalmopathy, orbital varices, arteriovenous fistula, and superior mediastinal syndrome (superior vena cava obstruction). The angle in these disorders is characterized by the frequent presence of blood in Schlemm's canal. In Sturge-Weber syndrome the presence of episcleral hemangiomas may account for the glaucoma. The glaucoma in the Sturge-Weber syndrome may develop at birth, during childhood or adolescence, or in adulthood.

Secondary Glaucomas

Secondary glaucomas, in childhood occur from similar conditions found in adults, such as inflammation, trauma, tumors, and even pigment dispersion.

Age of Onset

Childhood glaucoma can be further classified according to the age of onset of the glaucoma. According to Shields, cases occurring during the first few years of life are referred to as *primary infantile glaucoma* and cases occurring later in childhood or in early adulthood are referred to as *juvenile glaucoma* (2). Shields considers three years of age as the dividing point between the two because "the eye no longer expands in response to elevated IOP [intraocular pressure]" after this age (2). Hoskins and colleagues classify the time sequence

into congenital, infantile, and juvenile. *Congenital glaucoma* exists before or at birth, *infantile* from birth to age 2, and *juvenile* from 2 to 16 years of age (4). A recent study indicates that young, black, myopic patients are more susceptible to glaucomatous damage from juvenile glaucoma than whites (14).

The terms *buphthalmos* ("cow's eye"), referring to an eye enlarged from elevated IOP, and *hydrophthalmia* (excessive fluid volume in an enlarged eye) are older terms referring to childhood glaucoma; they are descriptive and generally are not used today.

Primary Congenital Glaucoma

Primary congenital glaucoma is rare, estimated to affect less than 0.05% of ophthalmic patients (8). In one study, it was found to occur in 22.2% of all childhood glaucomas and in another over 50% of all forms of developmental glaucoma (1,15). It is usually diagnosed within the first year of life but may present later in childhood. The incidence is greater in males and is bilateral in 75% of cases. The majority of cases are sporadic, with about 10% inherited in an autosomal recessive fashion (3). In North America, it is more likely a polygenic or multifactorial pattern of inheritance (16). The risk to siblings or children of an affected patient is 4% to 5% (17).

Signs and Symptoms

The signs and symptoms in the infant of tearing, photophobia, blepharospasm, increased corneal diameter, corneal edema, tears in Descemet's membrane (Haab's striae), and myopia should make clinicians suspicious of the presence of infantile glaucoma. These are not specific for childhood glaucoma, but evidence of these findings requires examination to rule out this disease. The tearing, photophobia, and blepharospasms are probably related to the epithelial breakdown secondary to the IOP-induced corneal edema (Table 8.2).

Corneal Diameter

The average corneal diameter at birth is 10.5 mm. The increase in IOP results in the enlargement of the corneal diameter so that a horizontal diameter of 12.0 mm during the first year of life is considered suspect (2). Most of the corneal enlargement occurs before the age of three (6).

Some observers have used axial length enlargement as a means for diagnosing congenital glaucoma (18,19). Kiskis and colleagues, however, found that, in their study comparing axial length and corneal diameter in 31 eyes with congenital glaucoma, the axial length measurements had a low sensitivity for diagnosing glaucoma. They found that a number of the studied eyes had falsely normal axial length values. They concluded that when compared to corneal diameter measurements, the axial length measurement provided no additional useful information. They further concluded that the corneal diameter was simpler to measure and was more sensitive for identifying congenital glaucoma (20,21). They reasoned that the elevated IOP causes the corneal diameter to increase more

TABLE 8.2

Other causes of corneal enlargement
  Megalocornea
  High axial myopia

Other causes for Haab's striae
  Forceps delivery trauma
  Sclerocornea
  Corneal clouding
  Metabolic diseases
    Cystinosis
    Hurler's syndrome
    Macroteaux-Lamy syndrome
  Posterior polymorphous dystrophy
  Congenital hereditary endothelial dystrophy
  Obstetrical trauma rupturing Descemet's membrane
  Inflammatory keratitis and iridocyclitis

Other causes of photophobia and tearing
  Nasolacrimal duct obstruction
  Ocular surface disease (blepharitis, conjunctivitis, keratitis)
  Meesman's or Reis-Buckler's dystrophy

Adapted from Hoskins HD Jr, Kass MA, *Becker-Shaffer's diagnosis and therapy of the glaucomas.* 6th ed. St Louis: CV Mosby, 1989.

than the axial length because of a weakness at the limbus. They describe and recommend measuring the corneal diameter with a transparent plastic gauge with calibrated holes (20).

Corneal Edema

As the cornea enlarges, Descemet's membrane and the corneal endothelium stretch, which may lead to ruptures of Descemet's membrane, resulting in sudden increases of corneal stromal and epithelial edema and, if chronic, eventual corneal scarring. Haab's striae do not usually appear until the cornea has reached 12.5 mm in diameter (6). Early in the process, corneal edema is usually limited to the epithelium secondary to the elevated IOP (6). The raised IOP also induces an enlargement of the anterior chamber, optic nerve, scleral canal, lamina cribosa, and the entire globe (6). The increases in the axial length manifest a myopic and astigmatic shift in the refraction. This is considered a ''soft sign'' and, when observed in infants, should encourage measurements of IOP and evaluation for other signs of childhood glaucoma (22). This type of refractive change may also be a sign of a late-developing primary congenital glaucoma (after age three), the result of the elevated IOP continuing to stretch the posterior sclera rather than the cornea. Subluxation of the lens may also take place when the globe enlarges, and this may induce refractive changes as well (13).

Optic Nerve

Examination of the optic nerve, as in the adult, is critical. In one report, cupping greater than 30% was considered suspicious in children under the age of one (1). Cupping occurs more quickly in infant eyes and at lower IOPs than in adult eyes, and there may be increases in the scleral canal, which also can lead to an increase in the cup (21,23). The appearance of cupping in the infant eye is usually different than it is in the adult eye; it is steep walled, round, central, and

surrounded by pink tissue. Once the IOP is lowered and controlled, a decrease in cupping can occur very rapidly—within hours to days (21). Quigly, in his report of 18 children with glaucoma, found that the reversal of cupping occurred all within the first year after successful treatment and is due to a lack of collagen in the nerve heads' connective tissue, allowing a more elastic response to IOP than in the adult eye. He also recommends avoiding Neo-Synephrine® for dilation because of its pressor effects, resulting in elevated blood pressure in the child (23).

IOP

Tonometry should be performed using a hand-held applanation tonometer whenever possible; Schiotz or indentation tonometry may give an artificially elevated reading because of the steep radius of curvature and increased scleral rigidity in these eyes (6,24). With the child under general anesthesia, the IOP should be measured early in the anesthesia to reduce anesthesia-related errors (20,22). Under general anesthesia, the IOP is usually in the vicinity of 9 to 10 mm Hg, so a pressure of 20 mm Hg should be considered suspicious; however, the pressure may vary depending on the type of anesthesia used and the depth of anesthesia (24,25). The normal range of IOP in the unanesthetized infant is slightly lower than in the adult eye; however, 21 mm Hg should still be considered as the upper limit of normal (3). Radtke and Cohen found that in awake and struggling newborns, the mean IOP is around 28 mm/Hg, and in unrestrained, nonstruggling, awake newborns, the mean IOP is around 11 mm/Hg, with a range of 6 to 17 (24).

Gonioscopy

Gonioscopy should be done using the Koeppe small-diameter lens, 14 mm or 16 mm, or the Richardson lens (26). Gonioscopically, the infant eye appears different from the adult eye (Figure 8.1). Normally, the trabecular meshwork in the infant appears as a smooth, homogeneous membrane that extends from the iris to Schwalbe's line. The normal angle is covered by a somewhat transparent shagreenlike membrane, and the

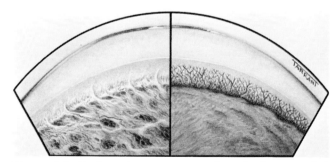

Figure 8.1 Gonioscopic appearance of angle in congenital glaucoma. Trabeculodysgenesis: Left, flat anterior iris insertion with prominent vessels. Right, concave iris insertion with prominent dense lacy meshwork. (From Kanski JJ, McAllister JA, eds. Glaucoma: A colour manual of diagnosis and treatment. *London: Butterworth-Heinemann, 1989.*

peripheral iris is thinner and flatter (27). The iris insertion is usually posterior to the scleral spur and flat since the angle recess is still unformed. During the first 6 to 12 months of life, the posterior movement of the uveal tissue and ciliary body creates the angle recess, which is usually present at 12 months. The trabecular meshwork is thicker and more translucent than the adult's and is nonpigmented, making it more difficult to identify. Also Schwalbe's line is less prominent. Retroillumination and specular reflection may improve detection of subtleties; however, the differentiation between the normal and the abnormal is often very difficult in the newborn's eye (5).

Walton notes that the uveal meshwork is the feature that differs most significantly in the infant and young child's eye when compared to the adult eye. In the normal infant eye, the uveal meshwork appears as a "smooth, homogeneous gossamer membrane" running from the iris periphery to Schwalbe's line (28). It appears translucent and glistening and, he notes, that it is so delicate that unless one focuses slightly away from the angle wall, the structure will not be obvious. At about one year, the meshwork may be observed to begin to become slightly pigmented. According to Walton, iris processes are seldom noted, but when present, they can be observed in front of the uveal meshwork. Walton also notes that the iris stroma is usually thinner; therefore, radial iris vessels are more visible as well as radial ciliary and circumferential ciliary band vessels. Normally, the anterior chamber depth of an infant is equivalent to approximately two corneal thicknesses. Thus, when a child has a deepened central chamber (similar to the normal adult eye) and an enlarged cornea, glaucoma should be suspected.

In primary infantile glaucoma, the angle may appear similar to the angle in the normal infant eye (6). It is open with a high or anterior insertion of the iris root, possibly into the trabecular meshwork. The iris insertion is usually flat, or it may be somewhat concave, with the anterior iris stroma sweeping forward as it inserts at the trabecular meshwork (21). The "membrane" Barkan referred to in the normal eye is more opaque, obscuring the angle wall details with evidence of traction pulling the iris anterior into the angle (29).

Pathogenesis of Glaucoma

Histological evidence of an actual membrane (Barkan's membrane) often assumed to represent corneal endothelium is lacking. Anderson believes the so-called membrane is really a thickened inner portion of the trabecular meshwork and that the thickened trabecular beams exert traction on the iris root, which prevents normal posterior movement of the ciliary body and iris root. It is this "premature or excessive formation of collagenous beams within the trabecular meshwork" that prevents the posterior movement of the uveal structures during the development of the eye, resulting in outflow obstruction, and is the primary defect in primary congenital glaucoma (25). Anderson notes that, in no normal eye does the posterior movement of the iris and ciliary body occur secondary to a presumed difference in growth rate of the

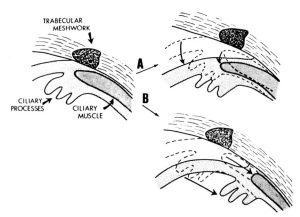

Figure 8.2 Process of exposing the trabecular meshwork during the anterior chamber development. (A) If the angle developed by cleavage or atrophy of tissue, the ciliary muscle would be extended into the iris, and the ciliary processes would be in back of the iris. (B) According to Anderson, the angle develops secondary to a differential growth rate of the angle tissue. The ciliary muscle and ciliary processes, which are initially located over the trabecular meshwork, end up posterior to it. (From Anderson DR. The development of the trabecular meshwork and its abnormality in primary infantile glaucoma. Trans Am Ophthalmol Soc. 1981;79:458–485.

angle tissue. The angle forms because of this, and not from any cleavage, atrophy, resorption, or rarefaction of angle tissue (Figure 8.2) (30,31). Thus, histologically, according to Anderson, the angle in infantile glaucoma is characterized by an anterior location of the iris and ciliary body, similar to the normal late-fetal location, resembling the angle at seven to eight months' gestation (6,29). Schlemm's canal is opened in early cases of primary congenital glaucoma and is not the primary site of aqueous outflow obstruction. Shields believes primary congenital glaucoma results from a developmental abnormality of the neural crest cell–derived angle tissue, which includes the corneal endothelium, corneal stroma, iris, ciliary body, sclera, and trabecular meshwork. This abnormal development affects the outflow mechanism, which leads to abnormal outflow occurring in eyes characterized by angle anomalies or with primary congenital glaucoma (2,32).

Treatment

In primary congenital glaucoma, gonioscopy has its major role in the treatment phase. Treatment consists of goniotomy, a superficial incision into the thickened trabecular meshwork. Specialized direct-view lenses such as the Hoskins-Barkan or Swan-Jacob lens are used to observe the angle. The incision into the trabecular meshwork (Figure 8.3) relieves the tension on the meshwork from the thickened uveal meshwork and allows the iris root to move posteriorly, accompanied by a posterior rotation of the scleral spur, thus opening the corneoscleral trabecular sheets. Early recognition and treatment are important; the longer the disease remains untreated, the greater the chance is for scarring and apposition of the trabecular sheets (8). The prognosis for surgical cure seems best in disease with onset at age 1 to 24 months, in eyes without

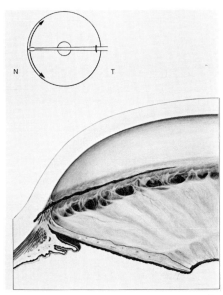

Figure 8.3 Top: A nasal goniotomy through a temporal corneal incision. Bottom: Illustration of goniotomy incision barely into the trabecular meshwork just below Schwalbe's line. (From Hoskins JD Jr, Kass, MA. Becker-Shaffer's diagnosis and therapy of the glaucomas, 6th ed. St Louis: CV Mosby, 1989.

associated ocular syndromes, and when the corneal diameter is less than 14 mm (23).

Trabeculotomy, trabeculectomy, filtration procedures, or cyclodestructive treatment may be effective if the goniotomy fails (33). Some surgeons prefer to perform a trabeculotomy *ab externo*, which enters the angle from the exterior. They feel the rate of success is similar to that of goniotomy (23). Others, however, feel that due to the excellent healing of the young, *ab externo* procedures generally have a poor prognosis and should be reserved for older children or in cases where corneal clouding prevents visualization of the angle (21). Trabeculotomy is considered less effective in eyes with cicatrized angles or with mesodermal dysgenesis; in these cases, trabeculectomy is the preferred treatment (34,35). Thermal sclerostomy has been recommended when corneal opacification precludes an adequate view for goniotomy as a means of lowering the IOP and reducing corneal clouding thus allowing a view of the angle to permit goniotomy. In some eyes, thermal sclerostomy is curative by itself (34). Stabilization and/or reversal of optic nerve cupping, stabilization of corneal diameter, decreased tearing and photophobia, and stabilization of myopia are useful criteria for evaluating whether adequate pressure control has been achieved (23).

When primary congenital glaucoma is suspected, a complete eye examination and general medical evaluation should be performed to search for a related ocular or systemic abnormality. After surgical remediation, prevention of amblyopia by proper lens prescription is imperative. Long-term medical management is challenging because of side effects and compliance issues, and it has been stated that successful treatment of congenital glaucoma always requires a surgical procedure (34). Hoskins and colleagues, however, showed an effective

response to timolol with as much as a 10 mm/Hg drop in IOP in 45% of eyes (36).

Developmental Glaucomas

According to Dickens and Hoskins (8) and Hoskins and colleagues (4), the developmental glaucomas can be classified based on anatomic maldevelopment of the visible iridocorneal structures, referred to as goniodysgenesis (4,8). This may manifest by a dysgenesis of the three major structures of the anterior chamber—the trabecular meshwork, the iris, and the cornea—either separately or in combination. The different presentations have different prognostic and therapeutic importance, so the correct identification of the abnormality will aid in the choice of therapy, provide prognostic information, and help avoid the use of confusing syndromes into which not all forms of developmental glaucoma will fit. Dickens and Hoskins and Hoskins and colleagues believe that "the malformation of the anterior segment is the hallmark of developmental glaucoma" and that all forms of developmental glaucoma have a maldevelopment of the anterior segment (3,4,8). This classification does not rely on histopathologic findings, age of onset, treatment responses, or inheritance patterns but rather on the clinical observation of defects to the iris, cornea, and/or trabecular meshwork (4). Surgical prognosis is best for eyes suffering only trabeculodysgenesis and poorer for eyes with additional developmental defects (4).

Trabeculodysgenesis

Isolated trabeculodysgenesis is the classical anomaly found in 50% of juveniles or infants with glaucoma (3). This may be an isolated abnormality, being synonymous with the Shaffer-Weiss classification of primary congenital glaucoma, or it may be associated with systemic diseases such as Sturge-Weber, Lowe's syndrome, and rubella, which is equivalent to the Shield's classification of developmental glaucomas. Trabeculodysgenesis is divided into two major clinical forms: flat iris insertion and a concave iris insertion.

The *flat iris insertion* is more common. Clinically, the flat iris appears to insert abruptly into a thickened trabecular meshwork, making a distinct angle between the iris and trabecular meshwork, or just behind the scleral spur as is shown on the left side of Figure 8.1. There may be variation in the height of the iris insertion in the same eye, from anterior to the spur to posterior to the spur (4). "The trabecula appears thickened and translucent," and small iris processes reach onto the trabecular meshwork (14). The iris stroma periphery may be thinned, and normal radial blood vessels may be visible. The trabecular meshwork may have a stippled orange peel appearance. The ciliary body band is usually hidden from view, but when the clinician uses a higher oblique vantage point, some portions of the ciliary body band may be visible through a thickened trabecular meshwork.

The *concave iris insertion* is a less common presentation. In this instance, the anterior iris stroma inserts just below Schwalbe's line as is shown on the right side of Figure 8.1.

This tissue appears to be wrapped around or pulled up over the trabecular meshwork, inserting anterior to the iris insertion and concealing the scleral spur and ciliary body. The anterior stromal tissue may be sheetlike, without conspicuous gaps, or it may be a dense, lacy, open network (4). The iris and cornea are otherwise normal.

Iridotrabeculodysgenesis

Iridotrabeculodysgenesis and corneotrabeculodysgenesis are categories often associated with glaucomas with congenital anomalies. This category is equivalent to the Shields classification of developmental glaucomas, with associated anomalies, as these conditions have "additional ocular and systemic anomalies" that aid in their characterization. Thus, the observation of this form of anterior chamber abnormality should encourage the examiner to search for other ocular or systemic anomalies.

Iris anomalies (iridotrabeculodysgenesis or iridodysgenesis) may present as an abnormal development of portions of the iris, with involvement limited to the anterior iris stroma, to the iris vessels, or to a full thickness involvement of the iris. There is an associated abnormal development of the trabecular meshwork in these eyes (3).

An absent or poorly developed anterior iris stroma is common in congenital glaucoma and in Axenfeld's and Rieger's anomalies (4). Thinning of this tissue may be secondary to a true hypoplasia or secondary to the stretching of the tissue from the increased IOP (4). Hoskins and colleagues consider an incomplete, poorly formed, or missing collarette as one of the signs of hypoplasia (4). The other sign is a thinned iris crypt layer, so thinned that the iris radial vessels, the sphincter muscle, and the iris pigment epithelium become easily visible. The sphincter muscle is quite prominent, making clinical identification easy. Gonioscopically, the iris inserts anterior at the scleral spur; the trabecular meshwork is thickened, and there may be anomalous circumferential vessels present in the angle (3,8).

Anomalous iris vessels may be present and are secondary to either persistence of the tunica vasculosa lentis, which appear as looping vessels into the pupillary axis, either in front of or behind the lens or because of the hypoplasia of the iris stroma, resulting in the presence of irregular superficial anomalous iris vessels. The presence of these anomalous iris vessels in developmental glaucoma indicates a poor prognosis. Because they are present at birth, they are not considered neovascular vessels (4).

Iris dysgenesis may result in aniridia or full-thickness iris holes with or without sphincter defects (Rieger's anomaly). Aniridia is a congenital absence of the iris; however, the peripheral portion of the iris is still visible on gonioscopy (5,37). It is a rare bilateral developmental disorder with an incidence of 1 in 80,000 and is most often a dominantly inherited defect that results in its occurrence over many generations in some families (18). It can occur as a mutation without any family history (7).

Hittner classifies aniridia into three genetic types: isolated autosomal dominant aniridia, which has an 85% prevalence;

autosomal dominant aniridia associated with Wilm's tumor, genitourinary anomalies, and mental retardation, which has a 13% prevalence; and autosomal recessive aniridia with cerebellar ataxia and mental retardation, which has a 2% prevalence (38). She ascribes the pathogenesis of aniridia to a primary developmental interruption of neuroectoderm and a secondary change in the various neural crest waves. Associated ocular findings may include microcornea, superficial peripheral corneal opacification (appearing clinically as pannus), cataracts, microaphakia, lens subluxation, macular and optic nerve hypoplasia, nystagmus, and glaucoma (38).

Glaucoma occurs in 50% to 75% of patients with aniridia (2,5,37). In contrast to primary infantile glaucoma, it usually occurs later in childhood, around the ages of 7 to 15, without corneal enlargement (39). In some cases glaucoma may not become obvious until adulthood (5). In contrast to eyes with primary congenital glaucoma, the development of glaucoma in aniridia is strongly associated with the gonioscopic angle appearance. The gonioscopic findings are different for aniridic eyes with glaucoma and without glaucoma. In glaucomatous eyes, the peripheral iris stump covers over the trabecular meshwork. According to Grant and Walton, eyes destined to develop glaucoma have progressive angle changes (37). Fine, irregular portions of iris stroma attach to varying locations on the angle wall, resembling sawtooth synechia. After several years, the attachments become denser, broadened, and they move anterior, obscuring portions of the angle wall, including the trabecular meshwork. In essence, they close the angle. In other eyes, a thin, amorphous, variably pigmented, avascular tissue increased in density becomes "more closely applied to the trabecular meshwork as the glaucoma worsens" (37). The observation of these types of progressive angle changes and the poor therapeutic response to medical and/or surgical treatment, once glaucoma develops, led Walton to suggest and perform prophylactic goniotomy surgery once the trabecular meshwork was covered more than half of its circumference (37,39).

Corneotrabeculodysgenesis

Corneal defects (corneotrabeculodysgenesis, corneodysgenesis) form the third group of anatomic imperfections. The corneal anomalies may be peripheral, midperipheral, or central and are associated with angle maldevelopment. The anomalies and syndromes of Axenfeld, Rieger, and Peter are examples of different forms of corneodysgenesis. Macro and microcornea abnormalities may also be present. In addition to Rieger's anomaly, microcornea is seen in nanophthalmos, rubella syndrome, and persistent hyperplastic primary vitreous (8).

Peripheral corneal defects are characterized by circumferential corneal involvement, concentric to the limbus and not extending more than 2 mm onto the cornea from the limbus. Clinically, they are typified as Axenfeld's anomaly (Plate 35), consisting of posterior embryotoxin with adherent iris strands (16). Axenfeld's anomaly differs from posterior embryotoxin. Posterior embryotoxin is an abnormal thickening and prominence to Schwalbe's line without iris attachments.

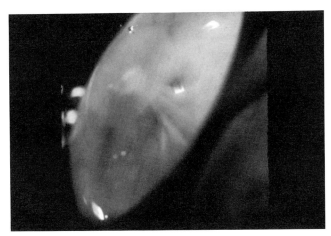

Figure 8.4 Mesodermal dysgenesis or Peter's anomaly. The iris tissue is adherent to the cornea. (Photo courtesy P. Ajamian, O.D.)

It is usually more noticeable along the horizontal meridians and is detectable on routine slit lamp examination (40). When this occurs in isolation, there is rarely any functional abnormality associated with it, and it is considered a variance of normal. *Axenfeld's anomaly* (Plate 35) is the term for those cases where the iris has attachments onto a prominent Schwalbe's line. Glaucoma may be associated with this finding when the trabecular meshwork is abnormal. Glaucoma occurs in about 50% of cases of Axenfeld's anomaly (3). When glaucoma manifests in early childhood, goniotomy or trabeculotomy is often effective. Glaucoma that develops in late childhood or adulthood should be managed initially by medical therapy.

Reiger's anomaly typifies the cases involving midperipheral corneal lesions. It includes the peripheral abnormalities associated with Axenfeld's anomaly with the addition of pupil abnormalities, hypoplasia of the iris stroma, and iris holes (2,22). Characteristically the iris tissue attaches to corneal opacities. Using Neodymium:YAG laser to lyse iridocorneal adhesions has been described for cases where the adhesions compromise vision and for reducing corectopia (41). Cases of Reiger's may display progressive iris thinning similar to what occurs in the ICE syndrome.

Rieger's syndrome manifests the same ocular findings as does Rieger's anomaly, but in addition, there are systemic abnormalities including dental abnormalities, maxillary hypoplasia, and umbilical hernia. More rarely visceral abnormalities occur such as congenital heart anomalies, middle ear deafness, and mental retardation (16). Glaucoma may develop later in childhood.

Peter's anomaly is an example of corneotrabeculodysgenesis involving the central cornea (Figure 8.4). Typically an opacified corneal defect (central leukoma) has adherent iris tissue located at its margin. Lens changes are also present and may consist of displacement into the anterior chamber, central opacification, or adhesion to the cornea.

Summary

Embryologically, it has been shown that the primary mesenchyme is formed by cells that accumulate circumferentially around the optic cup and surface ectoderm. The secondary mesenchyme is then formed by the addition of neural crest cells. Recent evidence suggests that the neural crest cell portion of the secondary mesenchyme, rather than the mesodermal portion, develops into corneal stroma, corneal endothelium, iris stroma, trabecular meshwork, and the other ocular and orbital structures (42). Apparently only the retina, lens, and corneal epithelium are not of neural crest origin (25).

The crest cells migrate in three waves. The first wave differentiates to form the endothelium and trabecular meshwork; the second wave into corneal keratocytes; and the third wave contributes to the development of the iris stroma (42). The extent to which each of these structures is involved by an abnormality of neural crest cells will determine the clinical signs and course of the disease (43).

The associated nonocular systemic anomalies observed in the developmental glaucomas may also be explained by neural crest abnormalities "as bones of the face, portions of the cranial fossa, dental papilla, are derived from neural crest cells. Neural crest cell migration also plays a part in the development of the smooth and striated muscle, cartilage and bone, meninges, and a variety of endocrine glands" (44).

Neural crest abnormalities of migration, proliferation, and final differentiation may explain corneal defects, such as megalocornea, microcornea and partial or total absence of iris stromal tissue. The latter leads to secondary developmental defects of the iris pigment and nonpigmented epi-

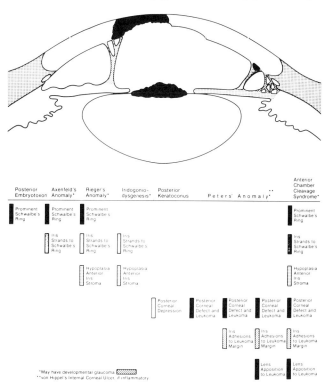

Figure 8.5 Composite illustration of the anatomic findings in the anterior chamber cleavage syndrome. The stepladder table demonstrates the spectrum of anatomic combinations and the terms by which they are commonly known. (Reproduced with permission from Waring GO et al. Anterior chamber cleavage syndrome. A stepladder classification. Surv Ophthalmol. 1975;20(1).

thelium, resulting in pupil abnormalities, and, if iris stroma defects are severe, adjacent lens and zonule development may be interfered with, resulting in ectopia lentis (44). Neural crest syndromes can be classified as deficiencies or insufficient cells, clinically exemplified as cyclopia. Deficient migration of cells are exemplified by congenital glaucoma, posterior embryotoxin, Axenfeld's anomaly and syndrome, Rieger's anomaly and syndrome, Peter's anomaly and sclerocornea; an abnormal neural crest cell proliferation is exemplified by the ICE syndrome, and an abnormal crest cell differentiation is exemplified by posterior polymorphous endothelial dystrophy, Fuch's endothelial dystrophy, and congenital hereditary endothelial dystrophy. Thus, the presence of angle abnormalities noted on gonioscopy in the developmental glaucomas should be considered a marker of neural crest abnormalities and alert the clinician to the possibility of other abnormalities, both ocular and systemic, that may be associated with the angle abnormalities (25).

Although this recent evidence suggests that the primary congenital and developmental glaucomas with their associated systemic and ocular anomalies all appear related on the basic neural crest embryological abnormalities, the abnormalities of the cornea, iris, and anterior chamber may be easier to conceptualize clinically by using Waring's stepladder table (Plate 47) (45).

References

1. Shaffer RN, Hetherington J Jr. The glaucomatous disc in infants. *Trans Am Acad Ophthalm Otol.* 1969;73:929.
2. Shields MB. *Textbook of glaucoma.* Baltimore: Williams & Wilkins, 1992.
3. Hoskins HD Jr, Kass MA. *Becker-Shaffer's diagnosis and therapy of the glaucomas*, 6th ed. St Louis: CV Mosby, 1989.
4. Hoskins HD Jr, Shaffer RN, Hetherington J. Anatomical classification of the developmental glaucomas. *Arch Ophthalmol.* 1984;102:1331.
5. Shaffer RN, Weiss DI. *Congenital and pediatric glaucomas.* St Louis: CV Mosby, 1970.
6. DeLuise VP, Anderson DR. Primary infantile glaucoma (congenital glaucoma). *Surv Ophthalmol.* 1983;28:1–19.
7. Walton DS. Aniridia with glaucoma. In Epstein D, ed. *Chandler and Grant's glaucoma*, 3d ed. Philadelphia: Lea & Febiger, 1986.
8. Dickens CJ, Hoskins HD Jr. Epidemiology and pathophysiology of congenital glaucoma. In Ritch R et al, eds. *The glaucomas*, vol 2. St Louis: CV Mosby, 1989.
9. Lewis RA, Riccardi VM. von Recklinghausen neurofibromatosis: Incidence of iris harmatomes. *Ophthalmology.* 1981; 88:348–354.
10. Perry HD, Font RL. Iris nodules in von Recklinghausen's neurofibromatosis. Electron microscopic confirmation of their melanocytic origin. *Arch Ophthalmol.* 1982;100:1635.
11. Grant WM, Walton DS. Distinctive gonioscopic findings in glaucoma due to neurofibromatosis. *Arch Ophthalmol.* 1968;79:127.
12. Yablonski ME, Podod SM. Glaucoma secondary to elevated episceral venous pressure. In Ritch R, Shields BM, eds. *The secondary glaucomas.* St Louis: CV Mosby, 1982.
13. Cibis GH, et al. Glaucoma in Sturge-Weber syndrome. *Ophthalmology.* 1984;91:1984.
14. Lotufo D et al. Juvenile glaucoma, race, and refraction. *JAMA.* 1989;261:249.
15. Barsoum-Homsy M, Chevrette L. Incidence and prognosis of childhood glaucoma. A study of 63 cases. *Ophthalmology.* 1986;93:1323.
16. Hoyt C, Lambert S. Childhood glaucoma. In Taylor D, ed. *Pediatric ophthalmology.* Cambridge, Mass.: Blackwell Scientific, 1990.
17. Demainis F et al. Congenital glaucoma genetic models. *Hum Genet.* 1979;46:305.
18. Nelson LB et al. Adiridia: A review. *Surv Ophthalmol.* 1984; 28:621.
19. Sampaolesi R, Caruso R. Ocular echometry in the diagnosis of congenital glaucoma. *Arch Ophthalmol.* 1982;100:574.
20. Kiskis AA et al. Corneal diameter and axial length in congenital glaucoma. *Can J Ophthalmol.* 1985;20(3):93–97.
21. Dickens CJ, Hoskins HD Jr. Diagnosis and treatment of congenital glaucoma. In Ritch R et al, eds. *The glaucomas*, vol 2. St Louis: CV Mosby, 1989.
22. Hoskins HD Jr et al. Developmental glaucomas: Diagnosis and classification. In Cairne JE et al., eds. Symposium on glaucoma: Transaction of the New Orleans academy of ophthalmology. St Louis; CV Mosby, 1981.
23. Quigly HA. Childhood glaucoma results with trabeculotomy and study of reversible cupping. *Ophthalmology.* 1982;89: 219–226.
24. Radtke ND, Cohen BF. Intraocular pressure measurement in the newborn. *Am J Ophthalmol.* 1974;78:501.
25. Beauchamp GR, Kneppere PA. Role of the neural crest in anterior segment development and disease. *J Ped Ophthalmol Strab.* 1984;21:209.
26. Richardson KT, Shaffer RN. Infant ophthalmoscopy and gonioscopy without general anesthesia. *Arch Ophthalmol.* 1965; 73:55.
27. Barkan O. Pathogenesis of congenital glaucoma. Gonioscopic and anatomic observation of the angle of the anterior chamber in the normal and eye and in congenital glaucoma. *Am J Ophthalmol.* 1955;40:1–11.
28. Walton DS. Considerations peculiar to infants and children. In Epstein D, ed. *Chandler and Grant's glaucoma*, 3d ed. Philadelphia: Lea & Febiger, 1986.
29. Anderson DR. The development of the trabecular meshwork and its abnormality in primary infantile glaucoma. *Trans Am Ophthalmol Soc.* 1981;79:459.
30. Allen L et al. A new concept in the development of the anterior chamber angle. *Arch Ophthalmol.* 1955;53:783.
31. Reese AB, Ellsworth RM. Anterior chamber cleavage syndrome. *Arch Ophthalmol.* 1966;75:307.
32. Tripathi BJ, Tripathi RC. Neural crest origin of human trabecular meshwork and its implications for the pathogenesis of glaucoma. *Am J Ophthalmol.* 1989;10:583.
33. Walton DS. Glaucoma. In Nelson LB, Calhoun JH, and Harley RD. *Infants and children in pediatric ophthalmology.* Philadelphia: WB Saunders, 1991.
34. Cadera et al. Congenital glaucoma with corneal cloudiness treated by thermal sclerostomy. *Can J Ophthalmol.* 1985; 20(3):98–100.
35. Luntz MH. Congenital, infantile and juvenile glaucoma. *Ophthalmol AAO.* 1979;86:793.
36. Hoskins HD Jr et al. Clinical experience with timolol in childhood glaucoma. *Ophthalmology.* 1985;103:1163.
38. Hittner HM. Aniridia. In Rich R et al, eds. *The glaucomas*, vol. 2. St Louis: CV Mosby, 1989.
39. Walton DS. Aniridic glaucoma: The results of gonio-surgery to prevent and treat this problem. *Trans Am Ophthalml Soc.* 1986;84:59.
40. Jerndal T. *Goniodysgenesis: A new perspective in glaucoma.* Copenhagen: Scriptor, 1978.

41. Chang JSM Jr, Lee DA, Christensewn RE. Neodynium:YAG laser lysis of iridocorneal adhesions in mesodermal dysgenesis. Letter in *J Am Ophthalmol*. 1984;108:548.

42. Bahn CF et al. Classification of corneal endothelial disorders based on neural crest origin. *Ophthalmology*. 1984;91:558–563.

43. Kupfer C et al. The contralateral eye in the iridocorneal endothelial (ICE) syndrome. *Ophthalmology*. 1983;90(11):1343–1350.

44. Kupfer C, Kaiser-Kupfer MI. New hypothesis of developmental anamolies of the anterior chamber associated with glaucoma. *Trans Ophthalmol Soc UK*. 1978;98:213.

45. Waring GO, Rodrigues MM, Laibson PR. Anterior chamber cleavage syndrome: A stepladder classification. *Surv Ophthalmol*. 1975;20:5.

Index